T0226875

Maxillofacial Reconstruction

Editor

PATRICK J. LOUIS

ORAL AND MAXILLOFACIAL SURGERY CLINICS OF NORTH AMERICA

www.oralmaxsurgery.theclinics.com

Consulting Editor
RICHARD H. HAUG

May 2013 • Volume 25 • Number 2

ELSEVIER

1600 John F. Kennedy Boulevard • Suite 1800 • Philadelphia, Pennsylvania, 19103-2899

www.oralmaxsurgery.theclinics.com

ORAL AND MAXILLOFACIAL SURGERY CLINICS OF NORTH AMERICA Volume 25, Number 2
May 2013 ISSN 1042-3699, ISBN-13: 978-1-4557-7130-1

Editor: John Vassallo; j.vassallo@elsevier.com
Developmental Editor: Teia Stone

Oral and Maxillofacial Surgery Clinics of North America (ISSN 1042-3699) is published quarterly by Elsevier Inc., 360 Park Avenue South, New York, NY 10010-1710. Months of issue are February, May, August, and November. Business and Editorial Offices: 1600 John F. Kennedy Blvd., Suite 1800, Philadelphia, PA 19103-2899. Periodicals postage paid at New York, NY and additional mailing offices. Subscription prices are $369.00 per year for US individuals, $543.00 per year for US institutions, $165.00 per year for US students and residents, $431.00 per year for Canadian individuals, $645.00 per year for Canadian institutions, $495.00 per year for international individuals, $645.00 per year for international institutions and $224.00 per year for Canadian and foreign students/residents. To receive student/resident rate, orders must be accompanied by name or affiliated institution, date of term, and the *signature* of program/residency coordinator on institution letterhead. Orders will be billed at individual rate until proof of status is received. Foreign air speed delivery is included in all *Clinics* subscription prices. All prices are subject to change without notice. **POSTMASTER:** Send address changes to *Oral and Maxillofacial Surgery Clinics of North America,* Elsevier Periodicals Customer Service, 11830 Westline Industrial Drive, St. Louis, MO 63146. Tel: 1-800-654-2452 (U.S. and Canada); 314-447-8871 (outside U.S. and Canada). Fax: 314-447-8029. E-mail: journalscustomerservice-usa@elsevier.com (for print support); journalsonlinesupport-usa@elsevier.com (for online support).

Reprints. For copies of 100 or more, of articles in this publication, please contact the Commercial Reprints Department, Elsevier Inc., 360 Park Avenue South, New York, NY 10010-1710. Tel.: 212-633-3812; Fax: 212-462-1935; Email: reprints@elsevier.com.

Oral and Maxillofacial Surgery Clinics of North America is covered in *MEDLINE/PubMed (Index Medicus)*, *Science Citation Index Expanded (SciSearch®)*, *Journal Citation Reports/Science Edition*, and *Current Contents®/Clinical Medicine*.

Printed and bound by CPI Group (UK) Ltd, Croydon, CR0 4YY

Transferred to digital print 2013

Contributors

CONSULTING EDITOR

RICHARD H. HAUG, DDS
Carolinas Center for Oral Health,
Charlotte, North Carolina

EDITOR

PATRICK J. LOUIS, DDS, MD
Professor and Residency Program Director,
Department of Oral and Maxillofacial Surgery,
University of Alabama at Birmingham; The
Kirklin Clinic, Birmingham, Alabama

AUTHORS

RUTH A. APONTE-WESSON, DDS, MS, FACP
Associate Professor, Department of
General Dental Science; Residency
Program Director, Maxillofacial
Prosthodontics, School of Dentistry,
University of Alabama at Birmingham,
Birmingham, Alabama

SHAHROKH C. BAGHERI, DMD, MD, FACS
Private Practice, Georgia Oral and Facial
Surgery, Marietta; Clinical Associate Professor,
Department of Oral and Maxillofacial Surgery,
School of Dental Medicine, Georgia Health
Sciences University, Augusta; Clinical
Assistant Professor, Division of Oral and
Maxillofacial Surgery, Department of Surgery,
School of Medicine, Emory University; Chief,
Division of Oral and Maxillofacial Surgery,
Department of Surgery, Northside Hospital,
Atlanta, Georgia

R. BRYAN BELL, DDS, MD, FACS
Medical Director, Oral, Head and Neck
Cancer Program, Providence Cancer Center;
Attending Surgeon, Trauma Service/Oral and
Maxillofacial Surgery Service, Legacy Emanuel

Medical Center; Clinical Professor, Department
of Oral and Maxillofacial Surgery, Oregon
Health and Science University, Portland,
Oregon

JUSTIN CLEMOW, DMD, MD
Department of Oral and Maxillofacial
Surgery; Chief Resident, Head and Neck
Oncology and Microvascular Surgery,
University of Florida – Jacksonville,
Jacksonville, Florida

RUI P. FERNANDES, DMD, MD, FACS
Associate Professor, Program Director,
Department of Oral and Maxillofacial Surgery
and Department of Surgery, Division of
Surgical Oncology, College of Medicine;
Fellowship Director, Head and Neck Oncology
and Microvascular Surgery; Chief, Section of
Head and Neck Cancer, Shands Hospital,
University of Florida – Jacksonville,
Jacksonville, Florida

SAVANNAH GELESKO, DDS
Resident in Training, Department of Oral and
Maxillofacial Surgery, Oregon Health and
Science University, Portland, Oregon

WILLIAM GIELINCKI, DDS
Private Practice, Jacksonville Center for
Prosthodontics and Implant Dentistry,
Jacksonville, Florida

RAÚL GONZÁLEZ-GARCÍA, MD, PhD
Staff Surgeon, Department of Oral and
Maxillofacial-Head and Neck Surgery,
University Infanta Cristina, Badajoz, Spain

RAJESH GUTTA, BDS, MS
Private Practice, Mountain State Oral and
Maxillofacial Surgeons, Charleston, West
Virginia; Visiting Assistant Professor, Division
of Oral and Maxillofacial Surgery, University of
Cincinnati, Cincinnati, Ohio

WOLFRAM M.H. KADUK, MD, DDS
Consultant, Maxillofacial Surgery/Plastic
Surgery, Oral Surgery and Orthodontics,
Department of Maxillofacial Surgery/Plastic
Surgery, Greifswald University, Greifswald,
Germany

DONGSOO D. KIM, DMD, MD
Professor of Oral and Maxillofacial Surgery,
Department of Oral and Maxillofacial Surgery;
Fellowship Director, Department of Head and
Neck Surgical Oncology and Microvascular
Reconstruction, Louisiana State University
Health Sciences Center, Shreveport,
Louisiana

NATHAN D. LENOX, DMD, MD
Fellow, Louisiana State University Health
Sciences Center, Shreveport, Louisiana

JOHN A. LONG, MD
Associate Clinical Professor, Department of
Ophthalmology, Alabama Ophthalmology
Associates, University of Alabama at
Birmingham, Birmingham, Alabama

PATRICK J. LOUIS, DDS, MD
Professor and Residency Program Director,
Department of Oral and Maxillofacial Surgery,
University of Alabama at Birmingham;
The Kirklin Clinic, Birmingham, Alabama

JOSHUA E. LUBEK, DDS, MD, FACS
Oncology Program, Department of Oral and
Maxillofacial Surgery, Greenebaum Cancer
Center, University of Maryland; Assistant
Professor and Fellowship Director,

Maxillofacial Oncology and Microvascular
Surgery, Department of Oral and Maxillofacial
Surgery, University of Maryland, Baltimore,
Maryland

MICHAEL R. MARKIEWICZ, DDS, MPH, MD
Resident in Training, Department of Oral and
Maxillofacial Surgery, Oregon Health and
Science University, Portland, Oregon

DANIEL J. MEARA, MS, MD, DMD
Chair, Department of Oral and Maxillofacial
Surgery and Hospital Dentistry; Program
Director, Oral and Maxillofacial Surgery
Residency, Christiana Care Health System,
Wilmington, Delaware

ROGER A. MEYER, DDS, MS, MD, FACS
Director, Maxillofacial Consultations Ltd,
Greensboro; Private Practice, Georgia Oral and
Facial Surgery, Marietta; Clinical Associate
Professor, Department of Oral and Maxillofacial
Surgery, School of Dental Medicine, Georgia
Health Sciences University, Augusta; Active
Medical Staff, Department of Surgery,
Northside Hospital, Atlanta, Georgia

ANTHONY B.P. MORLANDT, DDS, MD
Former Resident, Department of Oral and
Maxillofacial Surgery, School of Dentistry,
University of Alabama at Birmingham,
Birmingham; Currently, Fellow, University
of Florida, Microvascular Reconstruction
Fellowship, Department of Oral and
Maxillofacial Surgery, College of Medicine-
Jacksonville, Jacksonville, Florida

**ROBERT A. ORD, DDS, MD, FRCS,
FACS, MS**
Chairman and Professor, Oncology Program,
Department of Oral and Maxillofacial Surgery,
Greenebaum Cancer Center, University of
Maryland, Baltimore, Maryland

FRED PODMELLE, MD, DDS
Department of Maxillofacial Surgery/Plastic
Surgery, Greifswald University, Greifswald,
Germany

EBEN ROSENTHAL, MD
John S. Odess Professor of Surgery,
Otolaryngology Division Director, University
of Alabama at Birmingham, Birmingham,
Alabama

SOMSAK SITTITAVORNWONG, DDS, DMD, MS
Assistant Professor, Department of Oral and Maxillofacial Surgery, School of Dentistry, University of Alabama at Birmingham, Birmingham, Alabama

LUIS G. VEGA, DDS
Assistant Program Director, Oral and Maxillofacial Residency Program, Health Science Center at Jacksonville; Assistant Professor, Department of Oral and Maxillofacial Surgery, Health Science

Center at Jacksonville, University of Florida, Jacksonville, Florida

HILLIARY WHITE, MD
Head & Neck Surgery Center of Florida, Florida Hospital Celebration Health, Celebration; Assistant Professor of Otolaryngology Head and Neck Surgery, University of Central Florida College of Medicine, Orlando, Florida

JACOB G. YETZER, DDS, MD
Department of Oral and Maxillofacial Surgery, University of Florida, Jacksonville, Florida

Contributors

SOMSAK SITTITAVORNWONG, DDS, DMD, MS
Assistant Professor, Department of Oral and Maxillofacial Surgery, School of Dentistry, University of Alabama at Birmingham, Birmingham, Alabama

LUIS G. VEGA, DDS
Assistant Program Director, Oral and Maxillofacial Residency Program, Health Science Center at Jacksonville; Assistant Professor, Department of Oral and Maxillofacial Surgery, Health Science Center at Jacksonville, University of Florida, Jacksonville, Florida

HILLARY WHITE, MD
Head & Neck Surgery Center of Florida, Florida Hospital Celebration Health, Celebration; Assistant Professor of Otolaryngology Head and Neck Surgery, University of Central Florida College of Medicine, Orlando, Florida

JACOB G. YETZER, DDS, MD
Department of Oral and Maxillofacial Surgery, University of Florida, Jacksonville, Florida

Contents

Reconstruction of the Scalp, Calvarium, and Frontal Sinus 105

Somsak Sittitavornwong and Anthony B.P. Morlandt

Scalp and cranial deformities are common after trauma or ablative surgery. Local flaps and free flaps may be used in reconstruction of soft tissue defects, and autogenous bone or alloplastic bone substitutes may be used for cranioplasty procedures. Injuries to the frontal sinus, particularly when complicated by leak of cerebrospinal fluid or obstruction of the nasofrontal outflow tract, represent special challenges. Further studies are recommended to improve the multidisciplinary management of these complex, debilitating conditions, in anticipation of enhanced function and cosmesis, reduced donor site morbidity, and improved surgical outcomes.

Acquired Defects of the Nose and Naso-orbitoethmoid (NOE) Region 131

Daniel J. Meara

Nasal injuries coupled with midface fractures of the orbit and ethmoids constitute a nasoorbitoethmoid (NOE) fracture pattern, which is typically the most challenging facial fracture to repair. Hard and soft tissue defects of this region may require advanced reconstruction techniques, including local rotational flaps, free tissue transfer, and even prosthetics. The restoration of form and function dictates treatment, and the success of primary repair is paramount, because secondary correction is challenging in this area of the midface. Because of the complex nature of this region, this discussion is divided into hard tissue defects, with a focus on trauma, and soft tissue defects, with a focus on oncology.

Orbital, Periorbital, and Ocular Reconstruction 151

John A. Long and Rajesh Gutta

The repair and restoration of the eyelids and orbit can be a medical and surgical challenge. Inadequate orbital volume restoration could lead to poor functional and cosmetic defects. With advances in technology, our surgical techniques are constantly improving. This article focuses on ocular and orbital reconstruction following traumatic, iatrogenic, and acquired defects. Optimal outcomes can only be expected with appropriate diagnosis treatment planning in consultation with other specialists.

Zygoma Reconstruction 167

Michael R. Markiewicz, Savannah Gelesko, and R. Bryan Bell

Ideal reconstruction of the zygoma position is essential in restoring facial width, projection, and symmetry. Reconstruction should be focused on the zygoma's 4 articulations and restoring the vertical and horizontal pillars of the facial skeleton. This article describes the applied surgical anatomy as it relates to zygomatic deformities, surgical approaches, and reconstruction. The basis for diagnosing and classifying zygoma deformities as they relate to severity of injury and associated displacement, comminution, and comorbidities is also discussed. Traditional and contemporary concepts in posttraumatic, postablative, and esthetic reconstruction are also described.

Lip Reconstruction

Joshua E. Lubek and Robert A. Ord

This article discusses the reconstruction of full-thickness defects of the lower and upper lip. Although these may occur as a result of hereditary disorders (cleft lip) or trauma, reconstruction is described in relation to oncologic ablation for primary lip cancers. These defects will obviously be preplanned and most often of regular shape, unlike injuries sustained from penetrating trauma. Therefore, precise elective planning of reconstruction techniques must be undertaken.

Maxillary Reconstruction

Nathan D. Lenox and Dongsoo D. Kim

Postablative maxillary defects present a wide range of functional and esthetic challenges. Several classification schemes have added clarity to the subject, but the surgeon must maintain a clear vision of the defect and appreciate its reconstructive implications. Local tissue flaps remain valuable tools in the reconstruction of small isolated defects of the posterior maxilla and palate; however, microvascular free flaps have eclipsed prosthetic obturators as the mainstay of therapy in advanced postablative defects of the maxilla. Many excellent microvascular options exist and the overall objectives remain to preserve oral function in accordance with the needs of the patient.

Zygoma Implant Reconstruction of Acquired Maxillary Bony Defects

Luis G. Vega, William Gielincki, and Rui P. Fernandes

The reconstruction of acquired maxillary bony defects after pathologic ablation, infectious debridement, avulsive trauma, or previously failed reconstructions with zygoma implants represents a treatment alternative that is safe, predictable, and cost-effective. Still the single most important factor for treatment success of these complex reconstructions is the implementation of a team approach between the surgeon and the restorative dentist. The focus of this article is to review the surgical and prosthetic nuances to successfully reconstruct acquired maxillary defects with zygoma implants.

Reconstruction of Acquired Oromandibular Defects

Rui P. Fernandes and Jacob G. Yetzer

Acquired defects of the mandible resulting from trauma, infection, osteoradionecrosis, and ablative surgery of the oral cavity and lower face are particularly debilitating. Familiarity with mandibular and cervical anatomy is crucial in achieving mandibular reconstruction. The surgeon must evaluate which components of the hard and soft tissue are missing in selecting a method of reconstruction. Complexity of mandibular reconstruction ranges from simple rigid internal fixation to microvascular free tissue transfer, depending on defect- and patient-related factors. Modern techniques for microvascular tissue transfer provide a wide array of reconstructive options that can be tailored to patients' specific needs.

Various conditions are responsible for the development of acquired temporomandibular joint (TMJ) defects, the reconstruction of which represents a unique challenge, as the TMJ plays an important role in the functioning of the jaw including mastication, deglutition, and phonation. Autogenous reconstructions such as costochondral or sternoclavicular joint graft continue to be the best option in children, owing to their ability to transfer a growth center. In adults, alloplastic reconstructions are a safe and predictable option. Vascularized tissue transfers have also become a popular and reliable way to restore these defects.

Injuries to the ear can result in partial or complete loss of the external ear. Resection of the external ear may be necessary secondary to malignant tumor or infection. This article discusses the diagnosis and management of acquired defects of the external ear. Because autogenous reconstruction is not always possible, both autogenous and prosthetic reconstruction are presented as well as the indications for both. This information should help guide the clinician in the decision-making process. In the hands of experienced clinicians, reconstruction of the external ear can result in an excellent outcome, with improved quality of life for the patient.

Head and neck tumor surgery or traumatic injuries in the maxillofacial region often result in discontinuity defects of peripheral branches of the trigeminal (fifth cranial) nerve, causing loss of sensation to those areas of the face, mouth, or jaws supplied by this important nerve. Injuries to the peripheral branches of the trigeminal nerve can be repaired by microsurgical techniques, either at the time of the original injury or ablative operation if conditions are favorable, or at a later date. Repair of a peripheral nerve injury has a good chance of a satisfactory outcome if done in a timely fashion.

The patient with facial paralysis presents a daunting challenge to the reconstructive surgeon. A thorough evaluation is key in directing the surgeon to the appropriate treatment methods. Aggressive and immediate exploration with primary repair of the facial nerve continues to be the standard of care for traumatic transection of the facial nerve. Secondary repair using dynamic techniques is preferred over static procedures, because the outcomes have proved to be superior. However, patients should be counseled that facial movement and symmetry are difficult to mimic and none of the procedures described is able to restore all of the complex vectors and overall balance of facial movement and expression.

Navigational systems are paramount in solving today's traffic dilemmas, and have important applications in the human body. Current imaging must be diagnostic and is often dictated by the radiologist, but it is up to the surgeon to consider surgical procedures and to decide in which case surgical navigation (SN) has advantages. Knowledge of the surgical capabilities of SN is indispensable. The aims of this article are to support real-time image-guided SN, present routine and advanced cases with precise preoperative planning, and show the scientific capabilities of SN.

ORAL AND MAXILLOFACIAL SURGERY CLINICS OF NORTH AMERICA

THE CLINICS ARE NOW AVAILABLE ONLINE!
Access your subscription at:
www.theclinics.com

ORAL AND MAXILLOFACIAL SURGERY CLINICS OF NORTH AMERICA

FORTHCOMING ISSUES

August 2013
Anesthesia
Paul J. Schwartz, DMD, Editor

November 2013
Trauma and Reconstruction
David S. Precious, DDS, MSc, FRCD, Editor

February 2014
Sjögren's Syndrome
Michael T. Brennan, DDS, MHS, Editor

RECENT ISSUES

February 2013
**Current Concepts in the Management
of Pathologic Conditions**
John H. Campbell, DDS, MS, Editor

November 2012
The Orbit
Stephen A. Schendel, MD, DDS, FACS, Editor

August 2012
Pediatric Maxillofacial Surgery
Bruce B. Horswell, MD, DDS and
Michael S. Jaskolka, MD, DDS, Editors

RELATED INTEREST

Atlas of the Oral and Maxillofacial Clinics of North America
March 2013 (Vol. 21, No. 1)
Craniomaxillofacial Trauma
David A. Bitonti, DMD, CAPT DC, USN, Editor

THE CLINICS ARE NOW AVAILABLE ONLINE!
Access your subscription at:
www.theclinics.com

Preface
Maxillofacial Reconstruction

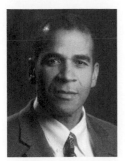

Patrick J. Louis, DDS, MD
Editor

Many oral and maxillofacial surgeons have been inspired to enter the field because of the reconstructive aspects of this specialty. This aspect of oral and maxillofacial surgery (OMS) has continued to grow through the use of new and innovative techniques, such as navigation, virtual surgery, and microvascular techniques. There are new and better biomaterials that continue to allow us to push the envelope of the reconstructive field. This allows us to offer our patients improved results.

There are many different types of insults to the human body that can result in facial defects. These insults include trauma from motor vehicle accidents, high-velocity weapons, and blunt objects. Surgical resection of diseased tissue due to neoplasms, infection, and necrosis is commonplace in the field of medicine and dentistry. Many of these defects involve both the hard and the soft tissue and are challenging to reconstruct. They require not only surgical skill but also knowledge of the normal and abnormal anatomy, knowledge of various surgical techniques, and available technologies that can help improve outcomes.

This issue of the *Oral and Maxillofacial Surgery Clinics of North America* focuses on reconstructive techniques for the maxillofacial region. Although there are some articles that are more heavily weighted toward acute trauma, the area that we have attempted to address is the delayed management of acquired facial defects and deformities. Each article addresses an anatomic subunit of the facial region and discusses techniques that can be used to reconstruct these areas. Both soft and, when appropriate, hard tissue problems are discussed. The last article addresses the use of navigation because it continues to grow in its application in resection and reconstruction.

I would like to dedicate this issue to my many mentors that have inspired me and previous and future generations in the area of maxillofacial reconstruction. As a resident I was inspired by my dedicated faculty, Dr Victor Matukas, Dr Charles A. McCallum, Dr Peter D. Waite, Dr Thomas Jones, Dr John Ballard, and my chief residents, Dr Gary Hudson, Dr Phillip Mitchell, and Dr "Joe" Mack. They nurtured and inspired me to become an OMS faculty member. As a young faculty member, I was mentored and inspired by many in the field of OMS, too numerous to mention, each of whom I consider a giant in their own way. Now, many of my own residents, some of whom are featured in this issue, inspire me to learn more with their dedication to teaching the next generation and pushing the envelope in the field of OMS. I hope this issue will impart some knowledge to the reader and help inspire you in your chosen career path and to improve patient care and inspire the next generation.

Patrick J. Louis, DDS, MD
Department of Oral and Maxillofacial Surgery
University of Alabama at Birmingham
1919 Seventh Avenue South
SDB 419, Birmingham, AL 35294, USA

The Kirklin Clinic
2000 Sixth Avenue South
Birmingham, AL 35233, USA

E-mail address:
plouis@uab.edu

Oral Maxillofacial Surg Clin N Am 25 (2013) xiii
http://dx.doi.org/10.1016/j.coms.2013.02.009
1042-3699/13/$ – see front matter © 2013 Published by Elsevier Inc.

Reconstruction of the Scalp, Calvarium, and Frontal Sinus

Somsak Sittitavornwong, DDS, DMD, MS[a],*,
Anthony B.P. Morlandt, DDS, MD[b,c]

KEYWORDS

- Scalp • Skull • Reconstruction • Defects • Flaps

KEY POINTS

- Scalp and cranial deformities are common after trauma or ablative surgery.
- Local flaps and free flaps may be used in reconstruction of soft tissue defects, and autogenous bone or alloplastic bone substitutes may be used for cranioplasty procedures.
- Injuries to the frontal sinus, particularly when complicated by leak of cerebrospinal fluid or obstruction of the nasofrontal outflow tract, represent special challenges.
- Further studies are recommended to improve the multidisciplinary management of these complex, debilitating conditions, in anticipation of enhanced function and cosmesis, reduced donor site morbidity, and improved surgical outcomes.

INTRODUCTION

Scalp and calvarial defects are common sequelae of trauma and ablative surgery. Surgical correction of acquired deformities, and of the scalp and calvarium in particular, is therefore critically important to the reconstructive maxillofacial surgeon. Although secondary healing (granulation), primary closure, and skin grafts may be used in selected soft tissue scalp defects, this article asserts local and free flaps as essential tools in the maxillofacial surgeon's armamentarium. Cranial reconstruction, with attention to modern cranioplasty techniques and management of the frontal sinus, is discussed as well.

Etiology: Trauma

Sharkey and colleagues[1] reported on the kinetic forces resulting in soft tissue laceration and skull fracture caused by falls and blunt trauma. The minimum force associated with the formation of a laceration is at least 4000 N, or the equivalent of 408.23 kg (900 pounds) moving at 1 m per second squared. Calvarial fractures were seen in a high percentage of cases involving simple falls (68%) and blows from blunt objects (75%).[1] Whittle and colleagues[2] reported similar findings, noting a minimum force of 2 to 10,000 N to sustain a complex scalp laceration.

PART 1: SCALP RECONSTRUCTION
Anatomy

Topography

Applying terminology commonly used when analyzing the face, the soft tissues of the scalp can likewise be subdivided into functional and aesthetic subunits. Those subunits commonly described are the forehead, vertex, occiput, and bilateral temporal zones (**Fig. 1**). Zones differ with respect to underlying anatomy and, correspondingly, vary greatly in their degree of relative elasticity and ease of manipulation. Flaps must be designed carefully, considering the underlying fascial architecture as well as adjacent critical

Dr Morlandt is now with University of Florida, Jacksonville, Florida.
a Department of Oral and Maxillofacial Surgery, UAB Medicine, 2321 Highway 150, Suite 113, Hoover, AL 35244, USA; b UAB Department of Oral and Maxillofacial Surgery, The Kirklin Clinic, 2000 Sixth Avenue South, Birmingham, AL 35233, USA; c University of Florida, Microvascular Reconstruction Fellowship, Department of Oral and Maxillofacial Surgery, College of Medicine-Jacksonville, Jacksonville, FL, USA
* Corresponding author.
E-mail address: sjade@uab.edu

Oral Maxillofacial Surg Clin N Am 25 (2013) 105–129
http://dx.doi.org/10.1016/j.coms.2013.02.004
1042-3699/13/$ – see front matter Published by Elsevier Inc.

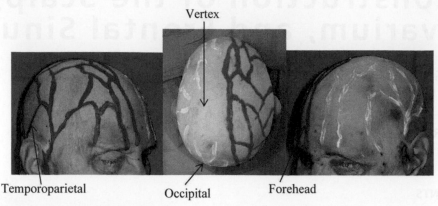

Fig. 1. (A–C) Topographic subunits of scalp.

structures such as the pinna of the ear or the brow. Although large expanses of scalp may be available for coverage, the distensibility of the skin to be mobilized can be an underappreciated but critical component of flap success.

Skin and fascia

Relaxed skin tension lines (RSTLs) course perpendicular to the direction of maximum skin extensibility and result from the arrangement of collagen and elastin bundles in the skin.[3] Placing incisions or suture lines appropriately within RSTLs allows for maximum skin mobility and decreased tension. In addition, wrinkles tend to fall in or are parallel to the RSTLs, and scars can be camouflaged in natural skin creases. These principles apply to closure of local rotational or advancement flaps as well: the donor site must be closed first, thereby exerting less tension at the distal margin of the flap. If excessive tension or distortion is noted, the surgeon must decide to back cut or further undermine the adjacent tissue margins.

The mnemonic SCALP describes the tissue planes seen during dissection (Fig. 2). In the temporal regions, the temporalis muscle and fascia are encountered as well.

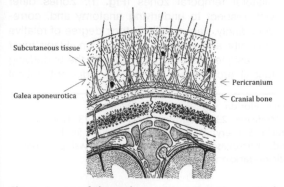

Fig. 2. Layers of the scalp at vertex. Superior sagittal sinus is seen in midline.

1. Skin
2. Connective tissue (tela subcutanea)
3. Aponeurosis (ie, galea aponeurotica/temporoparietal fascia)
   a. Contiguous inferiorly with the superficial musculoaponeurotic system and platysma
4. Loose areolar connective tissue (ie, Merkel space/innominate fascia/subgaleal plane)
   a. Contiguous inferiorly with superficial layer of deep cervical fascia
   b. In the lateral scalp, the temporalis muscle fascia and muscle are deep to loose areolar connective tissue
      i. Temporalis fascia fuses with periosteum to become pericranium above superior temporal line
      ii. Temporalis muscle
5. Pericranium
   a. Above superior temporal line laterally, below the temporalis muscle is known as periosteum

Vascular supply

In general, the blood supply of a given area of skin arises from segmental arteries (Fig. 3). Named vessels give off branches that supply overlying skin as either direct musculocutaneous or septocutaneous perforators or as part of the rich subdermal plexus. This pattern varies in the scalp, where many arterial end branches are invested in dense supragaleal tela subcutanea. The walls of these vessels are firmly attached to the fibrous tissue of the superficial fascial layer, resulting in profound bleeding as a result of the inability of the arteries to spasm and retract after surgical or traumatic disruption. The vascular supply of the scalp is derived from 5 pairs of arteries: 3 from the external carotid system and 2 from the internal carotid artery.

1. Internal carotid system:
   a. Ophthalmic

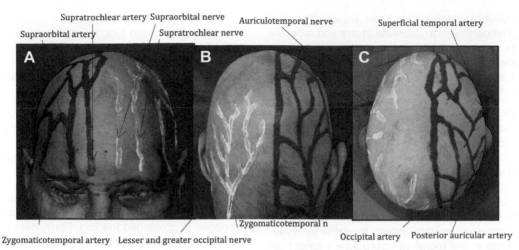

Supratrochlear artery Supraorbital nerve Auriculotemporal nerve   Superficial temporal artery
Supraorbital artery   Supratrochlear nerve

Zygomaticotemporal artery Lesser and greater occipital nerve   Zygomaticotemporal n

Occipital artery   Posterior auricular artery

Fig. 3. (*A–C*) Sensory innervation and blood supply of the scalp.

  i. Supratrochlear: ascends the forehead in the midline
  ii. Supraorbital: supplies the lateral forehead, scalp as far superiorly as the vertex
2. External carotid system:
  a. Superficial temporal
    i. Frontal
    ii. Parietal
  b. Occipital: supplies occipital aspect of scalp
  c. Posterior auricular: supplies skin above and behind the auricle

Neuroanatomy

The scalp is innervated by several sensory nerves originating from the trigeminal nerve (cranial nerve V) and the cervical spinal nerves (see **Fig. 3**). The supratrochlear and supraorbital branches of the ophthalmic division (V1), zygomaticotemporal branch of the maxillary division (V2), and the auriculotemporal branch of mandibular division (V3) arise from the trigeminal nerve (cranial nerve V). The supratrochlear and supraorbital nerves ascend vertically, supplying the forehead to the midvertex, and the zygomaticotemporal nerve runs along the lateral wall of the orbit and supplies the hairless temple. The greater occipital nerve (C2) ascends along the posterior scalp up to the vertex, and the lesser occipital nerve (C2, C3) supplies a patch of skin just posterior to the auricle.

Scalp Reconstruction

Healing by secondary intention

Although surgical repair is the mainstay of treatment of scalp defects, certain wounds may result in acceptable cosmesis and bone coverage if allowed to heal by secondary intention.[4] Heavily contaminated wounds, extensive tissue necrosis from ballistic injuries, or patients who are medically unfit for reconstructive surgery may benefit from meticulous wound care and watchful waiting. In oncologic defects, granulation allows for tumor surveillance.[5] It has been shown experimentally and clinically[6] that a delay in wound closure of 4 to 5 days increases the tensile strength of the wound as well as resistance to infection as a result of improved wound cleansing and lower bacterial counts.

Skin grafts

Split-thickness skin grafts (STSGs) and full-thickness skin grafts (FTSGs) are widely used for reconstructing simple scalp defects. Preauricular, postauricular, supraclavicular, and abdominal skin are common FTSG donor sites for use in head and neck defects. Skin grafts heal and are incorporated by way of 3 physiologic phases:

1. Plasmatic imbibition. Immediately on placement of the graft onto the recipient bed, the graft absorbs nutrients directly from the underlying tissues. Similar to a sponge, the graft takes up fluid by capillary action, shown by an increase of 20% in graft weight in the first 24 hours.[7,8]
2. Inosculation. After 48 hours, vascular buds start to align and anastomose. This process continues until there is a free interchange of nutrients between the vessels of the skin graft and soft tissue bed. For successful inosculation, intimate contact between the graft and the soft tissue bed is required, and the graft must be immobilized to prevent shearing of immature vessels. Fibrin, which initially acts to help adhere the skin graft to the recipient site, is infiltrated by fibroblasts, which form a fibrous attachment by the fourth or fifth day.[9]
3. Revascularization. By day 8 or 9, revascularization, with functional blood and lymphatic

draining systems, has been shown. The skin graft continues to decrease in size and recovers its original weight.[10] Lymphatics have been shown to revascularize by the fifth postoperative day, eliminating congestion and improving further nutrient exchange.[11]

FTSGs versus STSGs The FTSG, with a complete dermal layer, more closely resembles normal skin in color, texture, and the potential to maintain hair growth. There is a decreased risk of secondary contraction and hypopigmentation when FTSGs are compared with STSGs. For these reasons, FTSGs are preferred over STSGs for managing defects in the aesthetic zone. Thin skin grafts have more terminal capillary endings available for revascularization and therefore incorporate sooner than thick grafts. Care must be taken to place skin grafts over muscle, periosteum, perichondrium, or paratenon, because devascularized tissues such as bare bone, cartilage, or tendon do not provide adequate nutrients for graft survival. However, small grafts (<1 cm) can bridge over tendon or cartilage if adequate circulation is provided by adjacent capillaries. It has been reported that FTSGs can bridge denuded tissues more reliably than STSGs.[7,12,13]

Local flaps

Indications Local skin flaps are commonly used in craniofacial trauma and reconstruction. Using skin adjacent to the defect provides the best available color and texture match for reconstruction. With appropriate planning, excellent outcomes may be achieved.

Many factors drive the decision to use a local flap, including:

1. Topographic region of the scalp
   a. Forehead
   b. Temporoparietal zone
   c. Vertex
   d. Occiput
2. Defect factors
   a. Size of the defect
   b. Cause of defect
      i. Traumatic
      ii. Ablative
      iii. Ischemic/infectious
3. Patient factors
   a. Age: elderly patients have great skin laxity

b. Medical status of patient
c. Psychiatric and functional status
d. Patient/family desires
4. Surgeon preference
5. Lack of access to a microvascular surgeon (for large defects)

Skin flap physiology Although a comprehensive review of soft tissue flap biomechanics and physiology exceeds the scope of this article, an understanding of several key factors is critical for flap survival and successful reconstruction.

Stress relaxation and creep Stress relaxation occurs when soft tissue cellularity increases in response to prolonged loading. Permanent deformation with stretching of the skin occurs. Similarly, tissue creep results from extrusion of fluid from the dermis and breakdown of the dermal framework, which is the same phenomenon by which tissue expanders function. Physiologic advantages of stress relaxation and creep may assist in wound closure by providing additional flap tissue; however, a balance between tension and vascularity must be managed to prevent flap ischemia.

Flap delay A cutaneous or fasciocutaneous flap may be delayed to improve long-term survival. Flap delay involves incising and undermining the flap without simultaneous transposition to the recipient site. In the scalp and forehead, where there are no perforating vessels, incising the flap to the subgaleal plane without undermining is adequate for the delaying procedure. After 2 to 3 weeks of healing, the flap is then raised and transferred in the usual fashion. Timing of the transfer is important: after 3 weeks to 3 months the delay phenomenon is lost.[8]

Delaying flaps in this manner allows for:

- Improved blood flow
- Conditioning to tissue ischemia
- Closure of arteriovenous shunts

Flap design When a flap is designed, the surgeon must ask the following questions:

- Dimension
  ○ Is the flap similar in size and thickness to the defect?
- Configuration

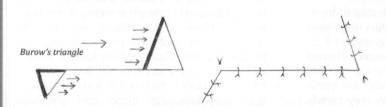

Burow's triangle

Fig. 4. Burow triangular advancement flap: a small triangle of soft tissue is excised, creating some soft tissue laxity for tension-free flap advancement and elimination of a dog-ear deformity.

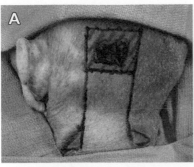
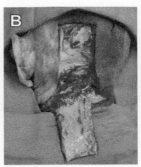
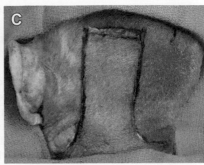

Fig. 5. (*A–C*) Advancement flap at occiput: the length/width ratio is typically limited to 2:1, although some cases have reported success with a ratio of 3:1. Two small Burow triangles are excised at the base of the flap. An important consideration when repairing defects overlying the nuchal ridge is maintaining tension-free closure when the patient flexes the neck to prevent wound dehiscence.

- ○ What is the most appropriate configuration?
  - ■ Rotation
  - ■ Advancement
  - ■ Transposition (see later discussion)
- Adjacent structures
  - ○ Will the flap distort eyebrows/lids, hairline, auricle?
  - ○ Will the incision cross vital structures (eg, temporal branch of VII)
- Vascularity
  - ○ Will the flap have sufficient vascular inflow and outflow?

- ○ Will the flap have a random (unnamed vessels) or axial (named) pattern?

Blood supply Skin flap survival depends on blood supply. Flap perfusion is based on the physical properties of its supplying vessels, perfusion pressure, and the metabolic demands of the flap.

Width of the flap pedicle The effect of decreasing the width of the flap base decreases the chance of the pedicle containing a large vessel. A wider random flap only adds subdermal arterioles,

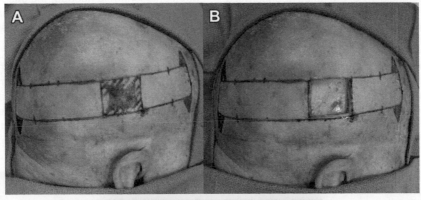

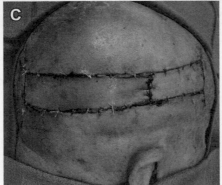

Fig. 6. (*A–C*) Bipedicled advancement flap: the H-plasty, or bilateral U-advancement flap, is a valuable flap. Double advancement flaps with Burow triangles are used in this cadaveric temporoparietal defect.

each carrying blood at the same perfusion pressure, because they are all based on the same feeding vessel. Therefore, 2 random flaps of equal length show similar survival regardless of width. When perfusion of the flap reaches a threshold, blood flow cannot be improved by widening the base of the flap. However, additional pedicle width does provide some benefit by allowing increased collateral circulation and improved venous outflow. A recommended length/width ratio used in head and neck advancement flaps is 3:1, although only 1:1 may be tolerated for trunk and extremity reconstruction.[14]

Tension When the skin is stretched beyond the limits of perfusion, circulation is compromised. The early sign is blanching with, eventually, distal necrosis of the flap tissue. Tension should be respected by the surgeon and care taken to minimize its effects.

Skin flap configuration

Primary closure Wide undermining may, in some cases, permit advancement and primary closure when defects are 3 cm in diameter or less.

Advancement flaps There are various types of advancement flaps, each with subtle differences in design and usefulness. These flaps are dependent on the extensibility of the galea aponeurotica. Therefore, an advancement flap is better suited for older patients with lax skin than for younger patients.

Burow advancement flap The Burow technique is a type of advancement flap. Burow triangles were first described in 1855 to treat the dog-ear deformity seen with flap advancement. Burow triangles allow excision of a dog ear, with reorientation into a favorable position in an RSTL. With

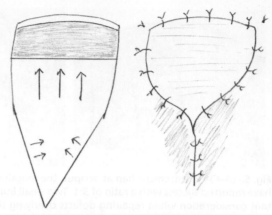

Fig. 7. Sliding advancement flap: The subcutaneous tissues are preserved to ensure flap viability.

double advancement flaps, an additional gain in tissue movement may be achieved (**Figs. 4–6**).

Sliding advancement flap The double opposed sliding flap was introduced by Lejour in 1975[15] and depends on a lateral subcutaneous pedicle for vascular supply, previously elucidated by Barron and Emmett.[16] The sliding flap is advanced as an island based entirely on subcutaneous tissues. The inelastic tissues of the vertex can be successfully repaired by this method (**Figs. 7** and **8**). If additional length is needed, the subcutaneous tissues may be judiciously divided along 1 margin, although risk of flap ischemia increases with this maneuver.

Rotational flaps Rotational flaps are a type of pivotal flap whereby a curvilinear arc is used to correct a triangular deformity. The base of the triangle forms a portion of the circumference of the circle, and the base of the flap is the radius of the large circle (**Fig. 9**). When the flap is elevated,

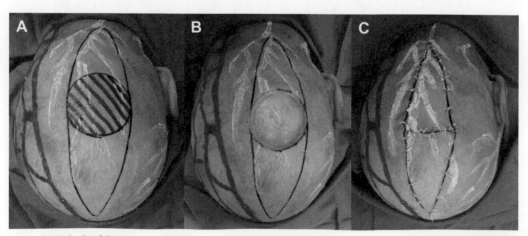

Fig. 8. (*A–C*) With double sliding advancement flaps, an additional gain in tissue movement may be achieved. Flaps are mobilized and pushed to repair this midline defect.

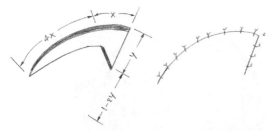

Fig. 9. The arc of rotational flap is made 4 times the width of the defect with a radius equaling 1 to 2 times its height. When there is an excessive skin or contour problems, a back cut or Burow triangle might be necessary. With a back cut, an incision is made toward the center of the circle. This technique decreases skin tension and allows for further rotation; however, it may violate the pedicle and result in flap ischemia.

it can be rotated to close the defect. These flaps are particularly popular in closing scalp defects because of the round shape of the scalp. The wide arc seen in rotational flaps often violates resting skin tension lines and aesthetic subunits when used in the face. However, in the scalp, these lines are less critical and can be crossed without a compromise in aesthetics. Ideally, the defect is designed with a height/width ratio of 2:1. The arc of rotation is then made 4 times the width of the defect, with a radius equaling 1 to 2 times its height. Although less tension may be seen on the final repair when extending the arc, no benefit has been shown when the length of arc is increased to greater than 4 times the width of the defect. In cases of defects involving the hair-bearing and glabrous skin, 2 separate flaps arising from their respective skin types are used to maintain continuity and cosmesis of the hairline (see **Fig. 9**; **Figs. 10** and **11**). Burow triangles are placed to avoid injury to vital neurovascular structures.

O-Z flap This flap consists of 2 rotation flaps designed to pivot in the same direction. Limbs are measured at 1.5 times the diameter of the defect and follow a 90° arc of rotation (**Fig. 12**). It is most commonly used in the vertex, occiput, or forehead regions. When used in the forehead, care must be taken to avoid distorting the anterior hairline.

Pinwheel flap A modification of the O-Z rotational flap, the pinwheel flap can be designed with 3 or 4 limbs to allow additional undermining and advancement for tension-free closure. To close circular defects the limbs are designed 1 to 1.5 times the diameter of the defect. This is an excellent flap for the vertex region, where the dense underlying galeal aponeurosis precludes monopedicled advancement or simple rotation flaps (**Fig. 13**).

Rhomboid/Dufourmentel First described by Limberg[17] in 1967, the rhomboid flap is used to repair defects with 2 equal, opposed 120° angles and 2 equal, opposed 60° angles. An incision perpendicular to the central axis of the defect is created, its length equal to the width of the defect (**Figs. 14** and **15**). A second incision parallels 1 of the lateral margins, with the pivot point at its extent. The flap is mobilized and rotated to close the wound. A variation described by Dufourmentel[18] places the first flap incision equally at a point bisecting the short diagonal span of the defect with 1 of the lateral margins, extending the length of 1 side of the defect margin. A second incision is parallel to the long diagonal span of the defect. In both cases, a standing cutaneous deformity must be excised at the base of the defect to prevent dog-ear formation. These flaps may be used to reconstruct the temporal or occipital regions.

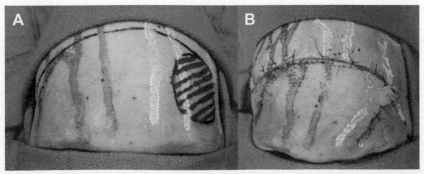

Fig. 10. (*A, B*) Rotational flap of the forehead: the skin of the forehead is loosely attached to the underlying fibrous pericranium, separated by the intervening frontalis muscle. However, near the hairline, dense galea aponeurotica fibers emerge from the belly of the frontalis in a vertical direction, resulting in tightness and minimal distensibility. Circular or triangular scalp defects may be repaired by simple advancement, but only in the loose zones of the forehead or vertex.

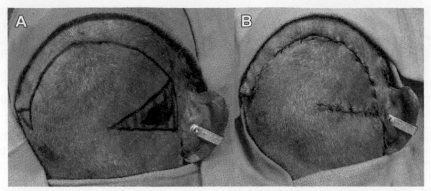

Fig. 11. (*A, B*) Rotational flap of occiput area: like the forehead, rearranging local flaps in the occiput region is aided by the occipitalis muscle, ensheathed in the fascia of the galea.

Multiple rhomboid Double or triple rhomboid flaps may be used to close large circular defects. The round defect is visualized as a hexagon, with each side equaling the radius of the circle. Incisions are designed radially at opposing corners of the hexagon, extending in length 1 radius from the border of the hexagon (see **Fig. 15**). A second incision parallels the border of the hexagon. Additional extensions may be added to increase laxity of the flaps, especially in the relatively immobile vertex and temporal regions. In the vertex area, the underlying galea is dense and thin, making mobilization of flaps in this area difficult. For this reason, flap mobility may be augmented by the incorporation of relaxing incisions in the galeal layer.

Microvascular surgery in scalp reconstruction

When primary closure, skin grafts, or local flaps are insufficient, microvascular techniques may be safely used in scalp reconstruction.[19] Microvascular tissue transfer is an effective modality, with reported success rates of up to 92% for ablative or traumatic scalp defects.[20] In ablative defects in which neoadjuvant or adjuvant radiotherapy is used, the ability to transfer distant, nonirradiated tissues makes free flap reconstruction an

attractive option.[21] Robust coverage offered by muscle-containing free flaps reduces the risk of dehiscence caused by radiation injury[21]; however, the risk of bone exposure increases over time as flap thinning from denervation atrophy occurs. Large traumatic scalp defects also present certain challenges, including vascular injury caused by high-energy forces, significant scarring from previous trauma or operations, and wound contamination.[20] Free flaps may be used to reconstruct soft tissue over alloplastic cranioplasty materials (see section on cranial reconstruction).[22] Although hair restoration techniques may be used, many patients require only soft tissue skull coverage and rely on wigs for hair replacement.[23,24]

Replantation Scalp reconstruction has been achieved by microvascular replantation since the first reported case by Miller in 1976.[25] When a patient is hemodynamically and neurologically stable for rapid transfer to the operating suite and the avulsed tissues are minimally traumatized, scalp replantation is recommended, because of the ability to reconstruct with tissue of identical texture, thickness, and color.[20] Cheng and colleagues[26] reported 20 cases of scalp replantation in which

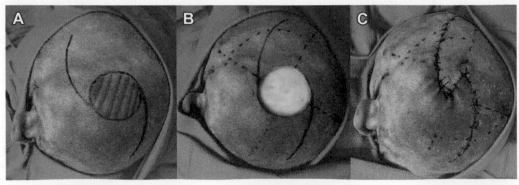

Fig. 12. (*A–C*) The O-Z flap follows the same principle of 2 rational flaps. Two curved incisions are made opposing each other. Both flaps are undermined and rotated centrally for primary soft tissue closure.

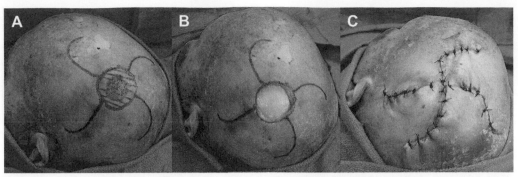

Fig. 13. (*A–C*) If a soft tissue defect cannot be closed without tension, the pinwheel flap can be designed with 3 or 4 limbs. The surrounding loose connective tissue of the pinwheel flap can be undermined to attain more mobility for primary closure of soft tissue.

75% or more of the scalp was completely amputated. These investigators cite extended warm ischemia time (>30 hours) and significant shearing vessel injury as contraindications to replantation of major scalp avulsions. Otherwise, it is recommended that an attempt should be made to repair these wounds immediately using microsurgical techniques, even in the case of pediatric trauma.[27] Temporary implantation of the scalp into the lower abdomen has been reported successfully in a case of significant recipient site injury with poor vessel availability.[28]

Free tissue transfer When avulsed tissues are unavailable for reanastomosis, or when ablative surgical defects are present, distant free tissue transfer is an option for total or subtotal scalp reconstruction. Chao and colleagues[29] reported 138 cases of microvascular free flap reconstruction for oncologic defects, 48 of which underwent

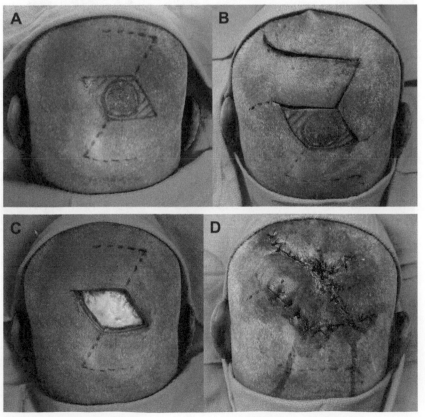

Fig. 14. (*A–D*) A rhomboid defect is created, which can be closed primarily. The rhomboid flap (*above*) or Dufourmentel modification (*below*) may be used.

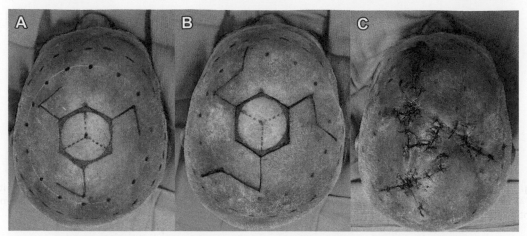

Fig. 15. (*A–C*) A hexagonal defect is approximated closely to cover a circular defect. The length of the radius is equal to the length of each side. The triple rhomboid flap may then be rotated into the hexagonal defect.

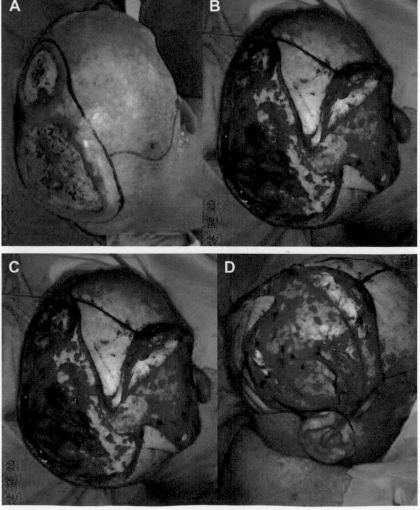

Fig. 16. (*A–G*) Extensive osteoradionecrosis of the calvarium, reconstructed with latissimus dorsi free flap and STSG. (*Courtesy of* Rui A. Fernandes, MD, DDS, FACS, Jacksonville, FL.)

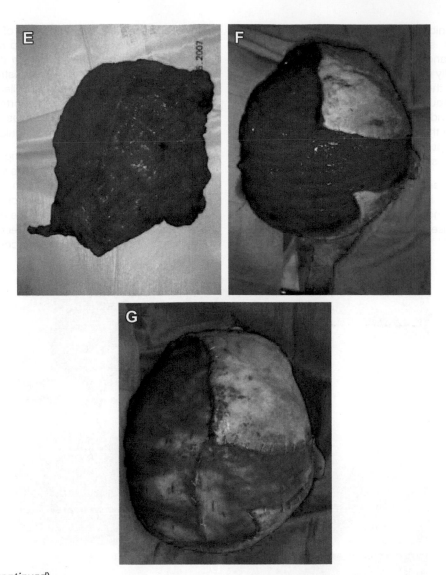

Fig. 16. (*continued*)

simultaneous alloplastic cranioplasty. Overall, major complications (reoperation within 30 days, readmission, death) were low (7.2%), suggesting microsurgery as a highly safe and effective technique in this population. In their retrospective review of patients with acquired scalp defects, Herrera and colleagues[20] reported successful replantation in 70% of cases, without need for further revision. Twin-twin allotransplantation of previously expanded scalp tissue has been reported with success in a limited number of cases by 1 institution.[30,31]

A variety of free flap types have been reported in the literature and include latissimus dorsi myocutaneous (LDM), radial forearm, anterolateral thigh (ALT), serratus anterior, free omentum,[20] rectus abdominus, scapula, and medial arm flaps.[32] In some cases, combinations of these flaps are required to achieve complete scalp coverage.[32–34] Outlined below are the 3 most commonly used microvascular flaps for scalp reconstruction: the LDM, radial forearm, and ALT.

LDM The LDM flap, introduced for use in the head and neck by Maxwell and colleagues in 1978,[35] has been the preferred free flap in several reviews of major scalp reconstruction.[19,20,29,36,37] Since its initial introduction in 1896,[38] the LDM has been cited for its large, broad available surface area, adequate pedicle length, and versatility. Calvarial bone exposure, a common problem after radiotherapy, may be mitigated when using the LDM flap by the vest over pants insetting maneuver with wide subgaleal undermining, advocated by Lipa and Butler.[39] To increase the pedicle length often necessary for scalp reconstruction, the

V-Y-I technique has been described, whereby the circumflex scapular or serratus branches are modified and used for anastomosis, instead of the typically used thoracodorsal artery.[40] Reinnervation of the frontalis muscle may be accomplished through preservation of the thoracodorsal nerve, providing mimetic activity to the forehead.[41] STSG over the latissimus dorsi muscle is used and may be kept unmeshed to enhance final skin contour and cosmesis (**Fig. 16**).[39]

Radial forearm free flap The radial forearm free flap (RFFF) is increasingly used by maxillofacial surgeons and is largely considered the workhorse flap for use in head and neck reconstruction (**Fig. 17**).[42] With its consistent pedicle length,

thin, pliable skin paddle, and ease of harvest, it has been the preferred flap for scalp reconstruction in several case series.[32,43–45] In their review of 28 cases of RFFF used to reconstruct mainly frontal scalp defects, Sweeny and colleagues[43] reported fewer complications and shorter length of hospitalization when the RFFF was compared with LDM, rectus abdominis, or scapula free flaps.

ALT free flap Introduced by Song and colleagues[46] in 1984, the ALT free flap is increasingly used in head and neck reconstruction. With a large skin paddle, ability to close the donor site primarily, and long vascular pedicle, the ALT flap offers excellent tissue for scalp reconstruction (**Fig. 18**).[47] Advocates cite lower cost as well,

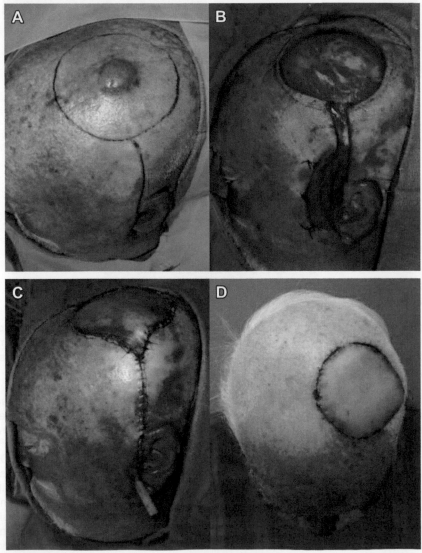

Fig. 17. (*A–D*) Angiosarcoma of the scalp, reconstructed with a fasciocutaneous RFFF. (*Courtesy of* Rui A. Fernandes, MD, DDS, FACS, Jacksonville, FL.)

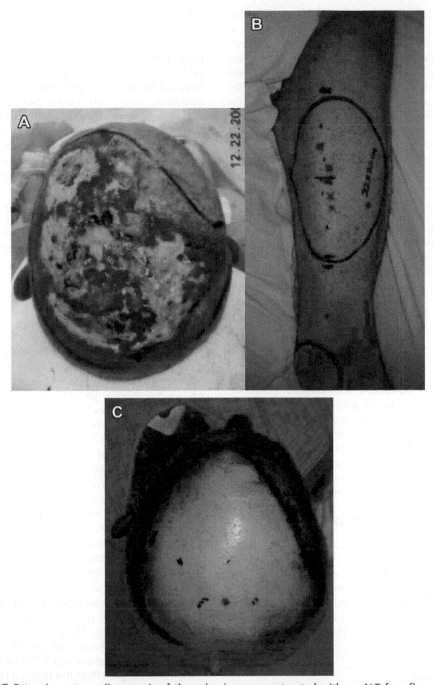

Fig. 18. (*A–C*) Extensive osteoradionecrosis of the calvarium, reconstructed with an ALT free flap. (*Courtesy of* Rui A. Fernandes, MD, DDS, FACS, Jacksonville, FL.)

because no preoperative imaging is typically required as in other perforator flaps.[48] Variability in the number of perforators and in their course through muscle, intermuscular septum, or both have been noted as limiting factors.[49] In their large review of 672 cases, Wei and colleagues[47] identified ALT flaps with musculocutaneous (87%) perforators, septocutaneous (12.9%), and only

6 cases without any skin vessels (0.09%). The perforators supplying the skin paddle typically arise from the transverse branch of the lateral circumflex femoral artery, and to a lesser degree from single perforators that come directly off the profunda femoris artery.[50] Extensive harvest of surrounding vastus lateralis or rectus femoris when dissecting musculocutaneous perforators

has been associated with increased postoperative pain and gait disturbance.[48] Initially popular in Asian reconstructive circles, the variable thickness of subcutaneous fat has limited use in the West when thin, pliable tissues are required, as in scalp and oral cavity reconstruction.[51] Flap thinning has been advocated by some groups[52–54] and may be accomplished to a total flap thickness of 3 to 4 mm,[55,56] but is not without risk to the skin paddle. In cases of extensive total scalp loss, bilateral ALTs may be harvested with minimal donor site morbidity and excellent coverage. Venous congestion in these cases is controlled by linking veins between the 2 flaps in the midline.[22]

Vascular principles The superficial temporal system provides the preferred recipient vessels used for anastomosis in most reports on scalp reconstruction.[20,39,57,58] Other arteries used include the facial artery, superior thyroid, supraorbital, postauricular,[20] external carotid (end-to-side), and occipital,[21] whereas veins typically used are typically the internal or external jugular or the occipital veins.[21] In scalp trauma, veins are typically injured to a greater degree than are the arteries, which may risk their availability for use in microsurgical anastomosis.[59] Cheng and colleagues[26] mention the novel technique of simultaneously applying vein grafts to the donor veins and recipient arteries using hand-sewn anastomoses to reduce operating time and improve outcomes. Vein grafts have been used successfully to increase pedicle length in cases involving the vertex, although they are associated with a higher risk of flap failure.[60]

PART 2: CRANIAL RECONSTRUCTION
Anatomy

Topography
The calvarium comprises contributions from the frontal, occipital, and the paired parietal and temporal bones (**Fig. 19**). Embryologically derived from desmocranium, the anterior and posterior fontanelles fuse between 18 and 24 months of

age. Inner and outer layers of bone are separated by the spongy cancellous diploe.

Bone thickness
In 1882, Anderson[61] reported on cranial bone thickness measured in 154 Irish cadavers. Todd[62] subsequently performed direct calvarial thickness measurements in 448 adult white men. Todd noted that the average thickness was 11.3 mm in the glabellar area, 5.7 mm at the opisthion (occiput), 5.98 mm at the vertex, and 3.6 mm at the euryion (the most lateral aspect of cranial outline in frontal projection).

Roche[63] suggested that the average cranial thickness of males exceeded that of females except at the euryion (the most lateral point of the skull). As a patient grows, the rate of increase in calvarial thickness decreases from 5 to 17 years. Skull thickness was also measured on lateral radiographs in 300 blacks and 200 whites observed in American general hospital emergency rooms by Adeloye and associates.[64] A rapid increase in skull thickness was observed during the first 2 decades of life followed by a less steep increase until a peak is reached in the fifth and sixth decades. Sexual differences were variable. It is difficult at best to ascertain if any basis for preoperative estimation of calvarial thickness exists. Pensler and McCarthy[65] analyzed 200 postmortem adult skulls, reporting that age and height had no statistical significance in the prediction of calvarial thickness, but that weight and race were significant variables for all measurements. However, sex was either significant or borderline for the various measurements. The study showed that mean value of skull thickness of parasagittal sinus suture from frontal to parietal area ranges from 6.80 to 7.72 mm for various points measured (minimum–maximum = 3.0–12.0 mm), with the parietal bone as the thickest area. These figures show the inherent risk in penetrating the inner table when harvesting an outer table calvarial bone graft (**Fig. 20**). By the time a child is 5 years old, the calvarium has reached 80% of its adult thickness, although it does increase in thickness for 15 more years.[66] The cranium follows the rapid growth of the brain; it reaches 80% development between 3 and 4 years of age, and 100% between 7 and 8 years. It then continues to grow in thickness but not in size, width, length, or height. The cranial sutures persist, although they become more or less fused with age.[67]

Vascular supply
Blood supply to the cranium arises from both intracranial and extracranial sources.[68,69] Internally, the principal blood supply is provided by the middle meningeal artery and its branches. An

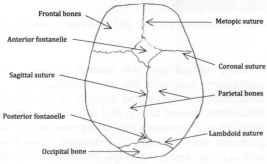

Frontal bones

Anterior fontanelle

Sagittal suture

Posterior fontanelle

Occipital bone

Metopic suture

Coronal suture

Parietal bones

Lambdoid suture

Fig. 19. Normal skull of the newborn.

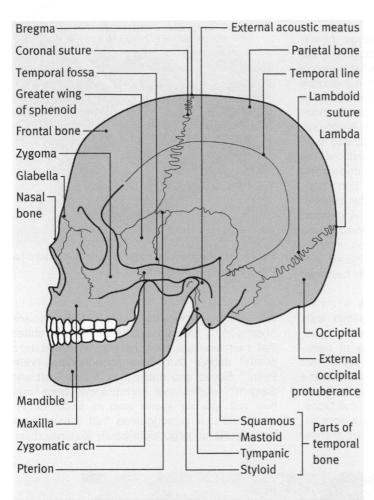

Bregma
Coronal suture
Temporal fossa
Greater wing
of sphenoid
Frontal bone
Zygoma
Glabella
Nasal
bone

External acoustic meatus
Parietal bone
Temporal line
Lambdoid
suture
Lambda

Mandible
Maxilla
Zygomatic arch
Pterion

Occipital
External
occipital
protuberance

Squamous
Mastoid
Tympanic
Styloid
Parts of
temporal
bone

Fig. 20. Lateral aspects of the skull. Danger areas of the skull: temporal line, coronal suture, and sagittal suture. The parietal calvarium shows the greatest thickness. (*From* Craven C. Anatomy of the skull. Anesthesia Intensive Care Medicine 2011;12(5):186–88; with permission.)

The external acoustic meatus (opening) is surrounded by the squamous and the tympanic parts of the temporal bone

extracranial anastomotic plexus arising from the superficial temporal occipital, supraorbital, and supratrochlear vessels sends perforators through the galea to the periosteum.

Cranial Bone Reconstruction

Cause of cranial defects
An estimated 50% of the 12 million annual traumatic wounds treated in emergency rooms across the United States involve the head and neck.[70] Motor vehicle collision (MVC) is the predominant cause, followed by blunt assault.[71] Protective devices decrease the incidence of facial fractures, whereas the lack of protective devices and the consumption of alcohol correlate positively with facial fractures. Facial fractures were found in 9.5% of restrained MVC patients compared with 15.4% of unrestrained patients. Nonhelmeted motorcyclists were 4 times more likely to sustain

facial fractures (4.3% vs 18.4%) than helmeted patients.[71] Shapiro and colleagues[71] noted twice as many legally intoxicated patients involved in MVCs compared with those injured by blunt assault. Men seem to be more involved in MVC and aggravated assault than women. In elderly patients, the chief causes of injury are falls, followed by MVC and assault.[72]

Autogenous bone graft reconstruction
During recent decades, the techniques of harvesting and using autogenous bone grafts have been refined, with new sources of donor bone frequently reported in the maxillofacial literature. Commonly harvested grafts include calvarial, iliac, costal, and tibial grafts. New instrumentation, updated techniques, and practitioner experience make graft harvest easier and faster for the surgeon and safer and less expensive for the patient.[73]

Cranial bone graft

Physiology With respect to embryologic formation, 2 basic types of bone are preferable for grafting. Membranous bones include the flat bones of the cranium, face, and mandible (the mandible has some endochondral component with Meckel cartilage association). These bones form by intramembranous ossification, in which embryonic mesenchymal cells differentiate directly into osteoblasts that synthesize a collagenous osteoid. The osteoid then becomes hard bone after undergoing mineralization by calcium phosphate. Endochondral bones are the long bones of the skeleton (including iliac and rib) as well as the petrous, occipital, ethmoid, mastoid, and sphenoid. These bones form by endochondral ossification, whereby cartilage growth occurs at an epiphyseal surface. It is replaced by osteoid, which becomes mineralized.

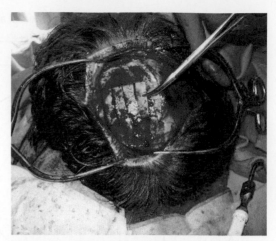

Fig. 21. An abundance of cranial bone is available for craniofacial reconstruction.

Membranous bone tends to have a thicker cortex and a denser, thinner cancellous layer than endochondral bone. There are several studies[74–80] that support the advantages of membranous bone. Zins and Whitaker[76] found that membranous bone grafts maintain their volume better than endochondral bone grafts when grafted on the rabbit snout. Hamilton and Mossman[81] have suggested that membranous bone ossifies in a more primitive and simplistic manner than endochondral bone. Peer,[74] Smith and Abramson,[75] and Zins and Whitaker[76] stated that membranous bone resists resorption to a greater degree than does endochondral bone. Peer,[74] Boyde and colleagues,[79] and Craft and Sargent[80] stated that membranous bone may heal with greater speed than its endochondral counterpart. It is suggested that membranous bone grafts undergo significantly less resorption

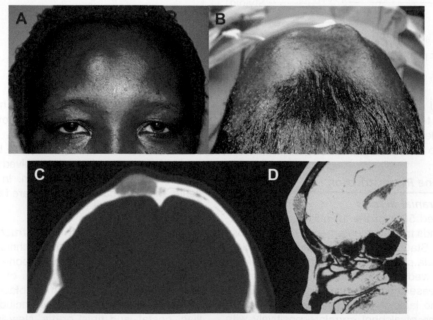

Fig. 22. (*A–M*) Central hemangioma affecting right forehead. Bone flap design outlined on frontal bone (*A–F*). Lesion was excised completely. The inner and outer tables of the frontal bone were separated (*G, H*). Inner table transposed to cover defect of the right forehead; outer table was repositioned. Ventriculostomy tube for intracranial pressure monitoring and CSF diversion (*I, J*). Postoperative 4 months: good facial appearance and projection without facial nerve or trigeminal deficit (*K–M*).

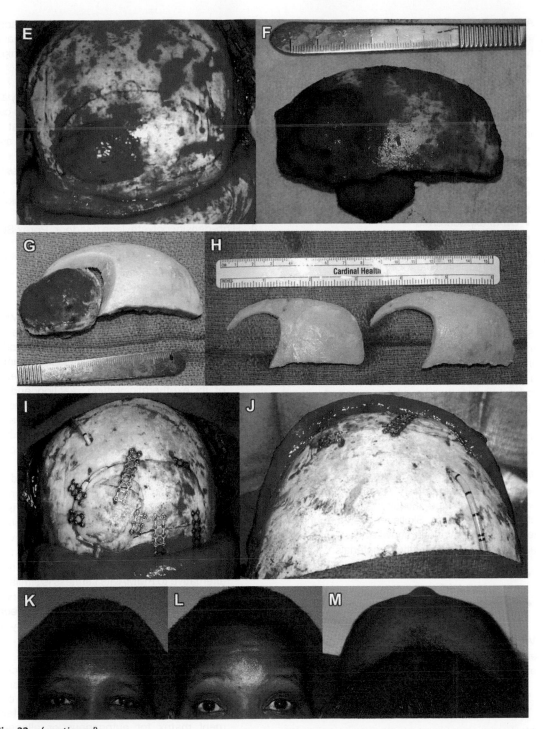

Fig. 22. (*continued*)

than endochondral bone grafts when applied to the craniofacial skeleton (**Figs. 21** and **22**).[76,82,83]

Several investigators[84–86] have theorized that a difference in microarchitecture is the basis for the differential resorption of bone grafts. Ozaki

and Buchman[85] noted that cortical bone grafts resorb significantly less than cancellous bone grafts and also concluded that bone graft resorption is determined by the microarchitecture rather than by its embryologic origin.

Advantages and complications of cranial bone graft harvest

Advantages:

- Dense bone
- Nonvisible scar
- Great quantity of bone graft available
- Minimal donor site pain

Complications:

- Scalp seroma/hematoma
- Alopecia
- Wound infection
- Paresthesias
- Bone contour irregularities
- Dural exposure/tear
- Intracranial hemorrhage
- Brain injury
- Cerebrospinal fluid (CSF) leak
- Meningitis
- Air embolism
- Death

Scalp seroma is the most common minor complication. Major complication rates range from 0% to 12%,[87–90] with most investigators citing rates of 0% to 2%. Two cases of postoperative subdural hematomas have been reported without violation of the inner cortex.[87,88] Both of these patients had previous closed head injuries, which may have placed them at increased risk for this complication.

Alloplastic cranial reconstruction

Brief history of cranioplasty A variety of materials have been used since antiquity to reconstruct defects of the calvarium. Skulls recovered during archeological excavations show evidence of early cranioplasty using a variety of materials:

- Nonmetallic (coconut shell, gourds, ivory, mica, celluloid)
- Bone xenograft (ape, canine, goose, rabbit, buffalo/ox horn)

World Wars I and II heralded the introduction of metallic sheets and plates to cover large surface areas caused by ballistic injuries.

- Metallic (lead, silver, gold, aluminum, vitallium, tantalum, platinum[91]

Modern cranioplasty techniques are intended to restore the shape and contour of the calvarium and provide protection for the brain. Some of the more well-known techniques are included below:

1. Custom-fabricated cranioplasty prostheses:
   a. Polyetheretherketone (PEEK)[92]
      i. A linear aromatic hydrocarbon, PEEK is resistant to heat and mechanical breakdown, nonallergenic, and does not create radiographic artifact. The implant may be easily modified intraoperatively using a high-speed cutting bur (**Fig. 23**).
2. Hard tissue replacement polymer[93]
   a. A substrate of polymethylmethacrylate (PMMA), sintered polyhydroxyethyl with calcium hydroxide coating may be fabricated. Its extensive porosity and negative surface charge allows for tissue ingrowth and bony attachment. It has high compressive strength and durability.
3. Computer-aided design and computer-aided manufacturing fabricated titanium plate
4. High-density polyethylene (Medpor, Porex Surgical, Newnan, GA)
   a. High-density polyethylene may be used with or without titanium reinforcement to maintain ideal contour (**Fig. 24**)
5. PMMA
   a. First introduced by Zander in 1940, PMMA remains one of the most widely used cranioplasty alloplasts. It is inexpensive and readily available. Disadvantages include potential thermal injury to adjacent tissues as a result of its exothermic setting reaction and its cytotoxic monomer. When placed adjacent to the frontal sinus, PMMA is associated with an increased incidence of infection.[94]
6. Kryptonite bone cement (Doctors Research Group, Southbury, CT)
   a. Kryptonite bone cement was approved by the US Food and Drug Administration in 2009 for use in cranioplasty applications. It is composed of calcium carbonate mixed with a proprietary preparation of hydroxyl terminated fatty acids. Kryptonite is marketed as a nontoxic, nonexothermic, porous alternative to PMMA. Its stiffness is similar to intact bone, and it bears a yield strength similar to PMMA. Recently, a voluntary recall of this product has limited its availability for use in the operative setting.
7. Resorbable materials
   a. Poly-L or poly-D lactic acid, polyglycolic acid, or a copolymer combining these forms is used in craniofacial reconstruction. In cranioplasty, it is typically used as a containment matrix for autogenous or allogenic bone graft material (**Fig. 25**).
8. Regenerative cranioplasty

Undifferentiated adult stem cells harvested from adult skeletal muscle have been used in cranioplasty to grow bone and recapitulate the native calvarium. Taub and colleagues[95] reported the use of adult skeletal muscle stem cells imbedded

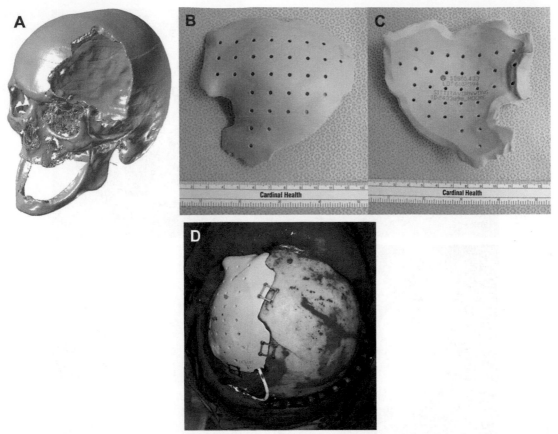

Fig. 23. (*A–D*) Reconstruction of a fronto-orbito-temporal defect using custom CAD-CAM PEEK prosthesis.

into polyglycolic acid mesh and implanted into rat calvarial defects. Recombinant bone morphogenetic protein (rhBMP-2) has been widely used in regenerative maxillofacial surgery. rhBMP-2 in a collagen sponge carrier resulted in statistically significant ossification when compared with both adipose-derived stem cells and adipose-derived stem cells induced with bone morphogenetic protein 2 in rabbit calvarial defects. Human trials are pending.[96]

9. Additional alloplastic materials:
   a. Hydroxyapatite cement
   b. Titanium mesh
   c. Silicone rubber
   d. Polytetrafluoroethylene
   e. Polyethylene

Frontal sinus reconstruction

Facial bone and soft tissue injuries are commonly encountered during automobile accidents, of which frontal sinus fractures comprise roughly 8%.[97] Most frontal sinus fractures are seen with midfacial injuries, particularly orbital fractures.[98] Managing

frontal sinus fractures depends on several factors, including dislocation/displacement of the anterior or posterior tables, dural involvement with CSF leakage, and injury to the frontal sinus drainage system (nasofrontal outflow tract [NFOT]). Indications for frontal sinus surgery include injury to or obstruction of the nasofrontal ducts, dural/cerebral involvement, and aesthetic deformity.

Displacement of the anterior table alone, if the NFOT is unobstructed, may be treated conservatively with oral and nasal decongestants.[98] However, clinical and radiographic surveillance with maxillofacial computed tomography (CT) scans should be considered at 6 weeks and 6 and 12 months to rule out the formation of frontal sinus mucocele with sinusitis, which typically occurs in the first 6 months after injury.[99] Assessment of the NFOT on facial CT scan is the most reliable and least invasive method.[100]

Questionable patient symptoms and frontal sinus opacification on CT scan could indicate NFOT obstruction, which is believed to occur in 25% to 50% of facial fractures.[101] In selected cases, endoscopic transnasal drainage (functional

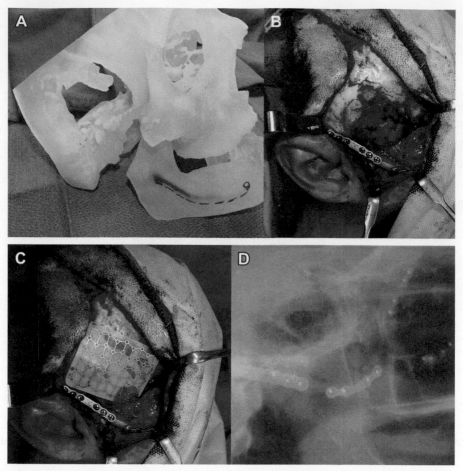

Fig. 24. (*A–D*) Reconstruction of pteryion defect with titanium-reinforced Medpor sheet. (*Courtesy of* Patrick J. Louis, DDS, MD, Birmingham, AL.)

endoscopic sinus surgery) may be attempted[101] with the placement of nasofrontal duct stents, although these are associated with a high failure rate (≤30%) for maintaining duct patency.[100] Open treatment of the injured frontal sinus and NFOT is currently the recommended standard, with careful attention to meticulous extirpation of the frontal sinus mucosa and vascular pits of Breschet, followed by obliteration of the frontal sinuses and NFOT.[98] The literature describes a variety of materials used for frontal sinus obliteration including autologous fat, cancellous bone, muscle, pericranial flaps, banked cadaveric tissue and synthetic materials (eg, polytetrafluoroethylene, methylmethacrylate, bioactive glass, and calcium phosphate cements).[102–120] Hardy and Montgomery reported overall complications of 18% after frontal sinus obliteration with abdominal fat, including donor site morbidity, wound complications, postoperative infections, fat necrosis, and recurring chronic sinusitis.[99] The pericranial flap is

also recommended for use in frontal sinus obliteration.[121] Shumrick and Smith[109] advocated the placement of cancellous bone rather than adipose tissue for formal sinus obliteration. Grahne[122] noted that frontal sinuses obliterated with autogenous bone showed complete ossification at 5-year follow-up. Hydroxyapatite and bioactive glass have been investigated for use in frontal sinus obliteration in several reports.[118,119,123,124] Peltola and colleagues[125] reported normal bone formation directly apposing surgically placed hydroxyapatite and bioactive glass, with no foreign body reaction. In addition, Stoor and colleagues[126] concluded that bioactive glass seems to have a broad antimicrobial effect on inhibiting of oral microorganisms. However, Tiwari and colleagues[98] recommended avoiding the use of synthetic resins for frontal sinus obliteration, citing the high potential for infectious complications when avascular media are used in reconstruction. In the case of severely displaced and comminuted frontal sinus

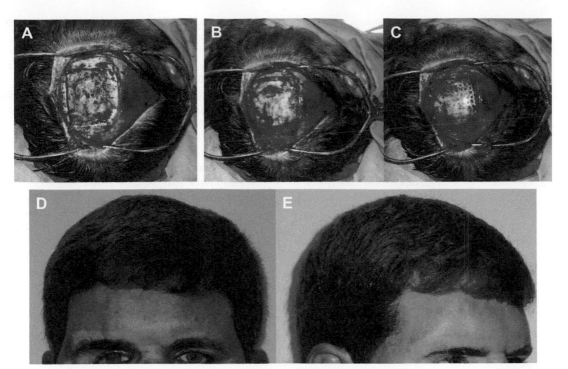

Fig. 25. (*A–E*) Cranial bone defect was reconstructed with allograft, biodegradable plate, and screws (*A–C*). Postoperative 1-month frontal and lateral views show good contour of facial bone (*D–E*).

fractures with significant posterior table damage, dural laceration and persistent CSF leak, cranialization must be considered. Endoscopically assisted frontal sinus repair, including fracture reduction and sinus obliteration, has been reported in several contemporary studies.[127–131] Although useful, the key determinant of successful frontal sinus treatment is careful removal of all sinus mucosa and obliteration of the frontal sinus and NFOT to prevent the formation of a mucocele or mucopyocele. Success in reconstructive surgery depends not only on the appropriate use of biomaterials, flaps, grafts, and so forth but also in the execution of the most appropriate operative technique.

SUMMARY

Scalp and cranial deformities are common after trauma or ablative surgery. Local flaps and free flaps may be used in reconstruction of soft tissue defects, and autogenous bone or alloplastic bone substitutes may be used for cranioplasty procedures. Injuries to the frontal sinus, particularly when complicated by CSF leak or NFOT obstruction, represent special challenges. Further studies are recommended to improve the multidisciplinary management of these complex, debilitating conditions, in anticipation of enhanced function and cosmesis, reduced donor site morbidity, and improved surgical outcomes.

REFERENCES

1. Sharkey EJ, Cassidy M, Brady J, et al. Investigation of the force associated with the formation of lacerations and skull fractures. Int J Legal Med 2011; 126(6):835–44.
2. Whittle K, Kieser J, Ichim I, et al. The biomechanical modelling of non-ballistic skin wounding: blunt-force injury. Forensic Sci Med Pathol 2008;4(1):33–9.
3. Pierard GE, Lapiere CM. Microanatomy of the dermis in relation to relaxed skin tension lines and Langer's lines. Am J Dermatopathol 1987; 9(3):219–24.
4. Deutsch BD, Becker FF. Secondary healing of Mohs defects of the forehead, temple, and lower eyelid. Arch Otolaryngol Head Neck Surg 1997; 123(5):529–34.
5. Moreno-Arias GA, Izento-Menezes CM, Carrasco MA, et al. Second intention healing after Mohs micrographic surgery. J Eur Acad Dermatol Venereol 2000;14(3):159–65.
6. Leaper DJ, Harding KG. Surgical wounds, wounds: biology and management. 1st Edition. Oxford (United Kingdom): Oxford University Press; 1998.
7. Rudolp R, Fisher JC, Ninnemann JL. Skin grafting. Boston: Little, Brown, and Company; 1979.

8. Harahap M. Principles of dermatologic plastic surgery: the delaying of skin flaps. New York: PMA Publishing; 1988.

9. Hynes W. The early circulation in skin grafts with a consideration of methods to encourage their survival. Br J Plast Surg 1954;6(4):257–63.

10. Smahel J, Clodius L. The blood vessel system of free human skin grafts. Plast Reconstr Surg 1971; 47(1):61–6.

11. Psillakis JM. Lymphatic vascularization of skin grafts. Plast Reconstr Surg 1969;43(3):287–91.

12. Gingrass P, Grabb WC, Gingrass RP. Skin graft survival on avascular defects. Plast Reconstr Surg 1975;55(1):65–70.

13. Camacho-Matinez F. Principles of dermatologic plastic surgery, skin grafts. New York: PMA Publishing; 1988.

14. Hammon RE. Principles of dermatologic plastic surgery: advancement flaps. New York: PMA Publishing; 1988.

15. Lejour M. Reconstruction of skin defects of the cheek with a large island flap (author's transl). Acta Chir Belg 1975;74(2):183–91 [in French].

16. Barron JN, Emmett AJ. Subcutaneous pedicle flaps. Br J Plast Surg 1965;18:51–78.

17. Limberg AA. Congenital cleft lip and palate. Stomatologiia (Mosk) 1967;46(1):11–5 [in Russian].

18. Dufourmentel C. Closure of limited loss of cutaneous substance. So-called "LLL" diamond-shaped L rotation-flap. Ann Chir Plast 1962;7:60–6 [in French].

19. Labow BI, Rosen H, Pap SA, et al. Microsurgical reconstruction: a more conservative method of managing large scalp defects? J Reconstr Microsurg 2009;25(8):465–74.

20. Herrera F, Buntic R, Brooks D, et al. Microvascular approach to scalp replantation and reconstruction: a thirty-six year experience. Microsurgery 2012; 32(8):591–7.

21. Hussussian CJ, Reece GP. Microsurgical scalp reconstruction in the patient with cancer. Plast Reconstr Surg 2002;109(6):1828–34.

22. Kwee MM, Rozen WM, Ting JW, et al. Total scalp reconstruction with bilateral anterolateral thigh flaps. Microsurgery 2012;32(5):393–6.

23. Leedy JE, Janis JE, Rohrich RJ. Reconstruction of acquired scalp defects: an algorithmic approach. Plast Reconstr Surg 2005;116(4):54e–72e.

24. Trignano E, Ciudad P, Fallico N, et al. Nodular cutaneous amyloidosis of the scalp reconstructed with a free anterolateral thigh flap: a case report. J Oral Maxillofac Surg 2012;70(8):e481–3.

25. Miller GD, Anstee EJ, Snell JA. Successful replantation of an avulsed scalp by microvascular anastomoses. Plast Reconstr Surg 1976;58(2): 133–6.

26. Cheng K, Zhou S, Jiang K, et al. Microsurgical replantation of the avulsed scalp: report of 20 cases. Plast Reconstr Surg 1996;97(6):1099–106 [discussion: 107–8].

27. Liu T, Dong J, Wang J, et al. Microsurgical replantation for child total scalp avulsion. J Craniofac Surg 2009;20(1):81–4.

28. Sanger JR, Logiudice JA, Rowe D, et al. Ectopic scalp replantation: a case report. J Plast Reconstr Aesthet Surg 2010;63(1):e23–7.

29. Chao AH, Yu P, Skoracki RJ, et al. Microsurgical reconstruction of composite scalp and calvarial defects in patients with cancer: a 10-year experience. Head Neck 2012;34(12):1759–64.

30. Buncke HJ, Hoffman WY, Alpert BS, et al. Microvascular transplant of two free scalp flaps between identical twins. Plast Reconstr Surg 1982;70(5): 605–9.

31. Valauri FA, Buncke HJ, Alpert BS, et al. Microvascular transplantation of expanded free scalp flaps between identical twins. Plast Reconstr Surg 1990;85(3):432–6.

32. Lutz BS, Wei FC, Chen HC, et al. Reconstruction of scalp defects with free flaps in 30 cases. Br J Plast Surg 1998;51(3):186–90.

33. Haddock MC, Creagh T, Sivarajan V. Double-free, flow-through flap reconstruction for complex scalp defects: a case report. Microsurgery 2011;31(4): 327–30.

34. Serra MP, Longhi P, Carminati M, et al. Microsurgical scalp and skull reconstruction using a combined flap composed of serratus anterior myo-osseous flap and latissimus dorsi myocutaneous flap. J Plast Reconstr Aesthet Surg 2007; 60(10):1158–61.

35. Maxwell GP, Stueber K, Hoopes JE. A free latissimus dorsi myocutaneous flap: case report. Plast Reconstr Surg 1978;62(3):462–6.

36. Shonka DC Jr, Potash AE, Jameson MJ, et al. Successful reconstruction of scalp and skull defects: lessons learned from a large series. Laryngoscope 2011;121(11):2305–12.

37. Furnas H, Lineaweaver WC, Alpert BS, et al. Scalp reconstruction by microvascular free tissue transfer. Ann Plast Surg 1990;24(5):431–44.

38. Tansini I. Spora il mio muovo processo di amputazione della per cancre. Riforma Med 1896;12(3) [in Italian].

39. Lipa JE, Butler CE. Enhancing the outcome of free latissimus dorsi muscle flap reconstruction of scalp defects. Head Neck 2004;26(1):46–53.

40. Karacalar A, Demir A, Guneren E. A pedicle-lengthening technique for free latissimus dorsi muscle flaps: the "Y-V-I" principle. J Reconstr Microsurg 2005;21(3):173–8.

41. Buntic RF, Horton KM, Brooks D, et al. The free partial superior latissimus muscle flap: preservation of donor-site form and function. Plast Reconstr Surg 2008;121(5):1659–63.

42. Kim DD, Fernandes R. Vascularized and nonvascularized hard and soft tissue reconstruction. In: Miloro M, Ghali GE, Larsen P, et al, editors. Peterson's principles of oral and maxillofacial surgery. Shelton (CT): People's Medical Publishing House; 2012.

43. Sweeny L, Eby B, Magnuson JS, et al. Reconstruction of scalp defects with the radial forearm free flap. Head Neck Oncol 2012;4(1):21.

44. Mateev MA, Beermanov KA, Subanova LK, et al. Shape-modified method using the radial forearm perforator flap for reconstruction of soft-tissue defects of the scalp. J Reconstr Microsurg 2005; 21(1):21–4.

45. Ioannides AP. The nurse teacher's clinical role now and in the future. Nurse Educ Today 1999;19(3): 207–14.

46. Song YG, Chen GZ, Song YL. The free thigh flap: a new free flap concept based on the septocutaneous artery. Br J Plast Surg 1984;37(2):149–59.

47. Wei FC, Jain V, Celik N, et al. Have we found an ideal soft-tissue flap? An experience with 672 anterolateral thigh flaps. Plast Reconstr Surg 2002; 109(7):2219–26 [discussion: 2227–30].

48. Kimata Y, Uchiyama K, Ebihara S, et al. Anatomic variations and technical problems of the anterolateral thigh flap: a report of 74 cases. Plast Reconstr Surg 1998;102(5):1517–23.

49. Yu P. Characteristics of the anterolateral thigh flap in a Western population and its application in head and neck reconstruction. Head Neck 2004; 26(9):759–69.

50. Lin DT, Coppit GL, Burkey BB. Use of the anterolateral thigh flap for reconstruction of the head and neck. Curr Opin Otolaryngol Head Neck Surg 2004;12(4):300–4.

51. Seth R, Manz RM, Dahan IJ, et al. Comprehensive analysis of the anterolateral thigh flap vascular anatomy. Arch Facial Plast Surg 2011;13(5):347–54.

52. Ross GL, Dunn R, Kirkpatrick J, et al. To thin or not to thin: the use of the anterolateral thigh flap in the reconstruction of intraoral defects. Br J Plast Surg 2003;56(4):409–13.

53. Koshima I, Fukuda H, Yamamoto H, et al. Free anterolateral thigh flaps for reconstruction of head and neck defects. Plast Reconstr Surg 1993; 92(3):421–8 [discussion: 429–30].

54. Alkureishi LW, Shaw-Dunn J, Ross GL. Effects of thinning the anterolateral thigh flap on the blood supply to the skin. Br J Plast Surg 2003;56(4): 401–8.

55. Kimura N, Satoh K, Hasumi T, et al. Clinical application of the free thin anterolateral thigh flap in 31 consecutive patients. Plast Reconstr Surg 2001; 108(5):1197–208 [discussion: 1209–10].

56. Kawamoto Y, Nakamura S, Nakano S, et al. Immunohistochemical localization of brain-derived neurotrophic factor in adult rat brain. Neuroscience 1996;74(4):1209–26.

57. Chang KP, Lai CH, Chang CH, et al. Free flap options for reconstruction of complicated scalp and calvarial defects: report of a series of cases and literature review. Microsurgery 2010;30(1): 13–8.

58. Kruse-Losler B, Presser D, Meyer U, et al. Reconstruction of large defects on the scalp and forehead as an interdisciplinary challenge: experience in the management of 39 cases. Eur J Surg Oncol 2006; 32(9):1006–14.

59. Gatti JE, LaRossa D. Scalp avulsions and review of successful replantation. Ann Plast Surg 1981;6(2): 127–31.

60. Kroll SS, Schusterman MA, Reece GP, et al. Choice of flap and incidence of free flap success. Plast Reconstr Surg 1996;98(3):459–63.

61. Anderson RJ. Observations on the thickness of the human skull. Dublin J Med Sci 1882;74:270–80.

62. Todd TW. Thickness of the male white cranium. Anat Rec 1924;27:245.

63. Roche AF. Increase in cranial thickness during growth. Hum Biol 1953;25(2):81–92.

64. Adeloye A, Kattan KR, Silverman FN. Thickness of the normal skull in the American Blacks and Whites. Am J Phys Anthropol 1975;43:23.

65. Pensler J, McCarthy JG. The calvarial donor site: an anatomic study in cadavers. Plast Reconstr Surg 1985;75(5):648–51.

66. Kohan D, Plasse HM, Zide BM. Frontal bone reconstruction with split calvarial and cancellous iliac bone. Ear Nose Throat J 1989;68(11):845–6, 48–50, 53–4.

67. Tessier P. Autogenous bone grafts taken from the calvarium for facial and cranial applications. Clin Plast Surg 1982;9(4):531–8.

68. Cutting CB, McCarthy JG, Berenstein A. Blood supply of the upper craniofacial skeleton: the search for composite calvarial bone flaps. Plast Reconstr Surg 1984;74(5):603–10.

69. Casanova R, Cavalcante D, Grotting JC, et al. Anatomic basis for vascularized outer-table calvarial bone flaps. Plast Reconstr Surg 1986;78(3): 300–8.

70. Singer AJ, Hollander JE, Quinn JV. Evaluation and management of traumatic lacerations. N Engl J Med 1997;337(16):1142–8.

71. Shapiro AJ, Johnson RM, Miller SF, et al. Facial fractures in a level I trauma centre: the importance of protective devices and alcohol abuse. Injury 2001;32(5):353–6.

72. Gerbino G, Roccia F, De Gioanni PP, et al. Maxillofacial trauma in the elderly. J Oral Maxillofac Surg 1999;57(7):777–82 [discussion: 782–3].

73. Tessier P, Kawamoto H, Matthews D, et al. Autogenous bone grafts and bone substitutes–tools

and techniques: I. A 20,000-case experience in maxillofacial and craniofacial surgery. Plast Reconstr Surg 2005;116(Suppl 5):6S–24S [discussion: 92S–4S].

74. Peer LA. Fate of autogenous human bone grafts. Br J Plast Surg 1951;3(4):233–43.

75. Smith JD, Abramson M. Membranous vs endochondrial bone autografts. Arch Otolaryngol 1974; 99(3):203–5.

76. Zins JE, Whitaker LA. Membranous versus endochondral bone: implications for craniofacial reconstruction. Plast Reconstr Surg 1983;72(6): 778–85.

77. Kusiak JF, Zins JE, Whitaker LA. The early revascularization of membranous bone. Plast Reconstr Surg 1985;76(4):510–6.

78. Sato K, Urist MR. Induced regeneration of calvaria by bone morphogenetic protein (BMP) in dogs. Clin Orthop 1985;(197):301–11.

79. Boyde A, Hendel P, Hendel R, et al. Human cranial bone structure and the healing of cranial bone grafts: a study using backscattered electron imaging and confocal microscopy. Anat Embryol (Berl) 1990;181(3):235–51.

80. Craft PD, Sargent LA. Membranous bone healing and techniques in calvarial bone grafting. Clin Plast Surg 1989;16(1):11–9.

81. Hamilton WJ, Boyd JD, Mossman HW. Human embryology. 4th edition. Baltimore (MD): Williams & Wilkins; 1972.

82. Zins JE, Kusiak JF, Whitaker LA, et al. The influence of the recipient site on bone grafts to the face. Plast Reconstr Surg 1984;73(3):371–81.

83. Longaker MT, Kawamoto HK Jr. Evolving thoughts on correcting posttraumatic enophthalmos. Plast Reconstr Surg 1998;101(4):899–906.

84. Hardesty RA, Marsh JL. Craniofacial onlay bone grafting: a prospective evaluation of graft morphology, orientation, and embryonic origin. Plast Reconstr Surg 1990;85(1):5–14 [discussion: 15].

85. Ozaki W, Buchman SR. Volume maintenance of onlay bone grafts in the craniofacial skeleton: microarchitecture versus embryologic origin. Plast Reconstr Surg 1998;102(2):291–9.

86. Chen NT, Glowacki J, Bucky LP, et al. The roles of revascularization and resorption on endurance of craniofacial onlay bone grafts in the rabbit. Plast Reconstr Surg 1994;93(4):714–22 [discussion: 723–4].

87. Frodel JL Jr, Marentette LJ, Quatela VC, et al. Calvarial bone graft harvest. Techniques, considerations, and morbidity. Arch Otolaryngol Head Neck Surg 1993;119(1):17–23.

88. Young VL, Schuster RH, Harris LW. Intracerebral hematoma complicating split calvarial bone-graft harvesting. Plast Reconstr Surg 1990; 86(4):763–5.

89. Jackson IT, Helden G, Marx R. Skull bone grafts in maxillofacial and craniofacial surgery. J Oral Maxillofac Surg 1986;44(12):949–55.

90. Powell NB, Riley RW. Cranial bone grafting in facial aesthetic and reconstructive contouring. Arch Otolaryngol Head Neck Surg 1987;113(7): 713–9.

91. Sanan A, Haines SJ. Repairing holes in the head: a history of cranioplasty. Neurosurgery 1997;40(3): 588–603.

92. Lai JB, Sittitavornwong S, Waite PD. Computer-assisted designed and computer-assisted manufactured polyetheretherketone prosthesis for complex fronto-orbito-temporal defect. J Oral Maxillofac Surg 2011;69(4):1175–80.

93. Eppley BL, Kilgo M, Coleman JJ 3rd. Cranial reconstruction with computer-generated hard-tissue replacement patient-matched implants: indications, surgical technique, and long-term follow-up. Plast Reconstr Surg 2002;109(3):864–71.

94. Azmi A, Latiff AZ, Johari A. Methyl methacrylate cranioplasty. Med J Malaysia 2004;59(3): 418–21.

95. Taub PJ, Yau J, Spangler M, et al. Bioengineering of calvaria with adult stem cells. Plast Reconstr Surg 2009;123(4):1178–85.

96. Smith DM, Cooper GM, Afifi AM, et al. Regenerative surgery in cranioplasty revisited: the role of adipose-derived stem cells and BMP-2. Plast Reconstr Surg 2011;128(5):1053–60.

97. Montovani JC, Nogueira EA, Ferreira FD, et al. Surgery of frontal sinus fractures: epidemiologic study and evaluation of techniques. Braz J Otorhinolaryngol 2006;72(2):204–9.

98. Tiwari P, Higuera S, Thornton J, et al. The management of frontal sinus fractures. J Oral Maxillofac Surg 2005;63(9):1354–60.

99. Hardy JM, Montgomery WW. Osteoplastic frontal sinusotomy: an analysis of 250 operations. Ann Otol Rhinol Laryngol 1976;85(4 Pt 1):523–32.

100. Rohrich RJ, Hollier LH. Management of frontal sinus fractures. Changing concepts. Clin Plast Surg 1992;19(1):219–32.

101. Stevens M, Kline SN. Management of frontal sinus fractures. J Craniomaxillofac Trauma 1995;1(1): 29–37.

102. Newman MH, Travis LW. Frontal sinus fractures. Laryngoscope 1973;83(8):1281–92.

103. Larrabee WF Jr, Travis LW, Tabb HG. Frontal sinus fractures–their suppurative complications and surgical management. Laryngoscope 1980;90(11 Pt 1): 1810–3.

104. Bergara AR, Itoiz AO. Present state of the surgical treatment of chronic frontal sinusitis. AMA Arch Otolaryngol 1955;61(6):616–28.

105. Goodale RL, Montgomery WW. Experiences with the osteoplastic anterior wall approach to the

frontal sinus; case histories and recommendations. AMA Arch Otolaryngol 1958;68(3):271–83.

106. Sessions RB, Alford BR, Stratton C, et al. Current concepts of frontal sinus surgery: an appraisal of the osteoplastic flap-fat obliteration operation. Laryngoscope 1972;82(5):918–30.

107. Wolfe SA, Johnson P. Frontal sinus injuries: primary care and management of late complications. Plast Reconstr Surg 1988;82(5):781–91.

108. Merville LC, Real JP. Fronto-orbito nasal dislocations. Initial total reconstruction. Scand J Plast Reconstr Surg 1981;15(3):287–97.

109. Shumrick KA, Smith CP. The use of cancellous bone for frontal sinus obliteration and reconstruction of frontal bony defects. Arch Otolaryngol Head Neck Surg 1994;120(9):1003–9.

110. Luce EA. Frontal sinus fractures: guidelines to management. Plast Reconstr Surg 1987;80(4):500–10.

111. Nadell J, Kline DG. Primary reconstruction of depressed frontal skull fractures including those involving the sinus, orbit, and cribriform plate. J Neurosurg 1974;41(2):200–7.

112. Parhiscar A, Har-El G. Frontal sinus obliteration with the pericranial flap. Otolaryngol Head Neck Surg 2001;124(3):304–7.

113. Thaller SR, Donald P. The use of pericranial flaps in frontal sinus fractures. Ann Plast Surg 1994;32(3):284–7.

114. Sailer HF, Gratz KW, Kalavrezos ND. Frontal sinus fractures: principles of treatment and long-term results after sinus obliteration with the use of lyophilized cartilage. J Craniomaxillofac Surg 1998;26(4):235–42.

115. Kalavrezos ND, Gratz KW, Warnke T, et al. Frontal sinus fractures: computed tomography evaluation of sinus obliteration with lyophilized cartilage. J Craniomaxillofac Surg 1999;27(1):20–4.

116. Schenck NL, Tomlinson MJ, Ridgley CD Jr. Experimental evaluation of a new implant material in frontal sinus obliteration: a preliminary report. Arch Otolaryngol 1976;102(9):524–8.

117. Manson PN, Crawley WA, Hoopes JE. Frontal cranioplasty: risk factors and choice of cranial vault reconstructive material. Plast Reconstr Surg 1986;77(6):888–904.

118. Peltola M, Suonpaa J, Aitasalo K, et al. Obliteration of the frontal sinus cavity with bioactive glass. Head Neck 1998;20(4):315–9.

119. Rosen G, Nachtigal D. The use of hydroxyapatite for obliteration of the human frontal sinus. Laryngoscope 1995;105(5 Pt 1):553–5.

120. Ross DA, Marentette LJ, Thompson BG, et al. Use of hydroxyapatite bone cement to prevent cerebrospinal fluid leakage through the frontal sinus: technical report. Neurosurgery 1999;45(2):401–2 [discussion: 402–3].

121. Kelly CP, Yavuzer R, Keskin M, et al. Treatment of chronic frontal sinus disease with the galeal-frontalis flap: a long-term follow-up. Plast Reconstr Surg 2005;115(5):1229–36 [discussion: 1237–8].

122. Grahne B. Chronic frontal sinusitis treated by autogenous osteoplasty. Acta Otolaryngol 1971;72(3):215–9.

123. Snyderman CH, Scioscia K, Carrau RL, et al. Hydroxyapatite: an alternative method of frontal sinus obliteration. Otolaryngol Clin North Am 2001;34(1):179–91.

124. Peltola M, Aitasalo K, Suonpaa J, et al. Bioactive glass S53P4 in frontal sinus obliteration: a long-term clinical experience. Head Neck 2006;28(9):834–41.

125. Peltola MJ, Aitasalo KM, Aho AJ, et al. Long-term microscopic and tissue analytical findings for 2 frontal sinus obliteration materials. J Oral Maxillofac Surg 2008;66(8):1699–707.

126. Stoor P, Soderling E, Salonen JI. Antibacterial effects of a bioactive glass paste on oral microorganisms. Acta Odontol Scand 1998;56(3):161–5.

127. Schubert W, Jenabzadeh K. Endoscopic approach to maxillofacial trauma. J Craniofac Surg 2009;20(1):154–6.

128. Ung F, Sindwani R, Metson R. Endoscopic frontal sinus obliteration: a new technique for the treatment of chronic frontal sinusitis. Otolaryngol Head Neck Surg 2005;133(4):551–5.

129. Shumrick KA. Endoscopic management of frontal sinus fractures. Otolaryngol Clin North Am 2007;40(2):329–36.

130. Yoo MH, Kim JS, Song HM, et al. Endoscopic transnasal reduction of an anterior table frontal sinus fracture: technical note. Int J Oral Maxillofac Surg 2008;37(6):573–5.

131. Chen DJ, Chen CT, Chen YR, et al. Endoscopically assisted repair of frontal sinus fracture. J Trauma 2003;55(2):378–82.

Acquired Defects of the Nose and Naso-orbitoethmoid (NOE) Region

Daniel J. Meara, MS, MD, DMD

KEYWORDS

- Acquired • Nose • Naso-orbitoethmoid • Fractures • Soft tissue defects • Reconstruction

KEY POINTS

- Because of the exposed and prominent position of the nasal complex, acquired hard and soft tissue defects of the nose are common.
- Nasal injuries coupled with midface fractures of the orbit and ethmoids constitutes a naso-orbitoethmoid (NOE) fracture pattern, which is typically the most challenging facial fracture to repair.
- For nasal fractures, important elements to minimizing revision surgery or secondary septorhinoplasty are timing of initial repair and septal position.
- NOE fracture patterns suggest the surgical treatment required and the access necessary.
- After NOE repair, a traditional adhesive-retained extranasal splint is often insufficient, and improved soft tissue outcomes are realized with padded hard splint compression plates, secured via transnasal wires.
- Correction of acquired soft tissue defects is best addressed via nasal subunits and requires a robust surgical armamentarium, including rotational flaps, autogenous grafts, alloplastic implants, and implant support prostheses.
- Long-term clinical outcomes are typically excellent if surgical principles are followed and these surgical techniques used.

Because of the exposed and prominent position of the nasal complex, acquired hard and soft tissue defects of the nose are common. Traumatic injury, as well as the elements of nature, increase the risk of sun damage, with associated neoplasm, frostbite, and burns. For instance, nasal fractures occur more than any other facial fracture and are one of the most common anywhere in the body. Further, when nasal injuries are coupled with midface fractures of the orbit and ethmoids, the result is a naso-orbitoethmoid (NOE) fracture pattern, which is typically the most challenging facial fracture to repair. Hard and soft tissue defects of this region, caused by trauma, neoplasm, infection, and inflammatory disorders, may require advanced reconstruction techniques, including local rotational flaps, free tissue transfer, and even prosthetics. The restoration of form and function dictates treatment, and the success of primary repair is paramount, because secondary correction is challenging in this area of the midface. Because of the complex nature of this region, this discussion is divided into hard tissue defects, with a focus on trauma, and soft tissue defects, with a focus on oncology.

Department of Oral and Maxillofacial Surgery and Hospital Dentistry, Christiana Care Health System, 501 West 14th Street, Wilmington, DE 19899, USA
E-mail address: dmeara@christianacare.org

Oral Maxillofacial Surg Clin N Am 25 (2013) 131–149
http://dx.doi.org/10.1016/j.coms.2013.02.006
1042-3699/13/$ – see front matter © 2013 Elsevier Inc. All rights reserved.

HARD TISSUE DEFECTS
The Nose

The nasal complex is a prominent facial structure, and as a result, it is the most common facial fracture to occur in both children and adults. The force necessary to fracture the nose is less than for any other facial bone.[1] Further, it is a central facial feature, with considerable aesthetic importance and functional necessity for breathing and olfaction.

Examination

History should determine the mechanism of injury to focus the physical examination and ascertain if any difficulty in breathing is noted. The examination should immediately assess for hemorrhage and rule out the presence of a septal hematoma or other soft tissue abnormalities. Bony abnormalities can then be documented for changes in cosmesis, although final assessment may require resolution of perinasal edema, to determine the need for surgical intervention.

Imaging

Imaging for isolated nasal complex fractures is not necessary, because the clinical examination should determine the appropriate treatment. However, in conjunction with other facial or head injuries, computed tomography (CT) allows assessment of the nasal pyramid and the nasoseptal position and curvature. Plain films are typically of limited value. Han and colleagues[2] developed a system of radiographic correlation to clinical management and outcomes. Based on axial CT images, the nasal bone was marked from base to top of the nose and then divided into upper, middle, and lower levels. Analysis of 125 patients treated showed that fractures occurring at the upper level resulted in lower frequency of complication and reoperation than fractures at the other levels, whereas total level or fractures below the lower level showed the highest complication and reoperation rate (**Fig. 1**). Such information can be beneficial in regards to patient treatment and education.

Classification Schemes

In an attempt to categorize and create uniformity in the diagnosis of nasal complex injuries, numerous classification schemes have been suggested. Haug and Prather[3] in 1991, Ondik and colleagues[4] in 2009, and Lee and colleagues[5] in 2010 created newer classification schemes, improving on schemes by Gillies and Kilner[6] in 1929, Harrison[7] in 1979, and Murray and colleagues[8] in 1986.

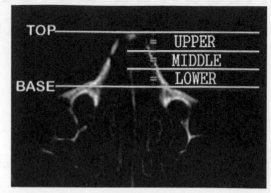

Fig. 1. Division of the nose for radiographic classification of nasal fractures and clinical application via axial CT. (*From* Han DS, Han YS, Park JH. A new approach to the treatment of nasal bone fracture: radiologic classification of nasal bone fractures and its clinical application. J Oral Maxillo Surg 2011;69(11):2841–47; with permission.)

Specifically, in 1991, Haug and Prather[3] created a study of nasal fractures solely for the purpose of providing a classification system of nasal bone fractures, with types I to IV and an S modification for fractures with septal involvement. Based on clinical evaluation, Ondik and colleagues[4] created criteria for evaluation of the nasal complex, including symmetry, septal status, and overall injury severity in the classification of nasal complex fractures (**Table 1**). Similarly, as a result of predictable fracture patterns of the nasal septum, in cadaver studies, Lee and colleagues[5] classified septal fractures into 3 types (types 1–3), with further detail as to whether the septum was intact on the nasal spine or if dislocation had occurred.

Treatment

Although not the focus of this article, appropriate acute nasal fracture management can minimize revision and reconstructive procedures. Reilly and Davidson[9] showed that an open approach can reduce potential revision rates in patients with an associated deformity of the septum. In an attempt to optimize clinical outcomes of nasal fracture management, Herford and colleagues[10] created an algorithm (**Fig. 2**). Fattahi and colleagues[1] reported that important elements to minimizing revision surgery or secondary septorhinoplasty are: (1) timing of initial repair and (2) septal position. Best results are achieved if closed reduction surgery is completed within the first 2 weeks, and the nasal septum must be positioned over the maxillary crest. Attention to these details results in a success rate of 89% to 91%, significantly higher than previous studies reporting success

Table 1
Classification of nasal and septal fractures

Type	Description	Characteristics
I	Simple straight	Unilateral or bilateral displaced fracture without resulting midline deviation
II	Simple deviated	Unilateral or bilateral displaced fracture with resulting midline deviation
III	Comminution of nasal bones	Bilateral nasal bone comminution and crooked septum with preservation of midline septal support; septum does not interfere with bony reduction
IV	Severely deviated nasal and septal fractures	Unilateral or bilateral nasal fractures with severe deviation or disruption of nasal midline, secondary to either severe septal fracture or septal dislocation. May be associated with comminution of the nasal bones and septum, which interfere with reduction of fractures
V	Complex nasal and septal fractures	Severe injuries including lacerations and soft tissue trauma, acute saddling of nose, open compound injuries, and avulsion of tissue

Data from Ondik M, Lipinski L, Dezfoli S, et al. The treatment of nasal fractures. Arch Facial Plast Surg 2009:11(5):296–302.

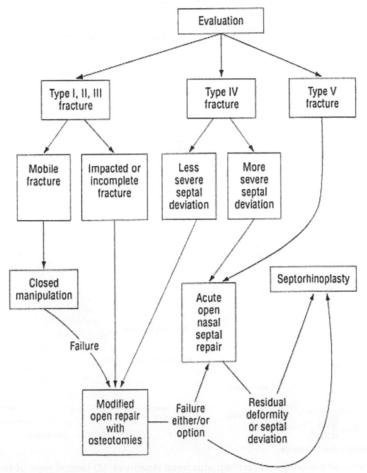

Fig. 2. Nasal fracture management algorithm. (*From* Ondik MP, Lipinski L, Dezfoli S, et al. The treatment of nasal fractures. Arch Facial Plast Surg 2009;11(5):296–302; with permission.)

as low as 70%. However, Ondik and colleagues[4] indicated that in their study, no statistical difference was noted between open repair and closed repair in terms of revision rate, surgeon postoperative evaluation scores, and patient satisfaction scores. However, their algorithm is designed to provide a guide to nasal fracture management based on the fracture classification type.

Rhinoplasty

Reconstruction of the nose is based on principles of rhinoplasty, which are presented in this section. Reconstruction of the nose is based on which subunit has been injured or deformed, and thus, the discussion addresses each subunit of the nose and the surgical techniques for correction.

Surface Anatomy and Nasal Subunits[11]
- Dorsum: radix to supratip break with lateral aspect merging with the nasal sidewalls
- Tip: central aspect of the nose bordered by the other subunits and formed by the lateral genu of the lower lateral cartilages
- Columella: middle and medial crura of the lower lateral cartilages extending from its junction with the upper lip philtrum superiorly to the nasal tip

- Alae: consists of the lateral crus of the lower lateral cartilage and the soft tissue extending to the nasolabial crease
- Sidewalls: extend from medial canthus to lateral edge of the nasal dorsum and lateral aspect merges with cheek skin; inferior aspect merges with the nasal ala and nasal tip
- Soft triangles: soft tissue depression inferior to the alar cartilage extending from apex of nasal aperture with no cartilage support

Deeper Anatomy of the Nasal Complex

The deeper anatomy of the nasal complex is a combination of bony and cartilaginous support, starting from the bony radix of the nose and extending inferiorly and posteriorly into the lower lateral cartilages and the septal cartilage, respectively. It is a complex structure that is composed of the nasal bones, upper lateral cartilages, lower lateral cartilages, and bony and cartilaginous septum (perpendicular plate of the ethmoid, the vomer, and quadrangular cartilage (**Fig. 3**).[11]

Perinasal Vascular Supply

The external blood supply consists of alar and septal branches of the maxillary artery, supporting

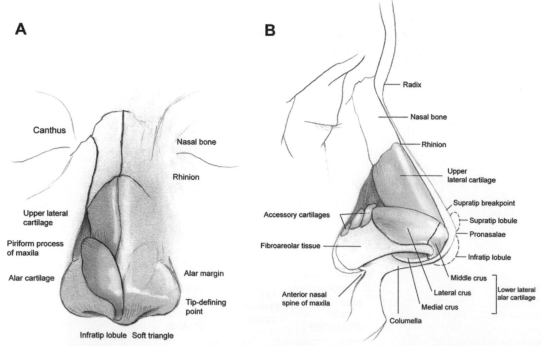

Fig. 3. (*A*) Frontal view of the bony and cartilaginous nasal structures. (*B*) Lateral view of the bony and cartilaginous nasal structures. (*From* Stevens MR, Emam HA. Applied surgical anatomy of the nose. Oral Maxillo Surg Clin North Am 2011;24(1):25–38.)

the nasal alae and septum. The dorsal and angular branches of the ophthalmic artery and the infraorbital branch of the maxillary artery support the nasal dorsum and sidewalls of the nose.[12] Intranasal blood supply is via an anterior and posterior anastomosis via the Kiesselbach plexus and Woodruff plexus, respectively. The main components are from the ethmoidal branches of the ophthalmic artery, the sphenopalatine branch of the maxillary artery, and the superior labial artery (**Fig. 4**).[12] Understanding of perinasal blood supply is essential if nasal reconstruction includes local or region flap design and the specific nasal subunit defect, which determine the flap type.

Patient Satisfaction

The 2 main criteria for patient satisfaction after nasal repair are aesthetics and functional nasal airflow. Love[13] suggests that aesthetics is more concerning to patients than the functional result, and that study shows 88% functional and 86% aesthetic outcomes, respectively. Patient satisfaction and postoperative surgeon evaluation determine the need for secondary revision; however, preexisting nasal deformities and the subjective nature of aesthetic evaluation can make the determination of success difficult.

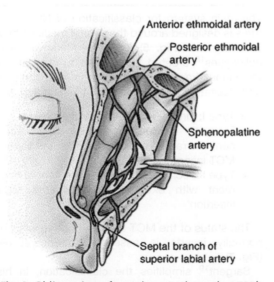

Fig. 4. Oblique view of septal mucosal vascular supply. The septal branch of the superior labial artery follows the lateral philtrum to enter the septal mucosa near the nasal spine, serving as the pedicle of the ipsilateral septal mucosal flap. The anterior ethmoidal artery provides the main contributions to the contralateral hinged flap. (*From* Tollefson TT, Kriet JD. Complex nasal defects: structure and internal lining. Facial Plastic Surg Clin North Am 2005;13(2):333–43.)

THE NOE COMPLEX

Acquired defects of the NOE complex are the most difficult area in which to restore form and function. Specifically, NOE fractures are both diagnostically and surgically challenging. Universal implementation of the automobile airbag restraint system has seemingly resulted in a reduction of such injuries as a result of less direct blows to the steering wheel or dash. Nonetheless, NOE fractures still occur and require a thorough knowledge of facial norms, surgical anatomy, and reconstruction techniques. Many of the principles of reconstruction of this region are based on the same principles of acute fracture management. Thus, acute fracture management of the NOE region is discussed first, followed by reconstruction techniques.

Pertinent Anatomy[14,15]
- NOE bony architecture: the confluence of the nasal bones, frontal process of the maxilla, nasal process of the frontal bone, lacrimal bone, lamina papyracea, ethmoid bone, and nasal septum
- Key NOE anatomic area: the central bone fragment of the medial orbital rim, the site of medial canthal tendon (MCT) insertion
- MCT: 3-limb structure with fan-shaped anterior limb, which inserts on the lateral surface of the nasal bones; the superior limb encompasses the lacrimal sac and attaches at the junction of the frontal process of the maxilla and the nasal process of the frontal bone; the posterior limb attaches to the posterior aspect of the lacrimal fossa
- Associated buttresses: horizontal in the forms of the (1) frontal bone and superior orbital rims, and (2) inferior orbital rims and zygomas; vertical comprises the paired central fragments of the NOE complex, including the frontal process of the maxilla and the nasal process of the frontal bone
- Separation of the anterior cranial fossa from the NOE or interorbital area is the cribiform plate, crista galli, and fovea ethmoidalis

Examination

NOE fractures require a significant amount of force. Understanding of the mechanism of injury as well as any associated injuries is crucial to the comprehensive care of the patient and often has surgical treatment implications, especially if associated with intracranial hemorrhage or cerebrospinal fluid leakage. Highlights of the physical examination include evaluation of intercanthal distance (normal = ~30–35 mm), medial canthal rounding and ligament laxity, condition of the nasofrontal junction and nasal dorsum, and assessment of the globe and its position.[15] In addition, globe injury should be ruled out and the condition of the associated soft tissues should be documented, with particular attention to the eyelid structures and lacrimal apparatus (**Box 1**). Specific examination techniques are used to assess the stability of the central fragment at the medial canthus, which is the landmark area of the NOE complex. The bowstring or traction test is a bimanual palpation, with placement of the index finger and thumb of 1 hand at the medial canthal region (posterior to the nasal bones), with the index finger of the opposite hand applying lateral traction at the lateral canthal region.[15] Any mobility with this maneuver suggests instability and likely need for surgical intervention. Another clinical examination technique is called the Furness test. A Kelly clamp is placed intranasally, in an anesthetized patient, against the medial orbital rim and the opposite index finger is placed in the medial

canthal area and again, any mobility palpated with movement of the Kelly clamp suggests instability.[16] Digital pressure is applied to the nasal dorsum to assess for collapse and loss of dorsal support, because posttraumatic edema may camouflage the extent of the deformity.

Imaging

Because of the complexity of the NOE injuries, maxillofacial CT imaging is the preferred modality to evaluate the fracture pattern, displacement, extent of comminution, nasoseptal status, and any other associated facial fractures. Volume-reconstruction three-dimensional images are desirable, allowing for a more global assessment of the injuries, which can be particularly useful in the surgical planning and sequencing of repair, especially in panfacial fracture surgery. Remmler and colleagues[17] show that three-dimensional and two-dimensional CT images together produce a higher diagnostic value in the evaluation of NOE fractures versus using either modality alone. Further, isolated NOE fractures or delayed repair cases may also benefit from surgical planning software as well as intraoperative navigation. Plain films have limited value in the diagnosis and treatment of NOE fractures.

Classification

The main system for classification of NOE fractures is designed around the central medial orbital wall fragment (**Fig. 5**). In 1991, Markowitz and colleagues[18] created the system to standardize the various fracture patterns of the NOE complex and facilitate surgical treatment planning (**Fig. 6**).

- Type I: single-segment central segment
- Type II: single-segment or comminuted central fragment fracture external to the MCT insertion
- Type III: comminution within the central fragment with extension beneath the MCT insertion

The status of the MCT and the bone to which it normally inserts is assessed intraoperatively (**Fig. 7**).

Sargent[19] simplifies the classification, in his 2007 review article, to:

- Unilateral or bilateral fractures and
- Simple or complex (comminuted) fracture segments

Such information is critical in surgical planning as to the extent of exposure and type of stabilization or fixation necessary.[19]

Box 1
Physical examination findings

Extranasal

Lacerations, edema, and ecchymosis of the periorbital and nasal regions

Loss of nasal projection and height

Flattening of the nasal dorsum

Telecanthus

Rounding of the medial canthus

Mobility of the central fragment

Intranasal

Lacerations of the septal mucosa

Dislocation of the septum

Fractures and comminution of the bony portion of the septum

Septal hematoma

Associated

Cerebrospinal fluid leak

Pneumocephalus

Anosmia

Vertical dystopia

Enophthalmos

Diplopia

Epiphora

Data from Vora N, Fedok F. Management of the central nasal support complex in naso-orbital ethmoid fractures. Facial Plast Surg 2000;16(2):181–91.

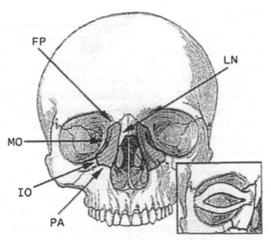

Fig. 5. Central fragment of NOE complex as defined by fracture through adjacent anatomic landmarks. FP, frontal bone; IO, inferior orbital rim; LN, lateral nose; MO, medial orbital wall; PA, piriform aperture. (*From* Remmler D, Denny A, Gosain A. Role of three-dimensional computed tomography in the assessment of nasoorbitoethmoidal fractures. Annals Plast Surg 2000;44(5):553–63; with permission.)

Another classification system was developed by Gruss in 1985[20] and characterizes NOE fractures as either isolated or in conjunction with other adjacent facial fractures, allowing for a broader view of the injuries and associated management issues.

Treatment

The surgical approach should be chosen based on the injury pattern and the appropriate exposure for reconstruction. Further, depending on the injury severity, a combination of approaches may be necessary.

Approaches for Access[19]
1. Coronal: exposes the NOE, frontal sinus, and superior and lateral orbital regions
2. Midline nasal: exposes the NOE region and is best for isolated NOE fractures, especially in balding patients and those with preexisting rhytids
3. Lower eyelid, including subciliary, transconjunctival, and transcaruncular: depending on surgeon preference and experience, the infraorbital rim and internal orbit can be accessed, and coupled with the transcaruncular incision, the medial orbital can be accessed
4. Maxillary vestibular: exposes the nasomaxillary buttress region at the piriform region
5. Facial degloving: exposes the maxilla, nasal complex, and NOE regions without any significant cutaneous incisions

Paranasal or Lynch incisions should be avoided because secondary soft tissue webbing often occurs and is not aesthetic. An existing laceration may be used and even extended, allowing for adequate access.

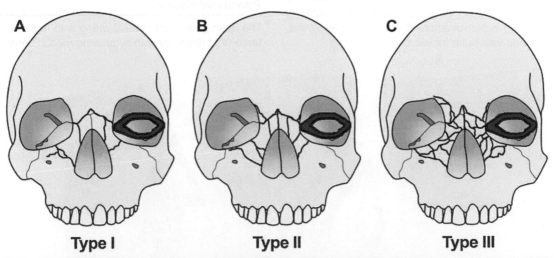

Type I   **Type II**   **Type III**

Fig. 6. NOE fracture classification system. NOE fractures are classified by the degree of comminution of the central fragment of the lower two-thirds of the medial orbital rim and the involvement of the MCT insertion. (*A*) Type I fractures: there is a single large central fragment that bears the MCT. (*B*) Type II fractures: there is comminution of the central fragment, but the MCT is attached to a fragment large enough to be stabilized. (*C*) Type III fractures: comminution extends beneath the insertion of the canthal ligament, and reconstruction of the canthal insertion point is necessary. (*From* Avery LL, Susarla SM, Novelline RA. Multidetector and three-dimensional CT evaluation of the patient with maxillofacial injury. Radiologic Clin North Am 2011;49(1):183–203.)

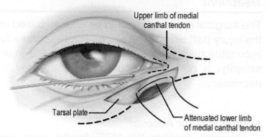

Fig. 7. Clinical anatomy of the MCT. (*From* Tyers AG, Collin JR. Ectropion. In: Colour atlas of ophthalmic plastic surgery. 3rd edition. London: Elsevier; 2008. p. 121–55; with permission.)

The NOE fracture pattern suggests the surgical treatment required and the access necessary.

Type I

The large single bony segment allows for rigid fixation without the need for transnasal wiring. As a result, depending on the segment stability, a vestibular incision alone may be adequate for fixation at the nasomaxillary buttress, and a midline nasal incision can be used to stabilize the fragment at the nasofrontal junction/superior orbital rim, if needed.[19]

Type II

Depending on the extent of comminution, the surgical plan and access can either be similar to a type I or type III, with type III NOE patterns requiring a combination of coronal, lower eyelid, and oral vestibular incisions.[19]

Type III

More extensive comminution and even loss of medial canthal attachment with the central bony fragment make repair of this injury pattern the most challenging. Unfettered access is required, so that the MCT can be reattached to the central bony fragment and normal intercanthal distance restored. The key with NOE fracture repair is the identification of the central bony fragment and the MCT. Sargent[19] suggests identification of this key landmark via a nasal side approach. Specifically, he suggests temporary dislocation of the nasal bones to allow enhanced exposure to the medial orbit (**Fig. 8**). Further, he states that the central bony fragment is more easily identified and the MCT is less likely to be erroneously released from its attachment during dissection.[19] Also, subsequent transnasal wiring is facilitated and is a necessary step in more comminuted type II and type III NOE patterns, because plate and screw fixation is typically inadequate to restore the intercanthal distance. Further, Young and Rice[21] emphasize that comminuted type II and all type III NOE fracture patterns are at risk for MCT destabilization during surgical exposure, even if the traumatic injury itself has not detached the MCT from the central bony fragment. In severely comminuted cases with no substantial central bony fragment, a bone graft as a new central bony fragment may be necessary to allow for MCT canthopexy.[14]

Transnasal Wiring

The main goal of transnasal wiring is to restore intercanthal distance with symmetric medial canthal

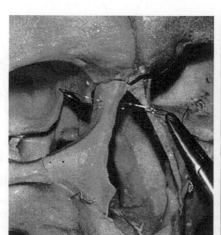
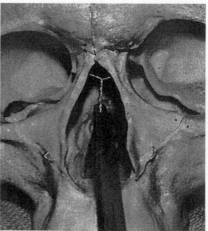

Fig. 8. Dislocation and temporary removal of the nasal bones for improved access and evaluation of the MCT as related to the central bony fragment. Also, facilitates proper transnasal wiring. (*From* Sargent LA. Nasoethmoid orbital fractures. Plast Reconstr Surg 2007;120(2):16S–31S; with permission.)

contours. The wires must be placed at the MCT attachment position of the central bony fragment as related to anterior-posterior and superior-inferior positions. Failure to accurately complete this step can result in flaring of the medial orbital bony segments and an unaesthetic result and continued telecanthus.[19] Sargeant[17] suggests 2 drill holes in each central bony fragment, approximately 4 mm apart, and 28-gauge wire or 3-O wire suture if the MCT needs to be reattached via canthopexy (**Fig. 9**). Slight overcorrection of the bony intercanthal distance is suggested, because the overlying soft tissue drape may create pseudotelecanthus, resulting in an imperfect result. Young and Rice[21] stressed caution in this region, to avoid intracranial or skull base encroachment. Anatomic landmarks to consider during transnasal wiring and canthopexy include anterior and posterior lacrimal crests, frontoethmoid suture line, anterior ethmoid artery, and the contralateral medial canthus (if not involved).[21]

Once transnasal wiring is complete and the MCT is attached to the central bony fragment and correct intercanthal distance is restored, plate and screw fixation can commence with low-profile titanium fixation.

Nasal Reconstruction in NOE Fractures

Typically based on the mechanism of injury and force required to create an NOE fracture pattern, the nasal dorsum sustains a debilitating loss of support, resulting in a pathognomonic appearance, with an upturned nasal tip, nasal foreshortening, an acute nasofrontal angle, and loss of septal support, particularly in the middle and distal thirds of the nose.[22] Physical examination further shows a depressable nasal dorsum to the nasal spine. Correction of the NOE complex and the nasal septum often do not correct the loss of support and the lack of nasal projection, and this can be achieved only with a dorsal graft.[22] Based on surgical access and natural compatibility, a bone graft is the ideal means of a cantilever correction. However, there are many alloplastic materials for nasal reconstruction, including silicone and porous polyethylene.[23] An outer-table calvarial graft is the natural choice for autogenous bone grafts, because if a coronal approach is used, the parietal bone is readily accessed.[22] The technique involves harvest of an approximately 4-cm × 2-cm outer-table cortical bone graft as least 2 cm lateral to the sagittal sinus (**Fig. 10**). The graft is then contoured and cantilevered at the nasofrontal junction to restore the correct nasal contours.[22] Shaping of the graft should avoid a widened dorsum and an excessively obtuse nasofrontal angle and plate fixation should be low profile.

Soft Tissue Management

Despite the optimal bony management of NOE fractures, the overall result can be compromised by the overlying soft tissues. As a result of the inherent NOE area contours, coupled with the soft tissue dissection during surgical correction, the final soft tissue drape can result in psuedotelecanthus and poor cosmesis. Thus, well-positioned incisions, controlled dissection, low-profile fixation

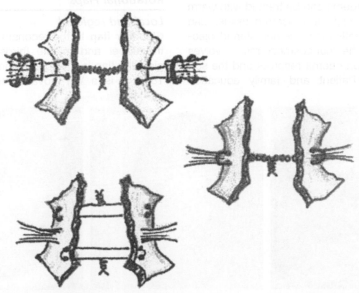

Fig. 9. Transnasal wiring technique based on clinical condition of central fragment and MCT. (*From* Sargent LA. Nasoethmoid orbital fractures. Plast Reconstr Surg 2007;120(2):16S–31S; with permission.)

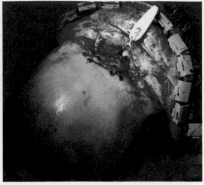
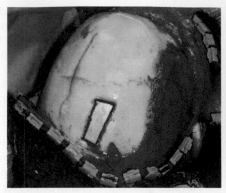

Fig. 10. Right parietal bone graft from outer calvarial table for dorsal nasal reconstruction. (Clinical pictures are *courtesy of* Dr Daniel J. Meara, Wilmington, DE.)

and perioperative tissue management and support are critical to surgical success. Further, dermal pexies secure the skin to the underlying bone or fixation materials, and NOE area bolsters are placed and secured to compress the overlying tissues against the bony skeleton in an attempt to prevent pseudotelecanthus.[19] A traditional adhesive-retained extranasal splint is often insufficient, and improved soft tissue outcomes are realized with padded hard splint compression plates, secured via transnasal wires (**Fig. 11**).[19] Compression for 10 to 14 days improves soft tissue contours and serves as a nasal splint for nasal bone healing. Appropriate soft tissue management can be the difference between cosmetic success or failure of surgical intervention for NOE fractures.

Postoperative Management

Persistent lymphedema can be treated with warm compresses and thickened, scarred tissues can be treated with gentle massage and steroid injections, if needed. The final cosmetic result evolves as remaining lymph edema resolves and the soft tissues mature. Patient and family education

regarding expectations, postoperative care and long-term soft tissue changes are paramount in the complete care of the NOE and nasal complex fractures.

ACQUIRED SOFT TISSUE DEFECTS

Traumatic injuries, such as those from dog bites or ballistics, or pathologic cutaneous lesions, such as basal cell carcinomas, often result in significant tissue distortion or even frank tissue loss. Correction of such defects of the nasal complex are best addressed via nasal subunits (**Fig. 12**)[24] and require a robust surgical armentarium, including rotational flaps, autogenous grafts, alloplastic implants, and implant support prostheses. Typically, defect size (greater or less than 1.5 cm) and location dictate the surgical technique.[25]

Rotational Flaps

Local and regional
Glabellar flap In the reconstruction of defects of the upper and middle thirds of the nose, the glabellar flap is a viable option. First described in 1818, it is a V-Y advancement flap based on

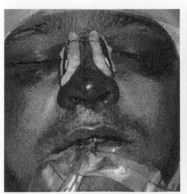
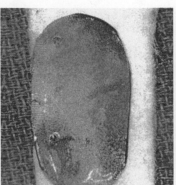
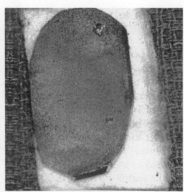

Fig. 11. Soft tissue management in NOE fractures to prevent pseudotelecanthus status after fracture repair. (*From* Sargent LA. Nasoethmoid orbital fractures. Plast Reconstr Surg 2007;120(2):16S–31S; with permission.)

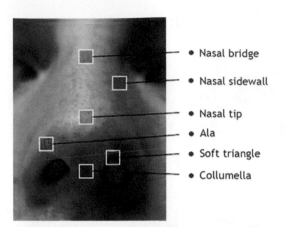

- Nasal bridge
- Nasal sidewall
- Nasal tip
- Ala
- Soft triangle
- Collumella

Fig. 12. Nasal subunits. (*From* Rahman M, Jefferson N, Stewart DA. The histology of facial aesthetic subunits: implications for common nasal reconstructive procedures. J Plast Reconstr Aesthetic Surg 2010; 63(5):753–6; with permission.)

a random blood supply, which uses redundant glabellar skin between the eyebrows for reconstruction.[26] The glabellar flap can be performed under local anesthesia and is an excellent skin match and allows for primary closure. The surgical technique includes (**Fig. 13**):

- Creation of an inverted V from the midpoint of the glabella region just above the brow
- Segment extension below brow with longer portion of the flap (side away from arc of rotation) extended to the most superior-lateral aspect of the defect
- Subcutaneous tissue dissection, followed by flap contouring and passive rotation into the defect, with V-Y closure of the donor site

Dorsal nasal flap In 1967, Reiger[27] first described the dorsal nasal flap for small to moderate-sized defects of the lower third of the nose, including the nasal tip, because the glabellar flap is for

defects of the upper and middle thirds of the nose. Initially, it was described as a rotational flap with a random pattern blood supply. Marchac[28] later modified the technique to base the flap off a defined axial pedicle based on blood vessels in the medial canthal area and the angular artery. The enhanced blood supply allowed the simplification of the flap design with greater rotation and is a reasonable skin match and allows for primary closure.[29] Midline defects can be reconstructed with a pedicle based on either medial canthus; otherwise, an ipsilateral-based pedicle allows for easier defect repair. The surgical technique includes (**Fig. 14**):

- The dorsal nasal flap pedicle is similar to the glabellar flap; however, the inverted V has less superior extension above the level of the brow.
- If axial blood supply is determined via branches of the angular or infratrochlear arteries, a more narrow pedicle is adequate, allowing for easier rotation and donor site closure

Alar flap Alar retraction deformities after trauma, disease, or infection often result in nasal asymmetry. Mild to moderate alar contraction can be addressed with cartilaginous reinforcement via grafting. However, severe alar retraction results in loss of normal alar soft tissues because of replacement by scar tissue. Thus, an alar rotational flap in conjunction with a cartilaginous alar batten graft allows reconstruction of the alar subunit and return of nostril symmetry.[30] The random pattern blood supply is robust and the skin match is excellent; the procedure can be accomplished in 1 stage. Alternative reconstruction options in the form of transposition flaps exist, but these require multiple surgeries and typically result in suboptimal tissue match. The surgical technique includes (**Fig. 15**):

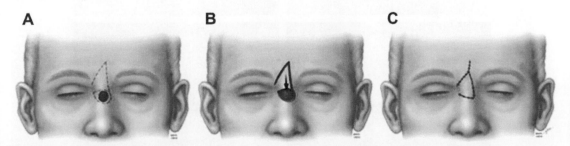

Fig. 13. Glabellar rotation advancement flap. (*A*) Defect marked for excision and proposed glabellar rotation advancement flap outlined. (*B*) Defect excised and flap being rotated into the defect. (*C*) Inset of the flap into the defect with closure of the secondary defect in a V-Y fashion. (*From* Koch CA, Archibald DJ, Friedman O. Glabellar flaps in nasal reconstruction. Facial Plastic Surg Clin North Am 2011;19(1):113–22.)

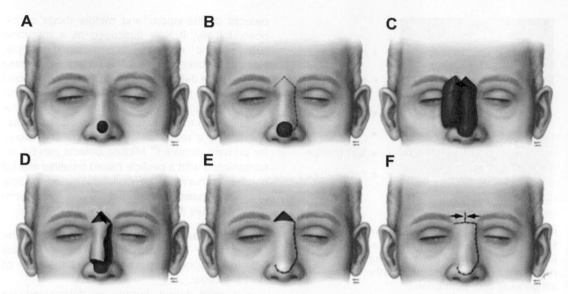

Fig. 14. Dorsal nasal flap. (*A*) Nasal tip defect to be excised. (*B*) Defect excised and proposed dorsal nasal flap outlined. (*C*) The flap is widely undermined. (*D*) The flap is rotated inferiorly into the defect. (*E*) The flap is inset within the defect and the resultant dog-ear deformity corrected. (*F*) The resultant secondary defect is closed in a V-Y fashion. (*From* Koch CA, Archibald DJ, Friedman O. Glabellar flaps in nasal reconstruction. Facial Plastic Surg Clin North Am 2011;19(1):113–22.)

- Intranasal marginal incision is extended onto the alar cutaneous crease, maintaining an intact alar base pedicle for perfusion and caudal rotation along the alar-facial groove
- Subcutaneous dissection should preserve residual alar cartilage, if present
- If deemed necessary, alar cartilage batten grafting is positioned at this stage, to

- support the underlying tissues and the repositioned ala
- Layered and passive closure is critical to minimize any cephalic migration, especially in large alar repositioning movements
- A key stitch is that aligning the alar rim, at the soft triangle area, so as to minimize the risk of webbing or notching

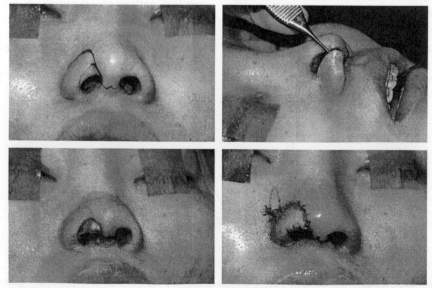

Fig. 15. Alar flap with rotation for correction of retraction. (*From* Jung DH, Kwak ES, Kim HS. Correction of severe alar retraction with use of a cutaneous alar rotation flap. Plast Reconstr Surg 2009;123(3):1088–95; with permission.)

Melolabial flap Defects often exist that are not amenable to primary closure or repair with local rotational flaps. For instance, large or composite defects of the nose and lips often require region flap reconstruction, and the melolabial flap is a workhorse flap for such cases. The flap has a random pattern blood supply, with survival most dependent on the perfusion pressure. The flap is capable of many design permutations, allowing for nasal tip, alae, columella, and internal lining reconstruction.[31] Also, the tissue match is acceptable for nasal reconstruction, with the donor scar well camouflaged in the melolabial crease. Three main melolabial flap types exist: (1) subcutaneous tissue pedicle, (2) cutaneous pedicle, and (3) advancement flaps, which are primarily used for cheek defects. The subcutaneous and cutaneous flaps require a second surgery, for flap division, at approximately 3 weeks after initial inset. The surgical technique for a subcutaneous flap is discussed and includes (**Fig. 16**):

- A nasal defect template is marked, with the inferior aspect of the flap design resting within the melolabial groove
- Inferior-lateral dissection proceeds to the superior-medial subcutaneous pedicle
- Clockwise rotation and inset into the defect
- Donor site primary closure

Bilobed flap First described by Esser,[32] the double-transposition flap is useful for nasal reconstruction of the distal third of the nose; however, involvement of the nasal ala precludes the use of this flap because of the likelihood of postoperative alar retraction.[33] The bilobed flap is a random pattern local flap, which can have a lateral or medial base. The geometric design is a most critical step to ensure proper rotation and defect reconstruction, without tension, which may result in postoperative nasal distortion. This geometric design spans a 90° arc of pivot, divided between the 2 lobes of the bilobed flap. The surgical technique includes (**Fig. 17**):

- Measurements determine the defect radius (r) with the arc of rotation based at 2 x r, within the alar groove at a distinct point
- The 2 lobes of this flap are then designed from this point, with 1 arc through the center of the defect and the second arc tangential to the most distal aspect of the defect
- Defect width is measured and duplicated for both reconstruction lobes between the 2 arcs
- Lobe height is equal to the distance between the 2 arcs for the first lobe, which is inset into the original defect; the second lobe is

approximately 2 times the height of the first, allowing for closure of the donor site
- Subcutaneous dissection, flap contouring, and inset complete the reconstruction, including the removal of a wedge of tissue within the alar groove to allow proper flap rotation

Rhomboid flap The rhomboid flap is a local flap based on a random blood supply that places wound tension perpendicular to the resting skin tension lines, the area of maximum extensibility.[34] At least 8 design variations exist for small defect nasal reconstruction; however, basic principles exist in all permutations. Specifically, the surgically created defect must be rhomboid, with internal angles of 60° and 120°, creating equilateral triangles, which are transposed to reconstruct the defect (**Fig. 18**).

Forehead flap Gillies and Millard[35] stated that, "the tint of forehead skin so exactly matches that of the face and nose that a forehead flap must be the first choice for reconstruction of a nasal defect." Because many local and regional flaps exist for nasal reconstruction, the forehead flap is particularly useful for larger defects. The paramedial forehead flap is an axial pattern flap based on the supratrochlear artery, which is capable of total nasal resurfacing.[36] Negatives include a second surgery for division and thickened tissues, which may result in increased bulk and imperfect tissue match. In 2012, after angiography in fresh cadavers, Kishi and colleagues[37] showed clinically the use of an alternative 1-step nasal reconstruction technique via an island paramedial forehead flap based on the angular artery with ligation of the supratrochlear artery at its base. The surgical technique includes (**Fig. 19**):

- Ipsilateral flap design allows for the most conservative design and Doppler can be used to verify the location of the supratrochlear vessels
- Flap width should be at least 1.0 cm; flap thickness is based on the extent of tissues to be reconstructed, and flap length depends on the location of reconstruction
- The flap is rotated into the defect and divided after at least 3 weeks, allowing time for vascular in-growth

Distant Flaps

Free tissue transfer with microvascular reconstruction

In cases of total nasal reconstruction of composite defects, free flap microvascular reconstruction

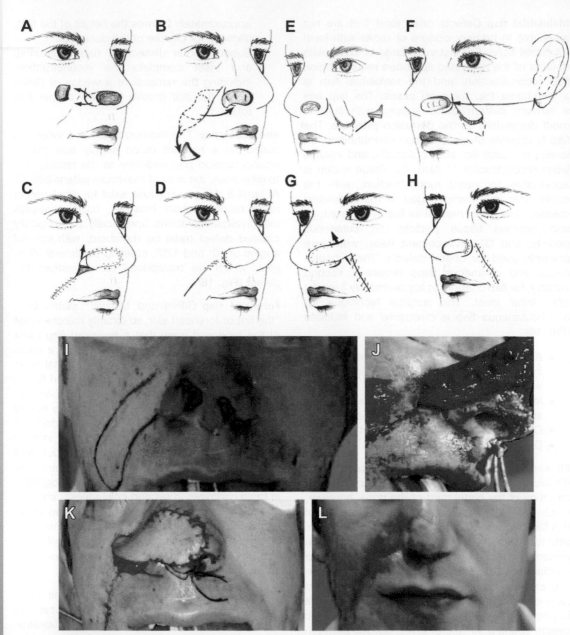

Fig. 16. The nasal alar defect is reconstructed with an interpolated melolabial subcutaneous pedicle flap. Because the alar defect is greater than 50% of the nasal subunit, the subunit excision is completed (*A*). The skin is incised, creating a cutaneous island, a fat pedicle developed, and the inferior triangle of skin excised to facilitate donor site closure. A cartilage graft is secured into the wound bed before flap transfer (*B*). The flap is inset, and the fat pedicle is left intact for 3 weeks. The superior triangle of skin is discarded during pedicle division (*C*). The completed second stage is shown with the pedicle divided, the lateral aspect of the flap contoured and inset, and the donor site closed (*D*). The nasal alar defect is reconstructed with an interpolated melolabial cutaneous pedicle flap. The flap is designed to anticipate the complete excision of the alar subunit. The flap is incised, and the inferior triangle of skin is discarded to facilitate donor site closure (*E*). The defect is enlarged to complete the alar subunit excision, because the original wound is greater than 50% of the nasal subunit. A conchal cartilage graft is then secured into the wound bed (*F*). The flap is inset and sutured into position, and the donor site closed (*G*). The completed second stage is shown with the pedicle divided, the lateral aspect of the flap contoured and inset, and the donor site closed (*H*). (*I–L*) Clinical example of cutaneous pedicle flap from design to initial healing status after pedicle division. ([*A–H*] *From* Yellin SA, Nugent A. Melolabial flaps in nasal reconstruction. Facial Plastic Surg Clin North Am 2011;19(1):123–39; Clinical pictures are *courtesy of* Dr Patrick Louis, Birmingham, AL.)

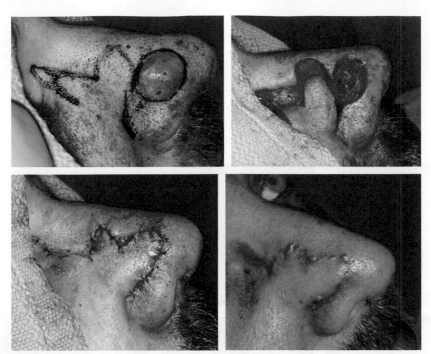

Fig. 17. Bilobed flap for reconstruction of nasal defect. (Clinical pictures are *courtesy of* Dr Daniel J. Meara, Wilmington, DE.)

provides a viable option. Variable free flap options exist for recreation of the skin, osteocartilaginous framework, and mucosal lining, such as the first dorsal metacarpal flap, the dorsalis pedis flap, the auricular helical flap, and the radial forearm flap (**Fig. 20**).[38] The decision to choose free flap microvascular reconstruction should be made only if regional flaps are not an option, prosthetic reconstruction is not desired by the patient, and reasonable cosmesis is attainable. A well-made

prosthetic nose is tolerable by the patient and often provides superior aesthetics, and any surgical reconstruction should be measured against prosthetic outcomes if undertaken for total nasal reconstruction.

Internal Nasal Lining

Septal pivot flap, septal mucoperichondrial hinge flap

In large or total nasal reconstruction, septal reconstruction in conjunction with a multistage paramedial forehead flap can be a reasonable treatment plan. The reconstruction of the septum can be accomplished via the septal pivot flap (SPF), which rotates the remaining nasal septum forward to create nasal support.[39] This procedure can also be modified for internal nasal lining reconstruction as a septal mucoperichondrial hinge flap.[34] The SPF and its modifications are axial pattern flaps, based on the superior labial artery. The surgical technique includes (**Fig. 21**):

- Incision through mucosa, perichondrium, and septal cartilage and bone for the pivot flap, maintaining at least a 1-cm anterior-inferior pedicle based on the superior labial artery; rotation can occur up to 90° and mucoperichondrium can be reflected for nasal passage lining
- Modified design includes only development of the mucoperichondrium and this can be

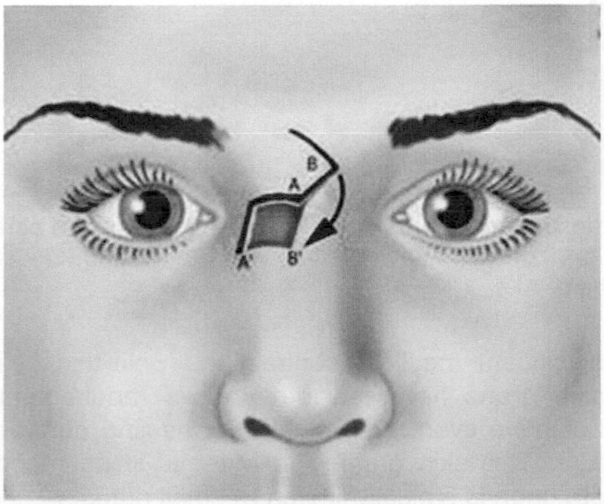

Fig. 18. Rhomboid flap from glabella. Closure of the defect with transposition of point A and B to A′ and B′, respectively. (*From* Lohuis PJ, Godefroy WP, Baker SR, et al. Transposition flaps in nasal reconstruction. Facial Plastic Surg Clin North Am 2011;19(1):85–106.)

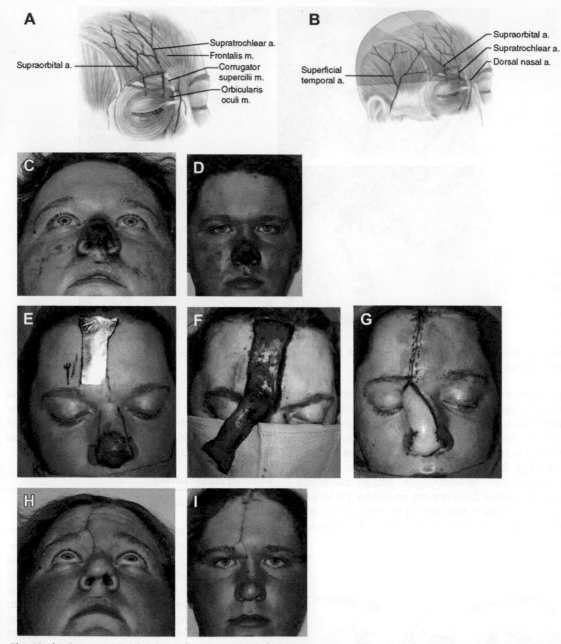

Fig. 19. (*A–I*) Paramedial forehead flap for nasal defect reconstruction. ([*A, B*] *From* Baker SR. Interpolated paramedian forehead flaps. In local flaps in facial reconstruction. London: Elsevier; 2007; with permission. Clinical pictures are *courtesy of* Dr Somsak Sittavorwong, Birmingham, AL.)

performed when septal support is adequate, but internal nasal lining is inadequate, as in composite alar defect cases.

Skin Grafts

Full-thickness skin grafts are available for the replacement of nasal lining as well as cutaneous coverage.[40] However, such grafts are incapable of cartilage graft coverage and tend to experience significant healing contraction. Split-thickness skin grafts have fewer metabolic requirements but have even more significant healing contracture. This skin grafting for internal lining reconstruction is typically limited to small defects.[41]

Other

Hinge flaps, bipedicle vestibular advancement flaps, and septal mucoperichondrial flaps are

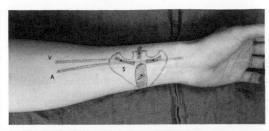

Fig. 20. Radial forearm cutaneous free flap with nasal specific design of skin paddle in reconstruction of large nasal defect. V, vein (venae comitantes); A, artery (radial artery); S, skin paddle with nasal design. (*From* Antunes MB, Chalian AA. Microvascular reconstruction of nasal defects. Facial Plastic Surg Clin North Am 2011;19(1):157–62.)

also surgical techniques for nasal lining reconstruction, because such flaps provide adequate nutrition for overlying tissues, have limited contraction, and do not obstruct nasal airflow.[25] Even the paramedian forehead flap can be considered via the modified Farina method.[42] Every flap choice has advantages and disadvantages and can be limited to certain anatomic locations (**Table 2**).

Osteocartilaginous Tissues

Bone grafting for nasal reconstruction is readily obtained from either cranial bone or iliac crest bone grafts, although costochondral grafts and tibial bone grafts have been readily used as well.[25,43,44] Cartilaginous harvest is from the nasal septum, but in cases of septal loss, additional cartilaginous support can be obtained from the conchal bowl of the ear, which is especially useful for lower lateral cartilage reconstruction.[25,43]

Alloplastic Materials

Alloplastic materials have been used in surgery dating back to the 1930s and more options are available each year. The ease of use and avoidance of an autogenous donor sites are clear benefits of such materials. The goal is for a material to be biocompatible, resistant to infection, removable, user-friendly, and cost-effective.[21] The main alloplasts in clinical use for nasal surgery are: silicone, porous polyethylene, proplast, Gore-Tex (W. L. Gore & Associates, Inc, Elkton, MD, USA), Mersilene (Ethicon Inc, Somerville, NJ, USA) mesh, and AlloDerm (Lifecell Corporation, Bridgewater, NJ,

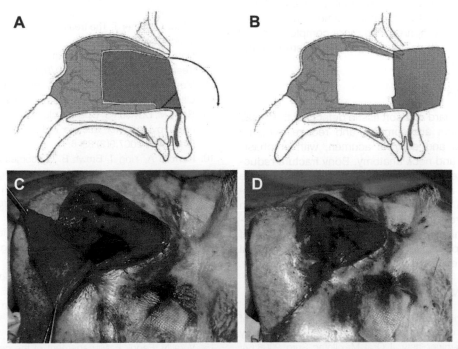

Fig. 21. (*A*) Rotation flap supplied by branches of the superior labial artery within 10-mm to 15-mm-wide mucosal bridge; rotation planned (*arrow*). (*B*) Rotation by 90°, axial pattern flap. (*C*) Ipsilateral septal mucoperichondrial flap shown before inset. Entire ala/sidewall defect was repaired with a unilateral hinged mucoperichondrial flap (*D*). ([*A, B*] *From* Quetz J, Ambrosch P. Total nasal reconstruction: a 6-year experience with the 3-stage forehead flap combined with the septal pivot flap. Facial Plast Surg 2011;27(3):266–75, with permission; [*C, D*] Weber SM, Wang TD. Options for internal lining in nasal reconstruction. Facial Plast Surg Clin North Am 2011;19(1):163–73.)

Table 2
Intranasal mucosal lining flaps

Flap	Defect Location	Advantage(s)	Disadvantage(s)
Bipedicled vestibular	Alar margin	Ease of dissection	Alar retraction if not caudally positioned
Septal mucosa (ipsilateral)	Ala, tip, lower vault	Bilateral flaps possible	May obstruct nasal airway
Hinged septal mucosal (contralateral)	Middle vault	Can be composite (lining and structure)	Septal perforation
Composite septal pivotal	Tip, columella middle vault	Bilateral lining	Difficult dissection Septal perforation
Interior turbinate	Caudal; occasional middle vault	When septal, mucosa absent Avoids septal perforation	Intranasal dissection Turbinate size Airway obstruction

Data from Tollesfson T, Kriet D. Complex nasal defects: structure and internal lining. Facial Plast Surg Clin North Am 2005;13:333–43.

USA).[21] Depending on the defect, alloplastic materials may be used alone or in tandem with autogenous grafts, to achieve optimal nasal reconstruction in the treatment of acquired defects.

Prosthetics

A nasal or midface prosthesis is another option in the reconstruction of significant acquired defects. Often the prosthetic reconstruction has superior aesthetics compared with more complex surgical repair, and thus, should be considered in the most severe cases.

SUMMARY

Acquired hard and soft tissue defects of the nasal/NOE region are complex and require accurate diagnosis and surgical acumen, with emphasis on head and neck anatomy. Bony fracture reduction, bone and cartilaginous grafting for hard tissue defects, and soft tissue flaps for optimal reconstruction of injured or missing elements are often all required to restore form and function. Long-term clinical outcomes are typically excellent if surgical principles are followed and these surgical techniques used.

REFERENCES

1. Fattahi T, Steinberg B, Fernandes R, et al. Repair of nasal complex fractures and the need for secondary septo-rhinoplasty. J Oral Maxillofac Surg 2006;64: 1785–9.
2. Han D, Han Y, Park J. A new approach to the treatment of nasal bone fracture: radiologic classification of nasal bone fractures and its clinical application. J Oral Maxillofac Surg 2011;69:2841–7.
3. Haug R, Prather J. The closed reduction of nasal fractures: an evaluation of two techniques. J Oral Maxillofac Surg 1991;49:1288–92.
4. Ondik M, Lipinski L, Dezfoli S, et al. The treatment of nasal fractures. Arch Facial Plast Surg 2009;11(5): 296–302.
5. Lee M, Inman J, Callahan S. Fracture patterns of the nasal septum. Otolaryngol Head Neck Surg 2010; 143:784–8.
6. Gillies H, Kilner T. The treatment of the broken nose. Lancet 1929;1:147.
7. Harrison D. Nasal injuries: their pathogenesis and treatment. Br J Plast Surg 1979;32:57.
8. Murray J, Maran A, Busuttil A, et al. A pathologic classification of nasal fractures. Injury 1986;7:338.
9. Reilly M, Davison S. Open vs closed approach to the nasal pyramid for fracture reduction. Arch Facial Plast Surg 2007;9(2):82–6.
10. Herford A, Ying T, Brown B. Outcomes of severely comminuted (type iii) nasoorbitoethmoid fractures. J Oral Maxillofac Surg 2005;63:1266–77.
11. Michelotti B, Mackay D. Nasal reconstruction. Clin Anat 2012;25:86–98.
12. Tollesfson T, Kriet D. Complex nasal defects: structure and internal lining. Facial Plast Surg Clin North Am 2005;13:333–43.
13. Love R. Nasal fractures: patient satisfaction following closed reduction. N Z Med J 2010;123:45–8.
14. Hoffmann J. Naso-orbital-ethmoid complex fracture management. Facial Plast Surg 1998;14(1): 67–76.
15. Vora N, Fedok F. Management of the central nasal support complex in naso-orbital ethmoid fractures. Facial Plast Surg 2000;16(2):181–91.
16. Papadopoulos H, Salib N. Management of naso-orbital-ethmoidal fractures. Oral Maxillofac Surg Clin North Am 2009;21:221–5.

17. Remmler D, Denny A, Gosain A, et al. Role of three-dimensional computed tomography in the assessment of nasoorbitoethmoidal fractures. Ann Plast Surg 2000;44:553–63.

18. Markowitz B, Manson P, Sargent L, et al. Management of the medial canthal tendon in nasoethmoid orbital fractures: the importance of the central fragment in classification and treatment. Plast Reconstr Surg 1991;87:843.

19. Sargent L. Nosoethmoid orbital fractures: diagnosis and treatment. Plast Reconstr Surg 2007;120(2):16S–31S.

20. Gruss J. Naso-ethmoid-orbital fractures: classification and role of primary bone grafting. Plast Reconstr Surg 1985;75:303.

21. Young P, Rice D. Management of a type II nasoethmoid orbital fracture and near-penetration of the intracranial cavity with transnasal canthopexy. Ear Nose Throat J 2007;86(6):344–60.

22. Potter J, Muzaffar A, Ellis E, et al. Aesthetic management of the nasal component of naso-orbital ethmoid fractures. Plast Reconstr Surg 2006;117:10e–8e.

23. Berghaus A, Stelter K. Alloplastic materials in rhinoplasty. Curr Opin Otolaryngol Head Neck Surg 2006;14:270–7.

24. Singh D, Bartlett S. Aesthetic considerations in nasal reconstruction and the role of modified nasal subunits. Plast Reconstr Surg 2003;111(2):639–51.

25. Woodard C, Park S. Reconstruction of nasal defects 1.5 cm or smaller. Arch Facial Plast Surg 2011;13(2):97–102.

26. Koch C, Archibald D, Friedman O. Glabellar flaps in nasal reconstruction. Facial Plast Surg Clin North Am 2011;19:113–22.

27. Reiger R. A local flap for repair of the nasal tip. Plast Reconstr Surg 1967;40:147–9.

28. Marchac D, Toth B. The axial frontonasal flap revisited. Plast Reconstr Surg 1985;76:686–94.

29. Zavod M, Zavod M, Goldman G. The dorsal nasal flap. Dermatol Clin 2005;23:73–85.

30. Jung D, Kwak E, Kin H. Correction of severe alar retraction with use of a cutaneous alar rotation flap. Plast Reconstr Surg 2009;123(3):1088–95.

31. Yellin S, Nugent A. Melolabial flaps for nasal reconstruction. Facial Plast Surg Clin North Am 2011;19:123–39.

32. Esser J. Gestielte locale Nasenplastik mit Zweizipfligem Lappen Decking des sekundaren Detektes vomersten Zipfel durch den zweiten. Dtsh Z Chir 1918;143:385 [in German].

33. Steiger J. Bilobed flaps in nasal reconstruction. Facial Plast Surg Clin North Am 2011;19:107–11.

34. Lohuis P, Godefroy W, Baker S, et al. Transposition flaps in nasal reconstruction. Facial Plast Surg Clin North Am 2011;19:85–106.

35. Gillies H, Millard D. The principles and art of plastic surgery. Boston: Little Brown; 1957.

36. Menick F. Nasal reconstruction with a forehead flap. Clin Plast Surg 2009;36:443–59.

37. Kishi K, Imanishi N, Shimizu Y, et al. Alternative 1-step nasal reconstruction technique. Arch Facial Plast Surg 2012;14(2):116–21.

38. Antunes M, Chalian A. Microvascular reconstruction of nasal defects. Facial Plast Surg Clin North Am 2011;19:157–62.

39. Quetz J, Ambrosch P. Total nasal reconstruction: a 6-year experience with the three-stage forehead flap combined with the septal pivot flap. Facial Plast Surg 2011;27:266–75.

40. Shaye D, Sykes J, Kim J. Advances in nasal reconstruction. Curr Opin Otolaryngol Head Neck Surg 2011;19:251–6.

41. Weber S, Wang T. Options for internal lining in nasal reconstruction. Facial Plast Surg Clin North Am 2011;19:163–73.

42. Parikh S, Futran N, Most S. An alternative method for reconstruction of large intranasal lining defects. Arch Facial Plast Surg 2010;12(5):311–4.

43. Saijadian A, Rubinstein R, Naghshineh N. Current status of grafts and implants in rhinoplasty: part I. Autologous graft. Plast Reconstr Surg 2010;125:40e–9e.

44. Garcia-Diez E, Guisantes E, Fontdevila J, et al. Cortical tibial bone graft for nasal augmentation: donor site short scar. J Plast Reconstr Aesthet Surg 2009;62:747–54.

Orbital, Periorbital, and Ocular Reconstruction

John A. Long, MD[a], Rajesh Gutta, BDS, MS[b,c],*

KEYWORDS

- Orbital reconstruction • Orbital fractures • Ocular injuries • Evisceration • Enucleation
- Orbital floor repair • Enophthalmos

KEY POINTS

- Re-excision and reapproximation is critical in the management of lid margin defects.
- In canalicular repair, the stents should be left in place for 2 months in both adults and children.
- When indicated, orbital floor fractures should be treated early to decrease postoperative complications.
- Precise reconstruction of the angle between the orbital floor and the medial wall is critical to prevent enophthalmos.
- The transconjunctival approach is associated with increased incidence of epiphora.
- Defects posterior to the equator of the globe are responsible for most posttreatment enophthalmic defects.
- Adequate volume replacement is critical to prevent poor esthetic outcomes in patients with anophthalmos.

EYELID LACERATIONS

Eyelid lacerations require evaluation and repair. The initial evaluation must include an ophthalmic evaluation of the globe. If the globe is lacerated or ruptured, the repair of the globe takes precedence over the eyelid repair. Eyelid lacerations may involve the eyelid margin, the canalicular system, or the eyelid only. Preoperative evaluation of eyelid trauma will determine plan for the repair.

1. Is the globe intact?
2. Is the canalicular system involved?
3. Is the margin involved?
4. Is the laceration full thickness?

EYELID MARGIN REPAIR

The integrity of the eyelid margin is necessary for the maintenance of ocular health. The function of the eyelid margin is to protect the eyeball and maintain the lubrication of the eyeball. The diagnosis of an eyelid margin laceration will lead to an eyelid margin repair. The repair can be performed in an emergency department setting, office, or an operating room, depending on the clinical situation.

The goal of eyelid margin repair is to maintain the alignment of the eyelid anatomy. There are several structures visible on the eyelid margin that aid in the alignment of the wound edges. The gray line is the junction between the skin and the conjunctival surface. It is the edge of the orbicularis muscle visible beneath the translucent eyelid margin. The linearity of the meibomian glands, the tarsus, and the eyelashes help with suture placement when repairing an eyelid margin. Approximation of the tarsus is necessary for an effective closure (**Fig. 1**). Performed correctly, the eyelid margin repair will restore the anatomic integrity of the eyelid. The initial 6–0 silk suture is

[a] Department of Ophthalmology, Alabama Ophthalmology Associates, University of Alabama at Birmingham, 1000, 19th Avenue South, Birmingham, AL 35205, USA; [b] Private Practice, Mountain State Oral and Maxillofacial Surgeons, 1215 Virginia Street East, Charleston, WV 25301, USA; [c] Division of Oral & Maxillofacial Surgery, University of Cincinnati, 231 Albert Sabin Way, Cincinnati, OH 45229, USA
* Corresponding author. 1215 Virginia Street East, Charleston, WV 25301.
E-mail address: rajeshg76@yahoo.com

Oral Maxillofacial Surg Clin N Am 25 (2013) 151–166
http://dx.doi.org/10.1016/j.coms.2013.01.005
1042-3699/13/$ – see front matter © 2013 Elsevier Inc. All rights reserved.

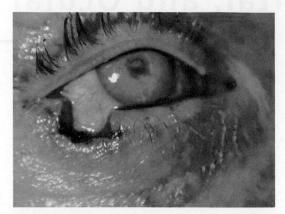

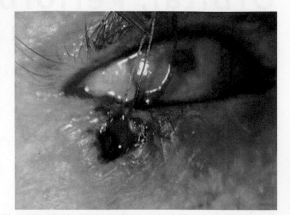

Fig. 1. This eyelid margin defect is a result of Mohs surgery without involvement of the canalicular system. The tarsus in the lower eyelid is approximately 4 mm in depth.

Fig. 3. Deep sutures.

at the gray line. The alignment of the eyelid depends not only on the placement of the suture at the gray line but also the depth of the suture (**Fig. 2**). With the silk suture on stretch, the eyelid margin should be aligned. This stitch will help with the placement of all further sutures. The initial suture can be placed and replaced until a perfect position is found. The eyelid margin is held in good position with an upward pull on the 6–0 silk suture. A 5–0 Vicryl (Ethicon Inc, Somerville, NJ) suture is placed through the tarsus. One or 2 deep sutures may be needed to reapproximate the tarsus (**Fig. 3**). Care should be taken to make sure the deep Vicryl sutures do not penetrate the full thickness of the eyelid. Vicryl sutures exposed on the conjunctival surface will result in ocular irritation. With the eyelid margin in good alignment and the tarsus closed, additional 6–0 silk sutures are used to reapproximate the skin. The 6–0 silk suture at the eyelid margin is incorporated into a skin suture to direct it away from the eyeball

(**Fig. 4**). The skin sutures can be removed in 1 week. Complications of eyelid margin repair can lead to a compromise of ocular health. A notched eyelid may cause a tear film problem that can lead to a corneal ulcer and the loss of an eye. Trichiasis from misdirected lashes can cause eye pain, irritation, and infection.

COMPLICATIONS OF EYELID MARGIN REPAIR

The early loss of the sutures, postoperative wound infection, or poor technique can complicate the healing of eyelid margin lacerations. Swelling during the perioperative healing period can be extreme with complicated eyelid and periocular trauma. When the eyelid margin separates, a notched eyelid or trichiasis may develop (**Figs. 5 and 6**). A notched eyelid may lead to a tear film problem and complaints of a dry eye. The asymmetric appearance can also be distressing for patients. Trichiasis caused by scarring of the eyelid margin can lead to pain and corneal infection. The late repair of eyelid margin irregularities involves a re-excision and reapproximation of the

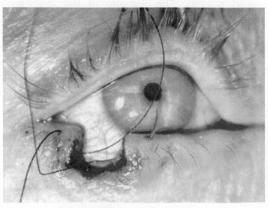

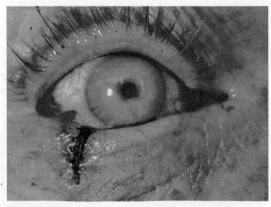

Fig. 2. Alignment of the eyelid margin.

Fig. 4. Closed eyelid margin defect.

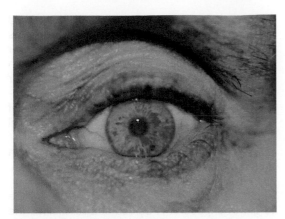

Fig. 5. Notched eyelid.

eyelid margin. The notched or trichiatic eyelid is re-paired after all the swelling from the initial injury has subsided. Preoperative assessment will deter-mine if there is adequate horizontal laxity to perform a block excision of the abnormal segment of the eyelid. The surgeon must keep in mind that the tarsus of the lower eyelid is 4 mm in width. The depth of excision only needs to be 4 mm to correct lower eyelid margin defects. A small notch or area of trichiasis involving the upper eyelid may require a greater amount of skin excision because the full height of the tarsus must be excised in the area of the abnormal eyelid.[1] In the mid aspect of the upper eyelid, the tarsus is 10 mm in height and the overlaying skin may need to be excised to improve the notch.

CRYOTHERAPY OF THE EYELID MARGIN

In cases when the eyelid margin is in good position but trichiasis is present, cryotherapy is an option.[2] Cryotherapy will selectively eliminate the eyelashes and should not damage the eyelid margin. Cryo-therapy has 2 main drawbacks. The incidence of recurrent trichiasis in the area of treatment is about 10%. The cryotherapy may need to be repeated if the eyelashes reappear. With cryotherapy, there

is unavoidable loss of adjacent eyelashes. Any hair follicles in the area of treatment are usually permanently destroyed. If effectively used for the treatment of trichiasis, there will be an area of the eyelid margin that is denuded of lashes. The patients must be informed of this unavoidable side effect of treatment. The use of a cryoprobe requires the eyelid to be adequately anesthetized. The cryoprobe is directed to the area of trichiasis and activated. A 1-minute freeze is timed beginning when the ice ball on the eyelid margin forms (**Fig. 7**). The cryoprobe is left in place and not moved for 1 minute. Any shearing or movement of the cryo-probe may damage the eyelid margin. After 1 minute, the ice ball is allowed to completely thaw and the cryoprobe is reapplied for an addi-tional 30 seconds. After another complete thaw, the cryoprobe is removed and the trichiatic lashes are epilated. During cryotherapy, the eyeball must be protected at all times. The probe cannot come into contact with the eyeball.

EYELID RETRACTION

Eyelid retraction is a common oculoplastic problem. The most common medical cause of eyelid retraction is thyroid eye disease. The most common iatrogenic cause of eyelid retraction is the infraciliary blepharoplasty. The most common posttraumatic cause of eyelid retraction is the in-fraciliary approach to the orbital floor. The cause of both postblepharoplasty and postblowout repair retraction is the same. An infraciliary approach to the orbit or the orbital fat requires opening the orbital septum. The orbital septum can heal with contraction and scaring. A midlamel-lar scar connecting the lower eyelid tarsus and the inferior orbital rim may contract and pull down the lower eyelid margin. Lower eyelid retraction following an infraciliary blowout repair is diag-nosed by the presence of inferior scleral show (**Fig. 8**). Patients may notice eyelid asymmetry or

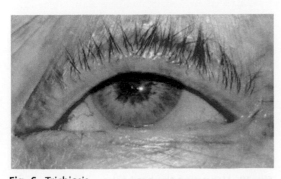

Fig. 6. Trichiasis.

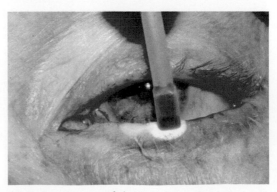

Fig. 7. Cryotherapy of the eyelid margin.

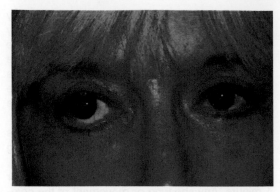

Fig. 8. Eyelid retraction after infraciliary blepharoplasty.

have symptoms of corneal exposure. The diagnosis of a midlamellar scar is confirmed by manually elevating the lower eyelid. A normal eyelid can be elevated to the superior limbus. Midlamellar scarring will prevent the elevation of the eyelid and a palpable restriction will be found.

REPAIR OF LOWER EYELID RETRACTION

Midlamellar scarring often causes posttraumatic eyelid retraction. The repair of this type of retraction involves the lyses of the midlamellar scar (**Fig. 9**). A transconjunctival approach is used to approach the lower eyelid retractor. In most cases of eyelid retraction, there is no deficiency of lower eyelid skin. The retraction is caused by shrinkage or scarring of the midlamella of the eyelid. The repair of lower eyelid retraction involves cutting the midlamellar scar, allowing the eyelid margin to elevate. With the release of the midlamella scar, a palpable elevation of the eyelid margin can be felt. The transconjunctival approach allows a buttress to be placed inside the eyelid.

In some cases, a spacer must be placed beneath the tarsus to form a buttress to hold up the eyelid margin. There are both autogenous and nonautogenous options for lower eyelid spacers. Preserved human and porcine dermis is available commercially and can be used for a posterior lamellar spacer. The most common autogenous material used for a posterior lamellar spacer is hard palate.[3–5] An autogenous hard-palate graft provides both the flexible rigidity of a tarsal substitute and conveniently has a mucosal lining that is well tolerated by the globe.

A hard-palate graft can be harvested both under general or modified local anesthesia. Before surgery, the hard palate is generously infiltrated with local anesthesia. A bite block is place to aid in exposure. A curved scalpel incises the full thickness of the hard palate (**Fig. 10**). An elliptical graft is harvested on either the left or the right side of the hard palate, avoiding the midline. The base of the donor site is cauterized, and pressure can be applied to aid with hemostasis. Wet gauze can be pressed into the donor site by the patient's tongue in patients who are cooperative. A hard-palate graft will not shrink after placement in the eyelid. The height of the graft should correspond to the elevation needed to remedy the eyelid retraction. Once the graft is harvested, the posterior surface is thinned in preparation for placement into the eyelid (**Fig. 11**). The length of the hard-palate graft should extend from the lateral canthus to the punctum. Typically, a hard-palate graft will be elliptical and measure 25 mm by 12 mm. The inferior portion of the graft is sutured to the conjunctiva and the lower eyelid retractor with a running 6–0 plain gut suture (**Fig. 12**). The superior edge of the graft is sutured to the inferior boarder of the tarsus with the same running suture. Complications of hard-palate grafts are usually related to pain in the mouth immediately after surgery and a foreign body sensation in the eye caused by the sutures and the rough mucous membrane on the hard-palate graft. Late ocular complications may include pyogenic granuloma formation that can be treated with either excision or steroid eyedrops.

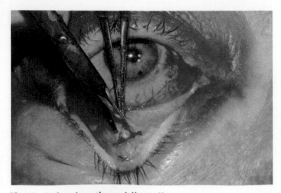

Fig. 9. Releasing the midlamellar scar.

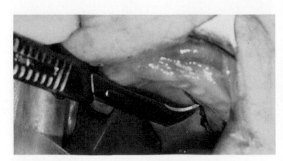

Fig. 10. Harvesting the hard palate.

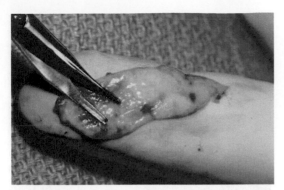

Fig. 11. Preparing the hard palate graft.

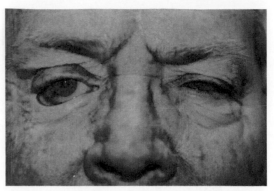

Fig. 13. Eyelid retraction caused by a loss of skin.

EYELID RETRACTION CAUSED BY SKIN LOSS

Eyelid retraction may be caused by the loss of skin (**Fig. 13**). Trauma, burns, or skin cancer surgery may lead to eyelid retraction caused by skin loss. When required, a full-thickness skin graft is usually harvested from the retroauricular area and placed on the eyelid where needed. The only indication to place a split-thickness skin graft on the eyelids is a shortage of skin available for grafting. A full-thickness skin graft can be harvested from many locations. The upper eyelid skin can be used for skin grafts. If a small amount of skin is needed and the removal of the skin graft will not compromise the eyelid function, then upper eyelid skin is a good choice. If a generous amount of skin is needed, then retroauricular skin is the best choice for thickness and color. The retroauricular area has sufficient skin for reconstructive purposes and the scar that develops in the donor site is not visible. Once the full-thickness skin graft has been placed into the recipient bed, it can be immobilized with either a bolster sewn over the graft or a tight pressure patch over the eyelids (**Fig. 14**). The bolster or the eye patch can be removed 4 or 5 days after surgery. Complications of full-thickness skin grafts include failure of the graft or graft shrinkage.

Patients that smoke or have diabetes are at increased rick for graft failure.

CANALICULAR REPAIR

The canalicular system is evaluated by placing a 0–00 Bowman probe through the dilated punctum. If the probe is visible in the wound, then a canalicular repair must be anticipated. Another technique to diagnose a lacerated canalicular system is to irrigate fluid through the punctum with a lacrimal cannula. If fluid is seen coming from the wound, then a canalicular laceration is present. The repair of the canalicular system requires an operating room and can be performed under general or modified local anesthesia. In the operating room, a cotton pledget soaked in 10% cocaine solution is placed under the inferior turbinate. This pledget provides both anesthesia and vasoconstriction. Pharmacologic shrinkage of the nasal mucosa allows for improved visualization. Canalicular repair involves passing a stent across the lacerated canalicular system (**Fig. 15**).[6–8] Identification of the cut canalicular system can be challenging at times. The canalicular system moves posterior to the eyelid margin as it courses more proximal. It can usually be identified with direct

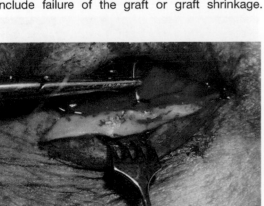

Fig. 12. Placement of the hard palate graft.

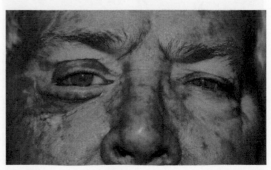

Fig. 14. Correction of eyelid retraction with a full-thickness skin graft.

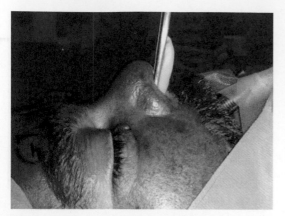

Fig. 15. Canalicular laceration repair.

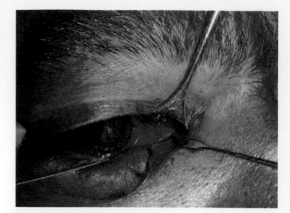

Fig. 17. Passing a stent across the cut canalicular system.

visualization (**Fig. 16**). Fluid irrigated into the superior punctum can aid with visualization. Usually a bicanalicular stent, such as a Crawford stent, is used. A bicanalicular stent is more stable and usually better tolerated that a monocanalicular stent.[7] A Crawford stent is used for bicanalicular intubation of the canalicular system. This stent has a small ball on the end of the metal stent. The small ball aids in the retrieval of the stent from under the inferior turbinate. Once the stent is passed across the cut canalicular system, it is threaded down the nasolacrimal duct and into the nose (**Fig. 17**). The Crawford stent is removed from beneath the inferior turbinate by hooking the little ball on the end of the stent with the Crawford hook. The hook will grasp the ball and allow for easy retrieval. The stent in the nose can often be seen by direct visualization, but many times it is felt and directed onto the Crawford hook with tactile senses (**Fig. 18**). The stent is grasped in one hand and the hook is held in the other hand. As the stent and the hook come into contact, they can be connected with proprioceptive skill.

Once a stent has been placed across the laceration, the wound is closed in a routine manner with a deep Vicryl suture at the medial canthal tendon and 6–0 silk or chromic sutures at the eyelid margin and skin. The metal stents that are connected to the silicone tubing are disconnected. The silicone tubing is tied in 4 overhand knots and allowed to retract into the nose. Usually 4 knots are sufficient to connect the silicone tubes. The tubes should not be sutured into the nose. There should be no tension on the silicone tubing, and the knot should rest at about the level of the inferior turbinate (**Fig. 19**). The canalicular system itself does not need to be repaired with sutures because the stent and the deep 5–0 Vicryl sutures will keep the cut edges of the canalicular system in good approximation. The skin sutures can be removed in 1 week. For both children and adults, the canalicular stent is left in place for 2 months. After 2 months, the stent is removed by pulling the silicone tubing laterally, away from the medial canthus. The silicone tubing is cut, and the cut stent is pulled from the eyelid.

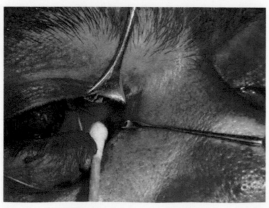

Fig. 16. Identification of the cut proximal canalicular system.

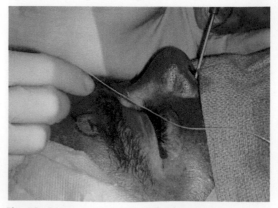

Fig. 18. Retrieval of the Crawford stent.

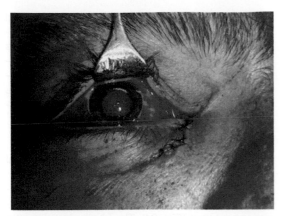

Fig. 19. Completed repair.

HARD TISSUE RECONSTRUCTION
Reconstruction of the Orbit

The orbit represents a critical functional and aesthetic component of the face. Because of its prominent location, the exposed position, and weak bony structure, the orbit is particularly susceptible to fractures. Traumatic orbital deformities can range from an isolated orbital blowout fracture to complex deformity involving the entire orbit (Figs. 20–22). Improper treatment can lead to complications, such as enophthalmos, ocular motility restriction, ocular or orbital dystopia, and associated soft tissue defects.

Evaluation

Operative management of orbital defects should be based on a comprehensive clinical and

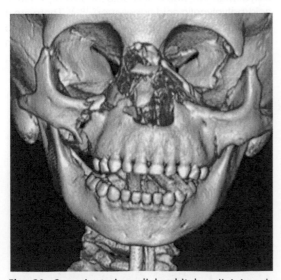

Fig. 20. Comminuted medial orbital wall injury in a 4-year-old patient.

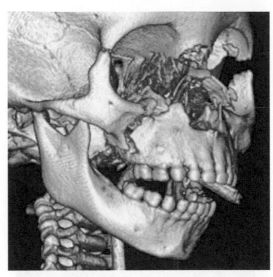

Fig. 21. Extensive injury involving both the medial and lateral orbital walls.

radiologic assessment. A comprehensive clinical examination should include ocular function, visual acuity, fundus examination, ocular movements, and pupillary function (Fig. 23). Appropriate ocular examination should be done in the acute and delayed presentations of patients in consultation with an ophthalmologist or an oculoplastic surgeon. Attention must be paid to subtle signs like the presence of a supratarsal sulcus deformity, which indicates the loss of support inferiorly and posteriorly. Computed tomography with axial and coronal scanning, supplemented with sagittal and 3-dimensional reconstructions, in selected cases provides optimal visualization of the orbital rim and walls.

Clinical indications

Treatment of such injuries is a demanding aspect of craniofacial fracture management. Based on

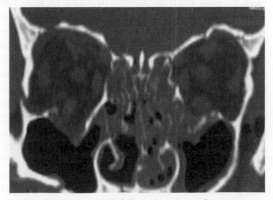

Fig. 22. Bilateral orbital floor blow out fractures.

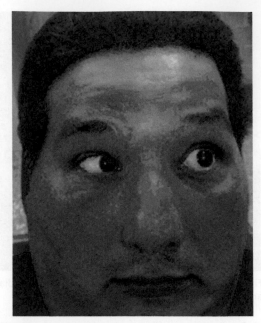

Fig. 23. Restricted ocular motility as a result of delayed orbital floor repair.

an evidence-based analysis, Burnstine[9] published clinical recommendations for the repair of isolated orbital floor fractures. An important consideration in the repair of orbital defects is not just continuity but support of the globe, restoration of function, and preventing facial asymmetry. Sometimes delaying surgery might be indicated to relieve periorbital swelling and, thus, facilitate exposure. However, others have reported that excessive delay in operative intervention might be associated with increased postoperative complications.[10,11]

Anatomic challenge

Contrary to the general belief, the orbital floor is not flat. In fact, the anatomy of the orbital floor is very complicated because the shape of the orbital floor ranges from sinusoidal to more or less flat configurations and differs within and between individuals. Appreciation of the anatomic configuration of the junctional area between the medial wall and floor in the posterior third of the orbit is particularly important. The upper portion of the maxillary antrum produces a characteristic bulge in this region, obliterating the angle between the orbital floor and the medial wall. Failure to precisely recreate this contour invariably leads to posterior globe displacement and eventual enophthalmos, even in the presence of small fractures.[12] Fractures of the orbit change the architecture of the posterior segment from conical to round because of enlargements. The posterior part of

the medial orbital wall together with the lateral orbital wall is the main support for a correct anterior projection of the globe. Hence, defects in this region are the main source of enophthalmos. According to Clauser and colleagues,[13] defects anterior to the equator of the globe do not influence the position of the globe and are usually not associated with the development of enophthalmos.

Surgical access

Depending on the type and location of the orbital defect, several surgical approaches have been described. Of these, the commonly used approaches are the transconjunctival and the subciliary approaches (**Fig. 24**). The choice between the transconjunctival and subciliary approaches is surgeon dependent. The preseptal transconjunctival approach takes more time for exposure of the orbital floor, and the postseptal transconjunctival approach has the burden of dealing with the herniated orbital fat. Studies showed a 20% incidence of ectropion associated with the subciliary approach versus 0% for the transconjunctival approach.[14,15] In contrast, there is a reported 22% incidence of epiphora in the transconjunctival approach compared with 13% in the subciliary approach.[14] Direct access is achieved through a laceration that is present overlying the fractures (**Figs. 25** and **26**).

Selection of reconstruction material

Many materials have been used for orbital reconstruction: autogenous bone, titanium mesh, silicone sheets, Gore-Tex (W.L. Gore and Associates, Inc, Elkton, MD), polypropylene, porous polyethylene, cartilage, lyophilized pericardium, polydioxanone, and resorbable mesh (poly L-lactic acid/polyglycolic acid copolymer).[15–17] There are 4 important variables that should be taken into account before the selection of a reconstruction material: (1) the size of the orbital floor defect,

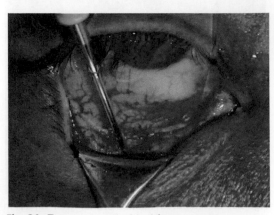

Fig. 24. Transconjunctival incision.

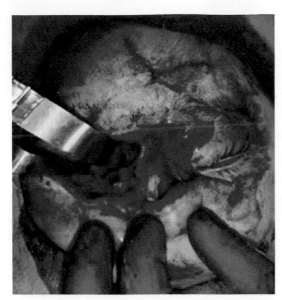

Fig. 25. Direct access to the medial orbital wall through the existing laceration in the same patient in **Fig. 20**.

(2) the mechanical properties of the implant material, (3) the thickness of the reconstruction material, and (4) the pressure load of the orbital content on the reconstruction material.[16] However, without proper guidelines, the onus is on the surgeon to choose an appropriate implant or graft material for the reconstruction of the orbit. Often the surgeon's experience and comfort plays a major role in determining the use of a particular reconstruction material.

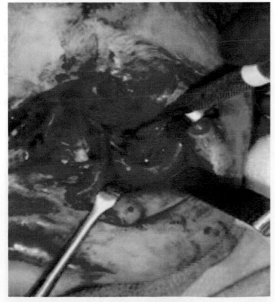

Fig. 26. Access to the lateral orbital wall through the laceration.

Autologous bone graft has been a mainstay of the treatment of repairing orbital defects. Because of the dense nature, the calvarium is perhaps the most recommended bone graft in the reconstruction of the orbit. Cranial bone graft offers several advantages. The scar is well hidden in the hair-bearing scalp, and the skull offers a large harvest site for grafts of varying geometric proportions. When compared with the ilium or the rib, cranial bone is one of the most dimensionally stable graft materials. The cranial bone graft can be shaped in such a way that the concave prominence can be placed into the orbital wall defect. This placement allows more accurate placement of the bone graft and provides more stability, thus resisting any shifting or soft tissue entrapment. The orientation of the implanted bone graft plays a part in the viability of cranial bone graft. The best result is achieved when the cancellous portion is placed in contact with the bone and the cortical portion with soft tissue.

A big disadvantage, however, is the limited malleability of the calvarial bone, which makes restoration of the correct anatomic situation of the orbit more difficult. When performing an acute or delayed enophthalmos correction, it is difficult to estimate the exact graft volume needed intraoperatively because of the swelling of the eyelids and intraorbital soft tissue. Precise thickness of the cranial bone is difficult to achieve, leading to volumetric asymmetry compared with the opposite side. One study showed that the incidence of orbital dystopia and postoperative enophthalmos was higher in cases reconstructed with bone grafts. The globe retracts with an increase in orbital volume. If the surgeon relies on autogenous bone grafts to recover orbital volume, it could lead to imprecise reconstruction and subsequently lead to enophthalmos.[17,18] Another drawback is donor site morbidity. If access to the skull is not necessary, the surgeon must critically evaluate the risk of a second surgical site, increased operative time, and surgical trauma. Postoperative evaluation of the donor site has revealed diminished strength up to 50% in the area of calvarial bone graft harvest. At present, technological advances have afforded new materials for orbital reconstruction. This comparison of modern materials suggests that cranial bone graft may no longer be the gold standard for orbital floor reconstruction.

In cases of a greatly expanded orbit when both the floor and the medial wall have been fractured or when there is no stable anatomy, titanium implant may be a good choice. Titanium mesh may be molded into any shape, is easy to fixate, and is visible on postoperative computed tomography scans. Although titanium has excellent biocompatibility, it has the potential to cause scarring around the soft tissue. Porous polyethylene is another implant that has been designed to allow for vascular ingrowth and has been put forward as a material resistant to infection (**Fig. 27**). Porous polyethylene with titanium mesh was developed to combine the advantageous properties of both materials. Other orbital implants, like silastic implants (Dow Corning, Midland, MI, USA) or supramid, can be used (**Fig. 28**). However, these are indicated only for smaller defects. The implants should be fixed to the orbital skeleton to prevent migration inferiorly and posteriorly into the maxillary sinus (**Fig. 29**). Recent technological advances have presented new reconstructive materials for the treatment of moderate and large orbital defects. In light of these advances, the role for autogenous bone grafting particularly with a separate donor site becomes questionable. Recent biomaterial advancements also suggest that bone grafts may no longer be the gold standard for orbital floor reconstruction.

Orbital floor defects
small and medium defects anterior to the equator of the globe are reconstructed with silicone sheets, resorbable sheets, porous polyethylene, and titanium mesh. Moderate to large defects are reconstructed with titanium mesh and autogenous bone. In large defects involving the posterior part of the orbit, it may be difficult to locate a stable posterior edge. In such cases, a lateral canthotomy can be performed to obtain superior access to the floor. This technique allows for better access for repositioning the herniated orbital contents and

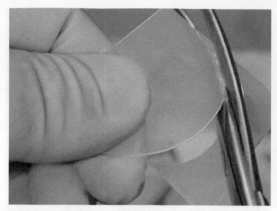

Fig. 28. Supramid implant.

precise placement of the implant material. Enophthalmos after a blowout fracture is caused by an increase in orbital volume rather than fat atrophy or fibrosis.[19] To avoid restriction of the inferior rectus muscle, attention has to be paid to the height of the posterior edge of the graft. With the fear of potential injury to the optic nerve, surgeons frequently do not perform adequate dissection to locate the posterior edge. This practice accounts for the placement of the graft/implant into the maxillary sinus rather than inclined upward along the orbital floor. However, one should remember that the optic canal is about 45 mm from the rim in a superior-medial direction. Defects posterior to the equator of the globe are responsible for most posttreatment enophthalmic defects. Hence, such defects should be managed aggressively and accurately. In the case of enophthalmos treatment, the bone graft should be placed behind the transverse axis of the globe. This placement allows for appropriate forward repositioning of the globe. A slight overcorrection is recommended to account for the potential intraoperative swelling of the soft tissue.

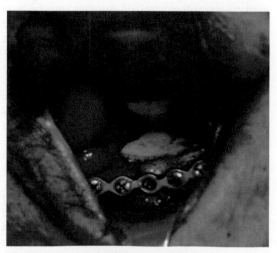

Fig. 27. Porous polyethylene implant on the floor of the orbit.

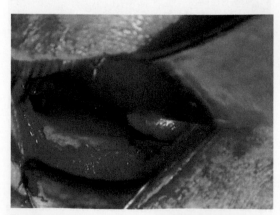

Fig. 29. Supramid implant in position in the orbit.

Medial wall defects

Medial wall reconstruction is extremely important, particularly in the face of an orbital blowout fracture. Defects in the medial orbital wall are often overlooked. Isolated blowout fractures at this site cause an increased orbital volume posterior to the globe axis as well as the enophthalmos. Higher complications are usually associated with complex orbital fractures and when the medial wall is unaccounted for.[20] In case of severe comminution, reconstruction of the medial orbital wall and medial orbital rim is necessary and bone grafting to restore continuity of the medial orbital wall is required (**Fig. 30**). Reconstruction of the medial orbital wall may precede reconstruction of the medial orbital rim when the medial wall disruption is extensive. In general, bone grafts should be stabilized to the bone to prevent movements. Grafts placed far posteriorly may be difficult to stabilize because of access. However, long pieces of bone used to reconstruct the medial orbital wall will extend to just behind the medial orbital rim and can be stabilized to the rim using lag screws, small bone plates, or wires. In rare instances, entrapment of the medial rectus muscle causes restricted ocular motility and retraction of the globe.

Orbital roof defects

Orbital roof fractures have an incidence of 3% to 9% of all facial fractures. Extensive upper face trauma sometimes leads to comminuted fractures of the orbital roof and the frontal sinus. In such cases, the loss of the posterior wall results in direct communication between the brain and the orbit and can lead to a pulsatile globe. In such cases, the orbital roof should always be reconstructed. There is no need to correct small fractures of the orbital roof if the posterior wall of the frontal sinus is intact. However, large roof defects should always be reconstructed either with cranial bone that is harvested through the coronal access or with titanium mesh and screws. These systems offer a near-ideal modality for orbital roof reconstruction. An upper eyelid incision has the benefit of not exposing patients to an intracranial procedure. In rare cases, intracranial access is indicated. After neurologic repair, the displaced orbital roof bone fragments should be removed and optic nerve decompression performed if a bone fragment is compressing the optic nerve. Failure to reconstruct large orbital roof defects can lead to herniation of the cranial contents, orbital encephalocele, impingement on the globe leading to vision loss, enophthalmos, and motility disorders.[21]

Lateral wall

In managing zygoma fractures, the lateral orbital wall must be exposed and the sphenozygomatic suture must be aligned (**Fig. 31**). This step is perhaps the most critical step in the treatment of extensive orbital complex deformities. A small misalignment in this region could lead to significant hypoglobus and enophthalmos. Studies have shown that a 1-cm^3 increase in orbital volume produces 0.8 mm of enophthalmos.[19] Malrotation of the lateral wall resulting from poor reduction of a zygomatic fracture is frequently observed and is a leading cause of posttraumatic enophthalmos.

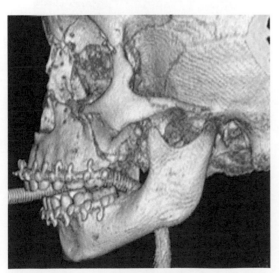

Fig. 30. Medial orbital wall repaired with a resorbable mesh.

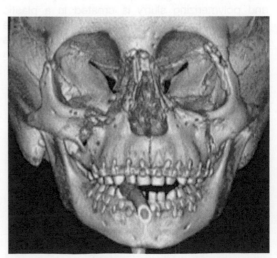

Fig. 31. Complex repair of the bilateral orbits involving lateral wall.

Late Orbital Volume Replacement

In some cases of late orbital reconstruction, cranioplast is a good choice for orbital volume augmentation.[22] Cranioplast is a methyl-methacrylate polymer that is mixed in the operating room and can be inserted into the orbit in a semi-liquid form. The polymer will quickly polymerize and form a thick permanent orbital floor implant that effectively elevates the orbital contents. The cranioplast orbital floor implant is especially useful in the anophthalmic socket because visual compromise and diplopia are not a problem. Orbital trauma with the loss of the eyeball is often extensive. With the initial attention placed on saving the eyeball, the repair of orbital fractures may be delayed. With the loss of the eyeball and especially if the orbit is expanded because of fractures, this is a good option for reconstruction. Cranioplast molds to the contours of the orbit and provides the ability to move the orbital contents superiorly and anteriorly. Augmenting the orbital volume with cranioplast can improve the appearance of anophthalmic enophthalmos. Cranioplast can also be used judiciously in patients with functioning globes.

Orbital volume augmentation with cranioplast begins with exposure of the orbital floor (**Fig. 32**). Either a transconjunctival or an infraciliary approach can be used. In patients with a shortage of conjunctiva and a contracted socket, the infraciliary approach is preferred. Exposure of the orbital floor is followed by exposure of the medial and lateral walls of the orbit. A potential space is created for the implant. A well-ventilated room is needed because the polymerization process releases annoying fumes. The cranioplast is prepared by mixing the liquid and the dry material, and polymerizing slurry is created in a plastic container (**Fig. 33**). After about 5 minutes, the material will begin to harden. At this stage, it is introduced into the orbit (**Fig. 34**). Cranioplast in

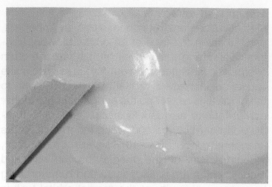

Fig. 33. Polymerization.

a semiliquid form can be digitally molded with light pressure to conform to the orbital bones in the previously created potential space. Once the hardening begins, the material will remain malleable for about 5 minutes. After molding the implant to fit the potential space of the orbit, all excess material is removed. The anterior lip of the implant should be behind the inferior orbital rim. The implant does not need to be sutured into the orbit because the shape of the final implant is a perfect reflection of the surrounding orbital bones and is held in place by its molded fit with the surrounding orbital bones (**Fig. 35**). With the cranioplast in good position in the floor of the orbit, the conjunctiva is closed and a conformer is placed (**Fig. 36**). The procedure provides excellent orbital volume augmentation. The main complication with cranioplast orbital implants is extrusion. The loss of an

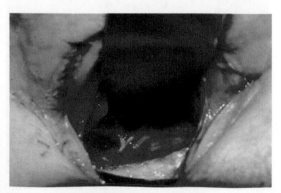

Fig. 32. Exposure of the orbital floor.

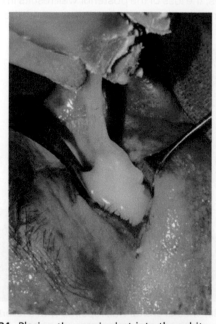

Fig. 34. Placing the cranioplast into the orbit.

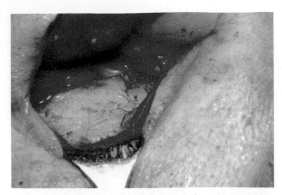

Fig. 35. Cranioplast orbital floor implant in position.

implant is very uncommon. The motility of the orbit is preserved, and infraorbital numbness caused by the procedure has not been noted.

Anophthalmos

The loss of an eyeball is a tragic event. The loss of an eyeball is also a reconstructive challenge. There are many indications for the removal of an eyeball. In patients with a history of trauma, often enucleation or the complete removal of the eyeball is the procedure of choice. Sympathetic ophthalmia is a rare immunologically mediated condition whereby the uninjured eyeball my loose vision because of uveitis. Many ophthalmologists prefer to enucleate blind injured eyeballs within a few weeks or months to prevent the development of sympathetic ophthalmia. During enucleation, the globe is disconnected from the extraocular muscles and the optic nerve is cut. Enucleation also injures the suspensory ligament of the orbit and may lead to dampened movement of the prosthetic eye and a superior sulcus deformity.[23] Patients with a distant history of trauma or blind painful eyeballs may be candidates for evisceration. Evisceration is the removal of the intraocular

contents along with the cornea. With this technique, the sclera and the extraocular muscles are left intact. The suspensory ligaments of the orbit are preserved. The long-term stability and appearance of the anophthalmic socket is better following an evisceration than an enucleation.

Orbital volume replacement is critical to maintain an acceptable appearance following the loss of an eyeball. An intact eyeball that is 24 mm in length contains 7.3 cm^3 of volume. When an eyeball is removed, an orbital implant is placed that may be only 16 to 18 mm in length (**Fig. 37**).[24] A prosthetic eye can replace about 3 cm^3 of volume. An orbital implant that is less than 20 mm (4.2 cm^3) in length will produce an orbital volume deficit. An orbital volume deficit will lead to a sunken appearance of the anophthalmic socket. In many cases, an ocularist will try to overcome the volume deficiency with increasingly larger prosthetic eyes. A larger and heavier prosthetic eye will put pressure on the lower eyelid and lead to ectropion. The difference between the size of the eyeball and the size of the orbital implant is a major contributor to orbital volume loss with the removal of the eyeball. In general, the largest implant that the orbit can accommodate is placed after the removal of the eyeball.

Enucleation

Enucleation is indicated when an intraocular tumor is present. Peritomy is the first step in enucleation (**Fig. 38**). Peritomy is performed releasing the conjunctiva and the Tenon capsule from the globe. Enucleation requires the extraocular muscle to be disarticulated from the globe. There are 6 extraocular muscles and each must be identified and cut. A Jameson muscle hook is used to elevate the extraocular muscle away from the globe. The muscle is cut with a needle tip cautery (**Fig. 39**). Scissors are introduced behind the eyeball, and the optic nerve is palpated. With the scissors spread

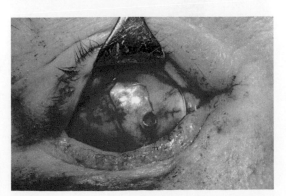

Fig. 36. Final appearance of socket with conformer in place.

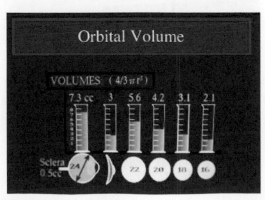

Fig. 37. Orbital volume.

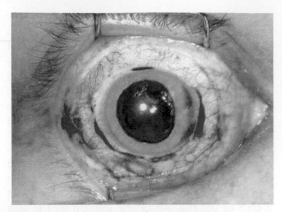

Fig. 38. Peritomy in an ocular melanoma.

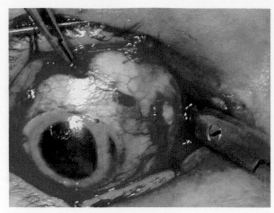

Fig. 40. Cutting the optic nerve.

slightly, the optic nerve is enveloped and cut behind the posterior sclera (**Fig. 40**). Care is taken not to damage the posterior eyeball. Once the optic nerve is cut, all connections between the eyeball and the orbit are lysed and the globe can be removed. Placing a 20- or 22-mm implant deep in the muscle cone will help restore the orbital volume after enucleation (**Fig. 41**).[25] Orbital implants are generally biocompatible. The ability for blood vessels to enter the orbital implant helps provide stability and reduces the risk of extrusion.[26] A layered closure with Vicryl sutures over the implant closes the anterior and posterior Tenon capsule. The conjunctiva is closed with a running 6–0 plain gut suture (**Fig. 42**). Over the closed conjunctiva, a plastic conformer is place between the eyelids. A firm pressure patch is left in place for 4 or 5 days.

Evisceration

An evisceration removes the intraocular contents of the eyeball and preserves the sclera and the extraocular muscles attached to the sclera. A scalpel is used to create a sclerectomy about 4 mm behind the limbus. A conjunctival peritomy has already been performed (**Fig. 43**). An evisceration spoon removes the intraocular contents (**Fig. 44**). The uvea is darkly pigmented and has generous blood supply. A scalpel is used to make a vertical incision in the posterior sclera (**Fig. 45**). Behind the posterior sclera is the intraconal space. Traditionally, an implant was placed inside the scleral shell; at best, a 16-mm implant could be placed. With this technique of evisceration, larger implants can be placed.[27] A 20-mm implant is visible behind the posterior sclera (**Fig. 46**). Forceps are gasping the edges of the posterior sclera. The vertical incision in the posterior sclera is closed vertically, and the anterior sclera is closed horizontally. The biocompatible implant will remain behind the posterior sclera and in the intraconal space. After closing the sclera and the conjunctiva, a conformer is placed behind the eyelids (**Fig. 47**). The conformer should remain in place until a prosthetic eye is made about 6 weeks after surgery. The conformer will help maintain the shape of the superior and inferior fornix.

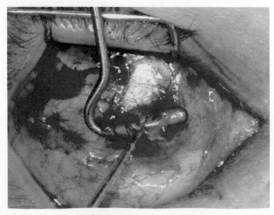

Fig. 39. Cutting the extraocular muscles.

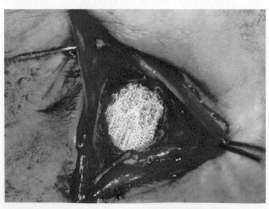

Fig. 41. Orbital implant in position in the muscle cone.

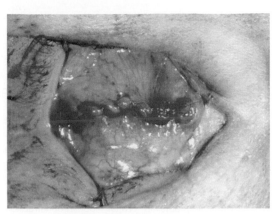

Fig. 42. Conjunctival closure.

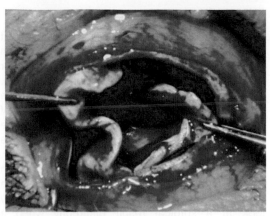

Fig. 45. Opening the posterior sclera.

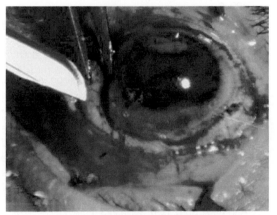

Fig. 43. Opening the sclera.

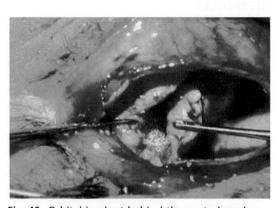

Fig. 46. Orbital implant behind the posterior sclera.

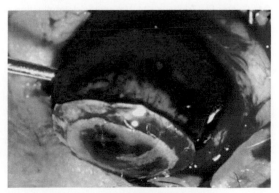

Fig. 44. Removing the intraocular contents.

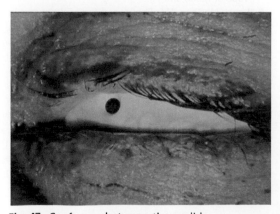

Fig. 47. Conformer between the eyelids.

SUMMARY

The repair and restoration of the eyelids and orbit can be a medical and surgical challenge. With advances in technology and equipment, our surgical techniques are constantly improving. The most important resource that any of us have is our teachers, colleagues, and mentors. All of the techniques that are described in this article are the authors' versions of material that has been described elsewhere and more eloquently. We teach and learn. We may look at a problem from a different perspective after a query from a medical student or a resident surgeon. We may look at a surgical result differently when a colleague shares his or her ideas and techniques with us. Collaboration is the way to improve our patient care. No one has a monopoly on knowledge. Together we can do better for our patients.

REFERENCES

1. Wojono TH. Lid splitting with lash resection for cicatricial entropion. Ophthal Plast Reconstr Surg 1992; 8:287–9.
2. Sullivan JH. The use of cryotherapy for trichiasis. Trans Am Acad Ophthalmol Otolaryngol 1977;83:708.
3. Siegel RJ. Palatal grafts for eyelid reconstruction. Plast Reconstr Surg 1985;76(3):411–4.
4. Bartley GB, Kay PP. Posterior lamellar eyelid reconstruction with a hard palate mucosal graft. Am J Ophthalmol 1989;107(6):609–12.
5. Cohen MS, Shorr N. Eyelid reconstruction with hard palate mucosa grafts. Ophthal Plast Reconstr Surg 1992;8(3):183–95.
6. Hawes MJ, Segrest DR. Effectiveness of bicanalicular silicone intubation in the repair of canalicular lacerations. Ophthal Plast Reconstr Surg 1985;1(3): 185–90.
7. Neuhaus RW. Silicone intubation of traumatic canalicular lacerations. Ophthal Plast Reconstr Surg 1989;5(4):256–60.
8. Long JA, Tann TM. Eyelid and lacrimal trauma. In: Kuhn F, Pieramici DJ, editors. Ocular trauma. Chapter 35. New York: Thieme; 2002. p. 373–80.
9. Burnstine MA. Clinical recommendations for repair of isolated orbital floor fractures: an evidence-based analysis. Ophthalmology 2002;109:1207–10.
10. Hawes MJ, Dortzbach RK. Surgery on orbital floor fractures. Influence of time of repair and fracture size. Ophthalmology 1983;90:1066–70.
11. Jordan DR, Allen LH, White J, et al. Intervention within days for some orbital floor fractures: the white-eyed blowout. Ophthal Plast Reconstr Surg 1998;14:379.
12. Antonyshyn OM. Rigid fixation of the orbital fractures. In: Yaremchuk MJ, Gruss J, Manson PN, editors. Rigid fixation of the craniomaxillofacial skeleton cap 23. Boston: Butterworth-Heinemann; 1992. p. 302–16.
13. Clauser L, Galie' M, Pagliaro F, et al. Posttraumatic enophthalmos: etiology, principles of reconstruction, and correction. J Craniofac Surg 2008;19(2):351–9.
14. Goldberg RA, Lessner A, Shorr N, et al. The transconjunctival approach to the orbital floor and orbital fat: a prospective study. Ophthal Plast Reconstr Surg 1990;6(4):241–6.
15. Villarreal PM, Monje F, Morillo AJ, et al. Porous polyethylene implants in orbital floor reconstruction. Plast Reconstr Surg 2002;109:877–85 [discussion: 886–7].
16. Kirby EJ, Turner BJ, Davenport DL, et al. Orbital floor fractures outcomes of reconstruction. Ann Plast Surg 2011;66:508–12.
17. Goldberg RA, Garbutt M, Shorr N. Oculoplastic uses of cranial bone grafts. Ophthalmic Surg 1993;24: 190–6.
18. Ramieri G, Spada MC, Bianchi SD, et al. Dimensions and volumes of the orbit and orbital fat in posttraumatic enophthalmos. Dentomaxillofac Radiol 2000; 29(5):302–11.
19. Whitehouse RW, Battebury M, Jackson A, et al. Prediction of enophthalmos by computed tomography after 'blow out' orbital fracture. Br J Ophthalmol 1994;78:618.
20. Ellis E. Sequencing treatment for naso-orbito-ethmoid fractures. J Oral Maxillofac Surg 1993;51: 543–58.
21. Martello JY, Vasconez HC. Supraorbital roof fractures: a formidable entity with which to contend. Ann Plast Surg 1997;38(3):223–7.
22. Neuhaus RW, Shorr N. The use of room temperature vulcanizing silicone in anophthalmic enophthalmos. Am J Ophthalmol 1982;94(3):408–11.
23. Dresner SC, Codere F, Corriveau C. Orbital volume augmentation with adjustable prefabricated methylmethacrylate subperiosteal implants. Ophthalmic Surg 1991;22:53.
24. Custer PL, Trinkaus KM. Volumetric determination of enucleation implant size. Am J Ophthalmol 1999; 128:489–94.
25. Thaller VT. Enucleation volume measurement. Ophthal Plast Reconstr Surg 1997;13(1):18–20.
26. Long JA, Tann TM, Bearden WH, et al. Enucleation: is wrapping the implant necessary for optimal motility? Ophthal Plast Reconstr Surg 2003;19: 194–7.
27. Long JA, Tann TM, Girkin CA. Evisceration: a new technique of trans-scleral implant placement. Ophthal Plast Reconstr Surg 2000;16:322–5.

Zygoma Reconstruction

Michael R. Markiewicz, DDS, MPH, MD[a],
Savannah Gelesko, DDS[a], R. Bryan Bell, DDS, MD[b,c,d],*

KEYWORDS

- Facial bones • Orbit • Zygoma • Maxillofacial surgery • Neuronavigation • Injuries
- Zygomaticomaxillary complex

KEY POINTS

- The most common error in reconstruction of acquired deformities of the zygoma is inadequate restoration of malar projection.
- Failure to adequately flatten the zygomatic arch and achieve optimal rotation of the zygomaticomaxillary complex results in flattening of the malar eminence and widening of the ipsilateral face.
- Modern digital technology may be used to optimize treatment outcomes in patients with complex deformities.
- Intraoperative navigation is used to assess malar projection and orbital implant position, and stereolithographic models are used to fit bone grafts or flaps at the time of inset.
- Modern mobile computed tomography scanners are helpful to evaluate the accuracy of the reconstruction and transfer the virtual plan into reality.

INTRODUCTION

The zygoma is a quadrangular structure composed of 4 articulations, commonly referred to as the zygomaticomaxillary (ZM), frontozygomatic (FZ), zygomaticotemporal (ZT), and the sphenozygomatic (SZ) sutures. Because the SZ is within the orbit, and the ZM and FZ articulations represent vertical buttresses of the face, accurate restoration of zygomatic anatomy is key to reestablishing facial projection, facial width, and orbital volume.[1] Knight and North[2] pointed out that the term zygoma fracture is misleading because there is usually no fracture of the zygoma bone, rather there are fractures of its neighboring sutures and their bones: the maxilla, the temporal bone, the sphenoid, and the frontal bone. Gruss and colleagues[3] recognized the importance of the zygoma in restoring

facial projection, symmetry, and orbital volume. Posterior-lateral displacement of the zygoma results in ipsilateral facial widening and facial flattening. Normal anatomic contour and position of the malar eminence and zygomatic body is critical to achieving favorable results in reconstruction of the midface, regardless of cause.

APPLIED SURGICAL ANATOMY
Soft Tissue

Soft tissues of the face depend on the underlying bony architecture for functional support and appearance. Muscular attachments to the zygoma include (1) the masseter muscle, which attaches to the temporal surface of the zygomatic arch and zygomatic tuberosity, and has an inferior vector from its origin; (2) the temporalis muscle and

Funding Support: None.
Financial Disclosures: The authors have no financial disclosures to declare.
[a] Department of Oral and Maxillofacial Surgery, Oregon Health and Science University, SDOMS, 611 Southwest Campus Drive, Portland, OR 97239, USA; [b] Oral, Head and Neck Cancer Program, Providence Cancer Center, Oregon Health and Science University, 4805 NE Glisan Street, Suite 6N50, Portland, OR 97213, USA; [c] Trauma Service, Legacy Emanuel Medical Center, Oregon Health and Science University, 2801 N Gantenbein Avenue, Portland, OR 97227, USA; [d] Department of Oral and Maxillofacial Surgery, Legacy Emanuel Medical Center, Oregon Health and Science University, Portland, OR, USA
* Corresponding author. 1849 Northwest Kearney, Suite 300, Portland, OR 97209.
E-mail address: bellb@hnsa1.com

Oral Maxillofacial Surg Clin N Am 25 (2013) 167–201
http://dx.doi.org/10.1016/j.coms.2013.02.005
1042-3699/13/$ – see front matter

temporalis fascia, which originate at the frontal process of the zygoma, passing beneath the arch and attaching to the coronoid process of the mandible; (3) the zygomaticus major and minor muscles, which insert to support the oral commissures; and (4) the zygomatic head of the levator labii superioris, which originates just above the infraorbital foramen. The temporalis fascia resists inferior displacement of the downward pull of the masseter muscles in zygoma fractures. Tendinous attachments to the zygoma include the medial and lateral canthal tendons, and the Lockwood suspensory ligament. Horizontal globe position is maintained by the Lockwood suspensory ligament, which attaches laterally to the Whitnall tubercle 1 cm below the FZ on the medial aspect of the frontal process of the zygoma, and medially to the posterior aspect of the lacrimal bone (**Fig. 1**). The medial canthal tendon maintains vertical globe position, and is divided into 3 limbs: anterior, superior, and posterior. The anterior limb attaches to the anterior lacrimal crest and nasal bone. The posterior limb attaches to the posterior lacrimal crest and lamina papyracea. Accurate repositioning of the posterior attachment of the medial canthal tendon is critical to achieving ideal position during canthopexy. Accurate resuspension of the lateral canthus similarly depends on the position of the lateral canthal tendon at its attachment to the Whitnall tubercle. Inferior displacement of the lateral canthal tendon in zygoma fractures often results in an antimongoloid (downward) cant of the lateral canthus and care must be taken to reduce both components if the canthal attachments are disrupted.

Sensory nerves that travel through the zygoma originate from the second division of the trigeminal

nerve and include the zygomatic nerve, which enters the orbit at the inferior orbital fissure and divides into its terminal branches; the zygomaticofacial nerve, which exits the orbit onto the face although the zygomaticofacial foramen; and the ZT nerve, which enters the temporal fossa through the ZT foramen on the deep surface of the zygoma. The zygomaticofacial and ZT nerves supply sensation to the skin overlying the malar prominence and the anterior temple area, respectively. The latter area is a focus of pain postoperatively after zygomatic trauma and reconstruction. Although the infraorbital foramen and nerve are often involved in zygoma fractures, they are located within the maxilla. The infraorbital nerve travels through the infraorbital groove and exits through the infraorbital foramen, 10 mm inferior to the rim and parallel to the lateral surface of the cornea in forward gaze. Before exiting the infraorbital foramen, its branches give sensation to the maxillary teeth, ipsilateral nose, upper lip, and lower eyelid. All these branches may be affected by zygoma fractures.

Hard Tissue

The facial skeleton is composed of low stress-bearing curved areas composed of thin bones that surround pneumatic cavities and sinuses positioned between high stress-bearing buttresses. The low stress-bearing thinner bony walls are more likely to show instability and comminution following fracture. Buttresses are architectural structures built against or projecting from a wall that serve to reinforce and support that wall. As in architecture, the buttresses of the face may support bony walls from the side, from directly beneath, or from the top (**Fig. 2**). Trusses are architectural units built of 1 or more triangular units that resist tensile, compressive, and shear loading forces. The nodes of the trusses are where all legs of the triangles connect. These are areas where external forces and reactions to these forces are applied. The structural pillars of the face act as an interconnecting network serving as both buttresses and trusses that connect the facial bones to the cranial base.[4] Bones adjacent to these pillars form the walls of cavities, including paranasal sinuses, and the orbits.[5] These bones are thin because of the minimal force placed on them, and provide support and portioning of soft tissues.

The buttresses of the facial skeleton represent areas of thicker bone that transmit chewing forces to the supporting regions of the skull. The vertical structural pillars of the midface as described by Sicher and Tandler[6] include vertical buttresses of the midface: the nasomaxillary (continues as

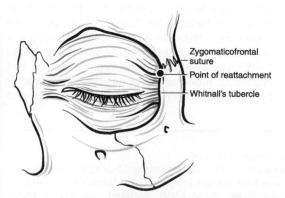

Zygomaticofrontal suture

Point of reattachment

Whitnall's tubercle

Fig. 1. Lockwood suspensory ligament attaches laterally to Whitnall tubercle, which is located on the zygoma approximately 1 cm below the FZ suture. (*From* Manson PN. Fractures of the zygoma. In: Booth PW, Schendel SA, Hausamen JE, editors. Maxillofacial surgery. 2nd edition. St Louis: Churchill Livingstone; 2006; with permission.)

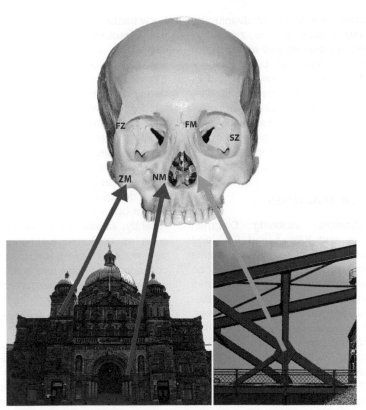

Fig. 2. Vertical facial support is provided by a series of buttresses including the zygomaticomaxillary (ZM) buttress, which is contiguous with the frontozygomatic (FZ) buttress and the nasomaxillary (NM) buttress, which is connected to the frontomaxillary (FM) buttress. These vertical pillars have been compared with those buttresses that provide support to large buildings (*bottom left*: Parliament Building, Victoria, British Columbia, Canada). These vertical pillars are stronger than surrounding areas, and bear tensile and compressive forces of multiple connecting limbs, which in engineering are known as trusses. The sphenozygomatic (SZ) (rarely fixated) and pterygomaxillary (not pictured and never accessed for fixation) sutures can be thought of as representing trusses, similar to those seen in bridges (*bottom right*: Broadway Bridge, Portland, OR). In addition, horizontal facial support is provided by the zygomatic arch and zygomaticotemporal (ZT) suture, both serving as the horizontal buttress in zygomatic reconstruction.

the nasofrontal) buttress medially, the ZM laterally (continues as FZ buttress), and the pterygomaxillary buttresses posteriorly. The infraorbital rim is often considered the fifth suture involved in zygoma reconstruction, and, along with the zygomatic arch and ZT suture, represents the horizontal facial buttress component in reconstructing the zygoma. The nasomaxillary and ZM make up the anterior buttresses and are the most accessible for stabilization (see **Fig. 2**; **Fig. 3**). No fixation of the pterygomaxillary buttress is needed because 4 anterior buttresses of the maxilla alone maintain maxillary position. The nasomaxillary buttress, which extends from the maxillary canine and the anterior maxillary alveolus along the piriform aperture, also extends along the medial orbit through the lacrimal crest and nasal process of the maxilla to the superior orbital rim and frontal region. The zygomatic

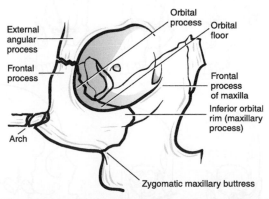

Fig. 3. Zygomatic articulations include the frontal process, the maxillary process, and the orbital process. (*From* Manson PN. Fractures of the zygoma. In: Booth PW, Schendel SA, Hausamen JE, editors. Maxillofacial surgery. 2nd edition. St Louis: Churchill Livingstone; 2006; with permission.)

buttress extends from the maxillary alveolus by the premolars and molars to the zygomatic process of the frontal bone, as well as the zygomatic process of the temporal bone (anterior portion of condylar fossa) and the sphenoid of the inferolateral orbital wall. The pterygomaxillary buttress is made up of 2 components: (1) the pterygoid component relates the maxillary alveolus to the cranial base via the pyramidal process of the palatal bone, and (2) the maxillary process relates to the cranial base via the sphenoid bone.

CLASSIFICATION OF FRACTURES

Numerous investigators, including Dingman and Native,[7] Rowe and Killey,[8] and Fujii and colleagues,[9] have described classification systems for fractures of the zygoma that are based on anatomic displacement and stability of the fractures following treatment. Fractures that are laterally displaced and comminuted are less stable than those that are medially displaced and noncomminuted (**Fig. 4**).[10–12] Perhaps the most popular classification system is that by Knight and North[2] in which the investigators studied the pattern of malar fractures within an 8-year period. The classification system was based on the anatomy of the fracture on the occipitomental radiograph (the Water view) and comprised 7 groups including (1) fractures with no displacement, (2) isolated zygomatic arch fractures, (3) unrotated depressed zygomatic

body fractures, (4) depressed and medially rotated body fractures, (5) depressed and laterally rotated body fractures, and (6), complex fractures (increased comminution). In their study, type IV fractures were associated with the highest incidence of diplopia (medial rotation), whereas isolated zygomatic arch fractures were associated with the highest incidence of trismus. However, most of these historical classification schemes were devised before the computed tomography (CT) scan era and before the development of rigid internal fixation. As a result, some of these traditional descriptors have lost relevance in the modern age of open reduction and internal fixation. More recently, newer classifications based on factors such as anatomic location, displacement, and comminution have been described by Zingg and colleagues,[27] Donat and colleagues,[13] Bächli and colleagues,[14] and Ozyazgan and colleagues.[15,16]

CRITICAL CONCEPTS OF ZYGOMATIC TRAUMA

Zygoma fractures usually occur from direct impacts and are most common at an area of prominence such as the malar eminence. This typically causes an in-bending at the area of contact and out-bending at an area of weakness away from the impact site, such as the ZM and FZ sutures as well as the zygomatic arch. The initial fracture is usually to the posterior maxillary sinus wall.

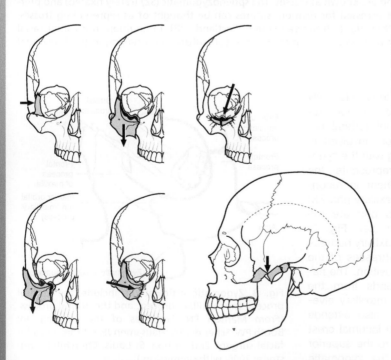

Fig. 4. Most classification schemes, such as this one by Rowe and Killey, are characterized by the degree of displacement and/or comminution, whether or not the fracture is medially or laterally displaced, fractures of the zygomatic arch or infraorbital rim in isolation, and the energy imparted at the time of injury (high or low velocity; ie, degree of comminution). (*From* Manson PN. Fractures of the zygoma. In: Booth PW, Schendel SA, Hausamen JE, editors. Maxillofacial surgery. 2nd edition. St Louis: Churchill Livingstone; 2006; with permission.)

Although most zygoma fractures have an orbital floor component, those that are most severe need decompression of the infraorbital fissure and foramen.

Isolated Zygomatic Arch Fractures

Nondisplaced or minimally displaced fractures of the zygomatic arch often require no treatment. The exception is in the thin-skinned, often older patient in whom minimal deformity is esthetically apparent. Two weeks should be given for resolution of swelling for final evaluation of esthetic deformity. Isolated zygomatic arch fractures often involve the ZT suture and posterior zygomatic arch. For noncomminuted zygomatic arch fractures, a straight rigid instrument such as a Dingman elevator can be used to run the arch. After reduction via techniques that are discussed later, the arch usually maintains its integrity. Only in the most severe, high-energy comminuted fracture does the ZT need to be exposed reduced and plated. In these injuries, the integrity of the periosteum is violated and therefore will not remain stable without fixation.

ZM Complex Fractures

Low-energy, nondisplaced ZM complex fractures

Low-energy fractures of the zygoma usually do not require repair. However, patients should always be followed for signs of progressive displacement, change in vision, extraocular dysfunction, and vertical or horizontal dystopia and enophthalmos. Any change in appearance should be noted.

Middle-energy, displaced, minimally comminuted fractures

Low-energy to middle-energy fractures are often displaced posteriorly, inferiorly, and medially. These fractures usually require open reduction and internal fixation. Ellis and Kittidumkerng[17] described an algorithm for middle-energy zygomatic fractures not requiring reconstruction of the orbit. In their study, Ellis and colleagues recommended the placement of a Carroll-Giard screw into the malar eminence transcutaneously. If reduction with the Carroll-Giard screw is unstable, open reduction and internal fixation of the ZM buttress should proceed. If still unstable, the FZ suture should be assessed and, if needed, reduced and fixated. Other investigators have recommended reduction of the infraorbital rim.

High-energy, complex comminuted fractures

High-energy fractures are commonly displaced posteriorly, inferiorly, and laterally. The force required to displace the zygoma 2.5 cm over a 1-second time period has been shown in a cadaver model to be a mean of 1826 N.[18,19] To permit this advanced lateral displacement, the zygomatic arch and its soft tissue attachments are usually disrupted. A variety of zygoma fracture combinations with other facial injuries may be seen with high-energy trauma.

Multiple approaches are required for repair when significant comminution of the anterior buttresses, zygomatic arch, and orbit is present, as in high-energy injuries. Particular attention should be paid to restoring orbital volume and facial projection. Posterior access (coronal flap) is often needed to access the zygomatic arch and possible associated fractures of the nasoorbitoethmoid complex, frontal sinus, nose, and superior orbits. Visualization of the orbital floor is often needed to assess the SZ suture and restore internal orbital volume and globe position.[19]

DIAGNOSIS
History and Physical

History
A clear chronologic history of events should be elicited from the patient. A timeline of pertinent events in the course of such changes in vision should be noted. The patient and witnesses should be queried for the mechanism, direction, vector, and force of the insulting blow to the face. Although insults to the front of the face usually result in posteriorly and inferiorly displaced zygoma fractures, blows to the side of the face may only result in fracture of the arch. A full secondary survey should be performed and associated injuries should be noted.

Signs
Before examining the patient, all blood and debris should be cleaned from the face and soft tissue lacerations should be examined carefully for extensions of bony fractures. However, physical examination findings are often masked by edema. Swelling is often significant enough to prevent passive eye opening. The surgeon should systematically examine and palpate the head and neck, performing full cranial nerve and ophthalmic examinations and viewing the patient superiorly, frontally, laterally, and inferiorly. Lacerations and ecchymoses should be noted.

The surgeon should begin by palpating the forehead, supraorbital rims, and FZ suture. Inferior displacement of the zygoma often results in an antimongoloid slant of the palpebral fissure and accentuation of the supratarsal fold. The inferior orbital rim may be palpated for a step deformity, which is often present medial to the fracture where the medial segment is generally superior to the lateral segment. All bony zygoma attachments and intraorbital surfaces should be palpated as well. From a bird's-eye view, malar depression from posterior displacement may be noted by placing index fingers on each malar eminence. The nasolabial fold may be more pronounced and there may be increased scleral show and ectropion on the fractured side caused by caudal ptosis of the facial soft tissues. Intraoral visualization and palpation may reveal edema, ecchymosis, and tenderness at the canine fossa indicating injury at the zygomatic buttress. The surgeon may be able to displace the zygoma in more severe fractures.

With the exception of isolated zygomatic arch fractures, subconjunctival and/or periorbital ecchymosis is almost always present caused by disruption of the orbital septum.[20] Zygoma fractures are often associated with painful or impeded maximum incisal opening, which results from edema within the muscles of mastication or tissue planes, and by medial depression of the zygomatic arch causing interference with the coronoid process. In more severe, laterally displaced zygomatic arches, mandibular opening is often not impeded. In severe posterior displacement of the zygoma, interference of the coronoid process with the malar eminence during the translation phase of opening may cause limitation in maximal incisal opening. If the origins of the zygomaticus muscles, or levator labii superioris, are disrupted, ptosis of the upper lip and commissure may be seen.

Eyelid position may be affected by displacement of the lateral canthal ligament when attached to a displaced zygoma fracture. The lateral canthal ligament attaches to the frontal process of the zygoma, therefore the eyelids move in the direction of the displaced canthal bearing frontal process. The Lockwood suspensory ligament and the lateral horn of levator, which are thickenings of the Tenon capsule, insert onto the Whitnall tubercle (see **Fig. 1**). The Lockwood inferior transverse suspensory ligament extends from the medial to lateral canthus. Inferior repositioning of this ligament combined with orbital floor expansion results in inferior orbital positioning. Posterior and inferior displacement of the zygoma may result in a variety of intraorbital soft tissue disruptions and may result in medial, lateral, or inferior displacement of the globe.[21–27]

A full ocular evaluation should be performed including visual acuity (with Snellen chart), the size of the pupils and their ability to accommodate to light symmetrically, extraocular movements, vertical and horizontal globe position, subconjunctival hemorrhage, blood in the anterior chamber of the eye (hyphema), and a fundoscopic examination. Epiphora may indicate damage to the lacrimal apparatus. Globe injury, significant extraocular muscle entrapment, afferent pupillary defects, or signs or symptoms of retinal injury should prompt an ophthalmologic consultation.

Symptoms

Patients may have a variety of complaints that include change in vision, restriction in mandibular opening, and paresthesia and anesthesia of the face. Most symptoms of zygoma fractures can be attributed to edema and hemorrhage.[28] Neurosensory complaints often include hypoesthesia or anesthesia along the distribution of the infraorbital nerve including the ipsilateral upper lip, maxillary teeth, nose, and eyelid. In addition, the patient may complain of a disturbance in sensation to the skin overlying the malar prominence and the anterior temple area respectively caused by injury of the zygomaticofacial and ZT nerves. In more severe injuries, contusion and weakness of the buccal branch of the facial nerve may be present.[29,30] Patients initially display exophthalmos caused by edema. This exophthalmos may persist because of medial impaction of the zygoma causing decreased orbital volumes or transition to enophthalmos caused by lateral displacement and/or associated blowout fractures causing increased orbital volumes.

The patient may complain of diplopia from extraocular muscle entrapment or contusion, or from entrapment of the musculofibrous ligament system.[31] Traumatic amaurosis may also be present in the case of orbital apex syndrome.

Radiographic Examination

Plain film radiographs

Plain film views such as the Caldwell, Waters, and submentovertex views were previously used to evaluate midfacial fractures in general, and fractures involving the zygoma in particular. They are now rarely used because CT images provide a more accurate representation of normal and abnormal anatomy.

Caldwell view This view is obtained by positioning the patient with the forehead against the film and the x-ray beam placed horizontally 13 mm below the occipital protuberance. The horizontal plane of the occiput is tilted downward 15° to 20°. This view is ideal for visualizing horizontal rotation of the zygoma, the infraorbital rim, the FZ suture, and the zygomatic buttress.

Waters (occipitomental) view The patient sits facing the radiographic base line with the head tilted at a 45° angle to the horizontal, with the chin resting on the cassette, and the x-ray beam centered horizontally over a 25-mm thick point above the occipital protuberance. It is the single best view for visualization of zygoma fractures and is especially useful for accessing the ZM and infraorbital rim as well as the petrous pyramids of the maxillary sinuses, the lateral orbits, and the infraorbital rims.

Submentovertex view This view, taken with the patient's back arched as much as possible so the skull base is parallel to the film and the x-ray beam is centered at midline between the angles of the mandible, is ideal for visualizing the zygomatic arches and symmetry of malar projection.

Orthopantogram Although useful in general evaluation for facial trauma, especially mandibular fractures, the panoramic radiograph is not particularly useful in zygoma fractures.

CT

CT is now the standard for the evaluation of zygoma, as well as all fractures of the craniomaxillofacial skeleton. Specific attention should be paid to commonly involved areas in zygoma fractures: the FZ, SZ, ZM, and ZT sutures; the zygomatic arches; and the infraorbital rims. Coronal views are preferable to evaluate the integrity of the orbital floor with or without associated tissue herniation into the maxillary sinus and possible extraocular muscle entrapment. Axial images are good for evaluating the malar projection and status of the zygomatic arch. Sagittal views are particularly helpful in evaluating the orbital floor and for

the accurate position of orbital implants in the postoperative setting.

PRIMARY MANAGEMENT OF ZYGOMA DEFORMITIES
Surgical Approaches

Surgical approaches to the zygoma are divided into anterior and posterior approaches.[16] Anterior approaches include those on the face to expose the zygomatic buttress, the FZ, and the infraorbital rim, with a posterior approach consisting of a coronal incision. In a study by Manson and colleagues,[32] abnormalities of the zygoma after repair were found in 48% of subjects. However, these deformities were minor. Most medially and posteriorly displaced zygoma fractures can be treated by an intraoral approach alone. Zygoma fractures with more severe medial arch dislocation and comminution were adequately managed by anterior approaches alone. When other facial fractures are present, or for fractures displaying lateral displacement, severe comminution, or severe dislocation of the zygomatic arch, management may take place with a combination of anterior and posterior approaches.

Keen (intraoral approach)

The Keen approach is an intraoral approach in which a mucosal incision is made from maxillary canine to first or second molar 3 to 5 mm above the mucogingival junction (**Fig. 5**A).[33] A full-thickness mucoperiosteal envelope flap is reflected around the pyriform rim and infraorbital nerve exposing the zygomatic buttress. An elevator

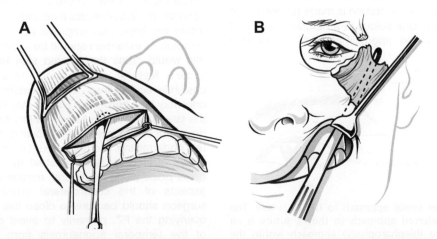

Fig. 5. Keen/transoral approach to the maxillary buttress. (*A*) Incision is made between the canine and first molar and a full-thickness mucoperiosteal flap is reflected. (*B*) Using a Dingman elevator, the zygoma is lifted in a bodily manner, anteriorly and laterally, while palpating the infraorbital rim for reduction. (*From* Manson PN. Fractures of the zygoma. In: Booth PW, Schendel SA, Hausamen JE, editors. Maxillofacial surgery. 2nd edition. St Louis: Churchill Livingstone; 2006; with permission.)

is then placed under the zygomatic arch and under the body of the zygoma being careful not to enter the orbit and violate the buccal fat pad. To reduce the fracture, the zygoma is lifted anteriorly and laterally while palpating the infraorbital rim (see **Fig. 5**B). A click is often heard as steady pressure is applied. An alternative intraoral approach involves mobilizing the zygoma by entering the maxillary sinus through a fracture site with an elevator placed beneath the body of the zygoma.

FZ buttress In any approach to the frontal process of the FZ there is partial stripping of the temporal aponeurosis attachment to the frontal process of the zygoma. The surgeon should strive to minimize detachment of the frontal process periosteum to avoid a temporal contour deformity.

Upper eyelid (blepharoplasty, supratarsal fold) In contrast with the supraorbital eyebrow incision, the upper eyelid incision offers access to most of the supraorbital rim and superior orbit and heals with an imperceptible scar (**Fig. 6**).[34–41] The orbital septum of the upper eyelid inserts and blends with the levator aponeurosis, which is located approximately 10 to 15 mm above the upper eyelid margin, which is unlike the lower eyelid, in which the orbital septum inserts onto the tarsal plate from its origin at the facial periosteum. As the levator palpebrae superioris extends anteriorly, it becomes aponeurotic as it passes superiorly to the equator of the globe. Deep to the orbital septum-levator aponeurosis complex lies the sympathetically innervated Müller muscle–tarsal complex, which originates from the inner surface of levator aponeurosis and inserts onto the superficial surface of the upper tarsal plate.

A 1-mm to 4-mm incision is made parallel to the superior palpebral sulcus in a naturally occurring skin line located approximately 10 to 14 mm

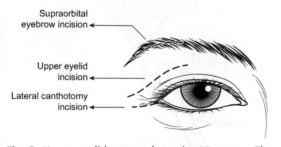

Fig. 6. Upper eyelid approach to the FZ suture. The authors' preferred approach to the FZ suture is an upper eyelid (blepharoplasty) approach within the upper eyelid fold, which is usually located 1 cm superior to the upper eyelid margin. (*From* Markiewicz MR, Bell RB. Traditional and contemporary surgical approaches to the orbit. Oral Maxillo Surg Clin North Am 2012;24(4):573–607.)

superior to the upper eyelid margin, or, in the case of edema masking a natural skin line, it may be made by comparison with the contralateral side.[41] For access to the lateral orbit and FZ, the incision may be extended laterally into the crow's feet for increased exposure staying 6 mm superior to the lateral canthus to avoid the frontal branch of the facial nerve. The senior author (RBB) has found this lateral extension to be unnecessary. The initial incision is made through skin and orbicularis oculi. As an alternative, a skin incision followed by scissor dissection through the orbicularis oris may offer an easier approach. A skin-muscle flap is then developed superiorly and laterally toward the FZ suture, staying deep to orbicularis oris and superficial to the orbital septum/levator aponeurosis complex.[36,40,42] While retracting the skin-muscle flap superiorly, a periosteal incision is made over the FZ suture. The incision should be closed in 2 layers: periosteum (4-0 polyglactin suture), and skin (running 6-0 fast gut).

Supraorbital brow (lateral brow) The supraorbital brow approach, also referred to as the lateral brow approach, offers direct access to the lateral supraorbital rim and FZ suture and carries the advantage of being a straightforward dissection.[43] However, the primary disadvantage is that the incision results in an unsightly scar, making it a poor choice when cosmetic approaches, such as the upper eyelid blepharoplasty, offer equivalent access and are imperceptible. For this reason, the lateral brow incision is not recommended, but is reviewed here for completeness.

The FZ suture is palpated and a 1-cm to 2-cm incision is made in trichophilic fashion on the lateral aspect of the eyebrow to the depth of the periosteum. Anteromedial extension of the incision within the brow may improve access; however, inferolateral extension should be avoided because this would cross the relaxed skin tension lines (crow's feet) at a 90° angle, resulting in an unsightly scar. Direct inferior extension in skin only may take place, but should stay 6 mm above the lateral canthus to prevent injury to the frontal branch of cranial nerve VII. Following supraperiosteal undermining, the periosteum overlying the FZ suture is incised. Subperiosteal dissection then takes place along the lateral, medial, and inferior aspects of the superolateral orbital rim. The surgeon should be sure to close the periosteum overlying the FZ, primarily to avoid detachment of the temporal aponeurosis from the frontal process of the zygoma, which preserves a flat contour to the temporal region.

Extended lower eyelid approach The extended lower eyelid approach provides additional access to the inferior and lateral orbits, greater wing of the sphenoid, and the lateral orbital rim to a point approximately 1 cm superior to the FZ suture.[34,44] For this technique, a subciliary incision is made and extended approximately 1 to 1.5 cm inferolaterally in a natural skin crease. A subtarsal incision does not allow as adequate a dissection up the lateral orbital rim as does the subciliary incision.[42] Supraperiosteal dissection of the lateral orbital rim is performed with scissors until just superior to the FZ suture, staying below the lateral canthal tendon. The anterior limb of the lateral canthal tendon is a thickening of fascia continuous with the fascia of the galea aponeurotica and temporal fascia lateral to the orbital rim on the posterior surface of the orbicularis oculi. The thicker, posterior limb of the lateral canthal tendon is more difficult to separate from the lateral horn of the levator palpebrae superior and Lockwood suspensory ligament. A periosteal incision from just superior to the FZ suture is made downwards connecting to the infraorbital incision. Subperiosteal dissection then takes place, stripping the orbital floor, orbital wall, posterior limb of the lateral canthal tendon, Lockwood suspensory ligament, and lateral cheek ligament from the Whitnall tubercle of the zygoma.[34] Lateral canthopexy is not required for lateral canthal tendon repositioning.[42] Only periosteal and skin closure is needed.

Infraorbital rim and orbit Numerous approaches to the orbit have been described and, although some have advantages compared with others, surgeons should generally use the approaches with which they are most comfortable, that provide for optimal cosmesis, and that result in minimal complications (**Figs. 7** and **8**).[45–52] The authors' preferred approach for most isolated orbital

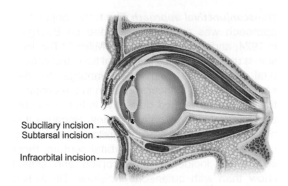

Fig. 8. The authors prefer a conjunctival fornix approach to the infraorbital rim and internal orbit. (*From* Markiewicz MR, Bell RB. Traditional and contemporary surgical approaches to the orbit. Oral Maxillo Surg Clin North Am 2012;24(4):573–607.)

fractures is a transconjunctival approach performed at the conjunctival fornix. A lateral canthotomy is not advised. Although once popular, the authors' experience is that the lateral canthotomy combined with transconjunctival incision for disarticulation of the lower lid often results in an unnatural appearance even when closed by an experienced surgeon. An isolated transconjunctival fornix approach combined with upper lid blepharoplasty typically provides adequate access to the orbit for most applications. A subtarsal approach is used for access to the orbit in some cases of acute trauma in which massive periorbital edema makes transconjunctival incisions technically difficult.

Although transconjunctival incisions are associated with a higher incidence of lower lid retraction, cutaneous approaches are associated with a higher incidence of scarring and, in some studies, a higher incidence of ectropion.[44,51,53] Although there are no formal meta-analyses on the topic, Ridgway and colleagues[54] reviewed the literature comparing subtarsal, subciliary, and transconjunctival incisions, and the incidence of ectropion was highest in subciliary incisions (12.5%), followed by subtarsal incisions (2.7%), with no reported cases in the transconjunctival group (0%). Entropion occurred in the transconjunctival group (4.4%), whereas there were no occurrences in the subtarsal and subciliary groups. Hypertrophic scarring most commonly occurred in the subciliary group (3.6%), once in the subtarsal group, and never in the transconjunctival group. However, similar studies have found as high as a 42% incidence of ectropion in the subciliary approach and superior esthetic results in those undergoing transconjunctival approaches.[47]

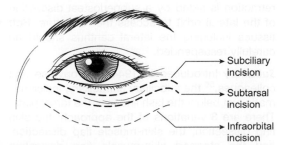

Fig. 7. Cutaneous lower eyelid approaches to the infraorbital rim and internal orbit. The subtarsal approach is the preferred transcutaneous approach to the infraorbital rim and internal orbit because it provides a balance between acceptable esthetics and minimal risk of complications. (*From* Markiewicz MR, Bell RB. Traditional and contemporary surgical approaches to the orbit. Oral Maxillo Surg Clin North Am 2012;24(4):573–607.)

Transconjunctival approach The transconjunctival approach was originally described by Bourguet in 1924, and later by Tenzel and Miller.[55] This incision is useful to access the orbital floor and infraorbital rim.[44] The primary advantage to this approach is that its scar is hidden in the conjunctiva and, if performed correctly, is imperceptible and rarely results in complications. Because it is not necessary to divide the pretarsal orbicularis muscle or interfere with the orbital septum, there is a lower incidence of ectropion and scleral show than with cutaneous incisions. Dissection may be performed in a preseptal or retroseptal fashion (**Fig. 9**).[56] In a retroseptal approach (fornix technique), a 15-blade or fine-tipped electrocautery is used to make an incision through the conjunctiva at the arcuate line within the conjunctival fornix. The incision may extend as medial as the lacrimal sac. At this point, orbital fat and contents extrude and should be retracted superiorly. With a Demars retractor positioning the lower eyelid forward, an incision is then made through the periosteum immediately posterior to the orbital rim. Periosteum is incised and a subperiosteal plane is then developed to access the orbital rim, anterior zygoma, and maxilla. In the preseptal approach, an incision is made 2 to 3 mm below the tarsal plate in the midportion of the lower eyelid in a plane anterior to the orbital septum. The thin cranial part of the capsulopalpebral fascia is dissected above the lower lid retractor muscles in a vector toward the orbital rim. The orbital septum is protected with a malleable retractor. Periosteum is incised and subperiosteal dissection is performed. The preseptal approach has been associated with an increased risk of entropion compared with other approaches. Closure of the periosteum is not warranted. The conjunctiva

may then be closed with a running 6-0 plain gut suture with the ends of the suture buried to avoid irritating the globe, or, as is the senior author's preference, the conjunctiva may be left unclosed.

Transconjunctival incision with lateral canthotomy (disarticulation of the lower eyelid) The lateral canthotomy incision may be combined with the transconjunctival approach to allow wide access to the inferior and lateral orbit.[57–59] Following a standard transconjunctival incision, lateral canthotomy is performed by using scissors to cut skin, orbicularis oculi, orbital septum, lateral canthal tendon, and conjunctiva a depth of 7 to 10 mm.[42] Cantholysis of the inferior limb of the lateral canthal tendon should then be performed such that the lower eyelid is detached from the lateral orbital rim. A pocket is made just posterior to the orbital septum to a point just posterior to the orbital rim. The transconjunctival and lateral canthotomy incisions are then connected. Following superior retraction of orbital contents, a periosteal incision is made. For closure, the inferior canthal limb and lateral portion of the tarsal plate are reapproximated. The conjunctival incision is then closed by tightening of the inferior canthopexy suture, which should be approximated more toward the FZ suture than its original attachment to the Whitnall tubercle to overcome forces that encourage inferior displacement. The lateral canthotomy incision is then closed with 6-0 fast gut suture.

When using this approach to access the FZ suture, a supraperiosteal dissection of the lateral rim may be performed to a point above the suture. The periosteum overlying the suture is incised from a point midway up the orbital rim to the most superior point of dissection. Orbital content retraction is aided by a subperiosteal dissection of the lateral orbit to access the FZ suture. Soft tissues including the lateral canthus should be carefully resuspended.

Subciliary Introduced in 1944 by Converse and colleagues,[56] the subciliary (infraciliary) incision is made just below the lash line over the tarsal plate. There are 3 variations of the approach: the skin flap dissection, the skin-muscle flap dissection, and the stepped skin-muscle flap dissection (**Fig. 10**).[51] The skin-only dissection dissects the thin eyelid skin from an incision inferior to the orbital rim where the orbicularis oculi and periosteum are incised; it is associated with severe complications such as ectropion, skin necrosis, and ecchymosis, and is thus rarely used.[35] The nonstepped skin-muscle flap incision is made through skin and pretarsal orbicularis oris until

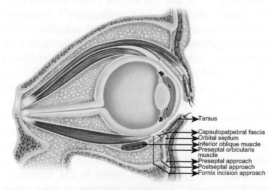

Tarsus
Capsulopalpebral fascia
Orbital septum
Inferior oblique muscle
Preseptal orbicularis muscle
Preseptal approach
Postseptal approach
Fornix incision approach

Fig. 9. Planes of dissection after transconjunctival incision may be preseptal or retroseptal. (*From* Markiewicz MR, Bell RB. Traditional and contemporary surgical approaches to the orbit. Oral Maxillo Surg Clin North Am 2012;24(4):573–607.)

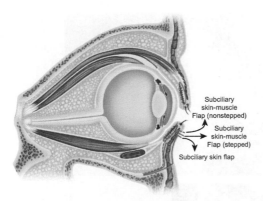

Subciliary
skin-muscle
Flap (nonstepped)
Subciliary
skin-muscle
Flap (stepped)
Subciliary skin flap

Fig. 10. Following a subciliary incision a skin-muscle (nonstepped), skin-muscle (stepped), or skin-only flap may be developed. (*From* Markiewicz MR, Bell RB. Traditional and contemporary surgical approaches to the orbit. Oral Maxillo Surg Clin North Am 2012;24(4):573–607.)

the tarsal plate is met. A preseptal plane is then dissected inferiorly to the orbital rim and a periosteal incision is then made just below the orbital septum. The stepped skin-muscle flap dissection divides the orbicularis oris muscle 2 to 3 mm below the skin incision leaving a strip of pretarsal orbicularis oculi to support the lower eyelid. Dividing the muscle below the initial skin incision leaves an intact innervated portion of muscle over the tarsal plate. This technique preserves the pretarsal orbicularis oculi fibers and limits scarring at the eyelid margin while maintaining normal vertical eyelid position and lessening the risk of ectropion, lid shortening, lid hypotonicity, and subsequent increased scleral show.[39,60] A preseptal plane to the orbital rim is advanced and an incision is made through periosteum onto the anterior face several millimeters below the infraorbital rim to avoid incising through orbital septum, which may result in vertical shortening of the eye lid. The levator labii superioris is dissected medially off its insertion onto the zygoma and maxilla, allowing visualization of the infraorbital foramen and nerve.

Subtarsal The subtarsal approach, as initially described by Converse and colleagues,[56] is similar to the subciliary approach in its anatomic dissection, but the incision is placed along the lower border of the tarsal plate in the subtarsal fold approximately 5 to 7 mm from the lower eyelid margin following an inferolateral vector to a point just past the lateral orbital rim (see **Figs. 7** and **8**).[47,51,61] A skin-muscle flap is then developed by using a blunt-tipped scissors to dissect and spread the orbicularis oris off the orbital septum in an inferior vector to the infraorbital rim. As in the subciliary approach, a plane

between orbicularis oris muscle and orbital septum should be dissected to the infraorbital rim. The orbital septum then merges with the periosteum of the anterior face. The surgeon should maintain dissection between the orbicularis oris and orbital septum; violation of either may cause vertical shortening of the lower eyelid. Dissection should then continue over the periosteum, avoiding any violation of the orbital septum to avoid shortening the septum. An incision should be made on the periosteum several millimeters below the orbital septum/periosteum interface. Fracture fragments are then dissected free from periosteum with medial dissection of levator labii superioris from its insertion on the zygoma and maxilla. Just as in an intraoral approach to the infraorbital rim, dissection of levator labii superioris allows visualization and protection of the infraorbital nerve.

Zygomatic arch and ZT suture Fractures of the zygomatic arch typically occur with minimal severity, with the fracture immediately springing back into position and necessitating no treatment. Goldthwaite[62] described an intraoral approach to the zygomatic arch that used stab incision to the buccal sulcus and the passing of a sharp elevator behind the maxillary tuberosity, elevating and reducing the arch. Quinn technique made a maxillary alveolar incision and dissected a plane along the ascending ramus to the lateral coronoid process to the zygomatic arch. A medially displaced fracture is then reduced by placing an elevator between the coronoid process and the zygomatic arch. More uncommon, but innovative, methods of reduction, such as towel clip reduction, are not discussed here.[63]

Gillies approach The zygomatic arch may be exposed and reduced with an approach described by Gillies and colleagues[64] (**Fig. 11**A). With this approach, an incision of no more than 2.5 cm parallel to the hair follicles is made within the temporal hairline down to the white glistening deep temporalis fascia. The temporal fascia divides approximately 2.5 cm above the zygomatic arch; therefore, 2 fascial layers with interlying syssarcosis fat may be encountered in more inferiorly placed incisions. The incision is then deepened to the temporalis muscle fibers. An elevator (Rowe elevator or urethral sound) is placed between the deep temporal fascia and muscle and advanced to beneath the zygomatic arch (see **Fig. 11**B). A lifting, but not rocking, motion should be used. Care must be taken not to fulcrum the elevator off the temporal bone to avoid inadvertent temporal bone fracture (see **Fig. 11**C). This approach may be used to reduce

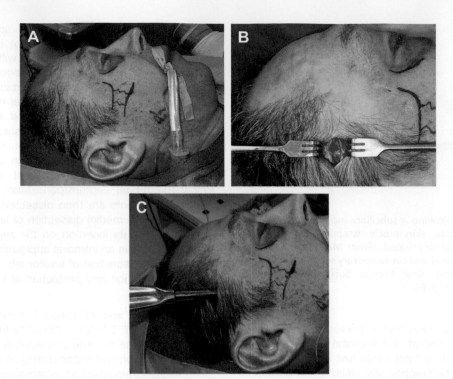

Fig. 11. Patient with isolated right zygomatic arch fracture (*A*). After incising down to the glistening white temporoparietal fascia, the fascia is incised down to the underlying temporalis fascia, immediately overlying the temporalis muscle (*B*). The arch is then elevated in a lateral bodily motion being careful not to fulcrum off the temporal bone (*C*).

the zygoma by advancing the elevator more anteriorly under the body of the zygoma.

Dingman approach This approach, as described by Dingman and Native,[7] can be used for not only reduction of the zygomatic arch but for the zygoma as well. In this approach, an incision is made just above the lateral eyebrow or as a blepharoplasty incision (**Fig. 12**). An elevator is passed beneath the temporal aponeurosis (attachment of deep temporal fascia to frontal process of zygoma). The elevator may be advanced anteriorly beneath the zygomatic arch or further beneath the zygoma and lifted laterally to reduce the arch and zygoma fracture respectively.

Coronal approach (posterior approach) Originally described by Tessier for an approach to the orbits, the coronal approach is useful not only for exposure of the zygomatic arches but for the superior orbits, FZ suture, and medial and lateral orbits.[65,66] One relative contraindication to this approach is a family history of male pattern baldness. Risks include injury to the temporal and zygomatic branches of the facial nerve, temporal hollowing, scalp hematoma, parietal scalp pain, paresthesia or anesthesia, infection, and nasal orbital hypertrophy.[67] The coronal approach is necessary to provide access to the zygomatic arch, but should be used selectively. Even with careful closure and technical modifications, a coronal approach

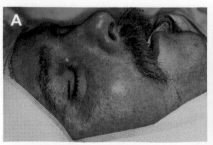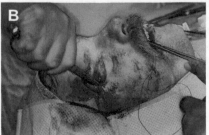

Fig. 12. Patient with fracture of right zygoma. Upper blepharoplasty approach to the zygoma (*A*). Elevator passed beneath the zygomatic arch and elevated in a bodily manner (*B*).

with subperiosteal dissection of the zygoma results in noticeable temporal hollowing. Its use therefore should be justified by the need to provide extensive exposure and open reduction and internal fixation of the zygomatic arch.

A comprehensive review of the regional anatomy is beyond the scope of this article and is described elsewhere.[68] However, clarification of the fascial and neuromuscular attachments pertinent to exposure of the zygomatic arch is useful. Beneath the temporoparietal fascia in the temporoparietal region lies an extension of the subgaleal fascia, which can be dissected as a separate layer in this area but is usually dissected as a continuance of the subgaleal plane in the coronal approach. The temporalis fascia (deep temporal fascia) arises superiorly from the superior temporal line where it fuses with pericranium and lies beneath the subgaleal fascia in the temporoparietal region. It is continuous with the pericranium above the superior temporal lines, the parotidomasseteric fascia below the level of the zygomatic arch, and the cervical fascia encasing the muscles of the neck. At the level of the superior orbital rim, the temporalis fascia divides into a superficial layer, which attaches to the lateral border of the zygomatic arch, and a deep layer, which attaches to the medial border of the zygomatic arch. The temporalis muscle arises from the deep layers of the temporalis fascia at the temporal fossa, passing medial to the zygomatic arch and inserting onto the coronoid process of the mandible.

The temporal branch (frontal branch) of the facial nerve exits the parotid gland just inferior to the zygomatic arch.[69,70] In general, the course of the temporal branch of the facial nerve is from a point 0.5 cm below the tragus to a point 1.5 cm above the lateral eyebrow,[70] and it crosses the zygomatic arch between a distance of 0.8 to 3.5 cm anterior to the anterior concavity of the external auditory canal at an average distance of 2 cm anterior to the anterior concavity of the external auditory canal. As it crosses the zygomatic arch it passes between the undersurface of the temporoparietal fascia and the fusion of the zygomatic arch, the superficial layer of the temporalis fascia, and the subgaleal fascia.[71]

The incision is made in a sinusoidal, sawtooth (zigzag, stealth), or a geometric broken-line pattern,[72,73] with a preauricular extension made only if exposure of the zygoma is necessary. In women, and men without potential for balding, incisions may be placed anteriorly at the vertex remaining 4 to 5 cm behind the hairline. The incision should be placed well behind the hairline in children because it will migrate with growth. The initial incision should be made between superior

temporal lines down to the loose areolar connective tissue of the subgaleal plane. This suprapericranial plane is dissected with ease. Incisions below the superior temporal line should be continuous with the subgaleal plane above the superior temporal line to the level below the temporoparietal fascia just before the superficial layer of the temporal fascia, which blends with the pericranium.

The flap is dissected anteriorly until within 3 to 4 cm of the supraorbital rims. When a pericranial flap is not planned, an incision through pericranium is made between the superior temporal lines. The incision is kept within the superior temporal lines to prevent unnecessary bleeding. A subperiosteal plane is developed toward the supraorbital rims. If the surgeon knows that a pericranial flap will not be used, then a subperiosteal plan may be developed posteriorly after the initial skin incision site. When planning to develop a vascularized pericranial flap, a suprapericranial (subgaleal), dissection is performed as described previously. Then an incision is made through pericranium from the most anterior aspect to most posterior aspect of the incision just above the superior temporal lines. A transverse incision through pericranium between the superior temporal lines is made, connecting the most posterior aspects of the sagittal incisions. Starting at the posterior aspect of the incision, pericranium is then elevated with a periosteal elevator. Following elevation of the anteriorly based pericranial flap, a subperiosteal dissection is continued toward the supraorbital rims.

The zygomatic arch is located between the superficial and deep layers of temporalis fascia, which are adherent to the lateral and medial arches, respectively. For access to the zygomatic arches and bodies, the superficial layer of temporalis fascia is incised at the root of the zygomatic arch just anterior to the ear and above the temporomandibular joint to the supraorbital rim in a vector paralleling the temporal branch of the facial nerve. The incision is continued in a superior direction at a 45° angle until it is combined with the transverse pericranial incision at the superior temporal line or where the pericranial flap has been elevated.

On incision of the superficial layer of temporalis fascia, the superficial temporal fat pad (contained between superficial and deep temporalis fascia) is exposed. Disruption of this fat pad is thought to contribute to temporal hollowing.[74] The mechanism of temporal hollowing is multifactorial, but can be partially attributed to disruption of branching perforators from the middle and deep temporal arteries that transverse the substance of the fat pad, and disruption of the septal network that suspends the temporal fat pad from the anterior temporalis fascia.[74,75] Staying immediately deep to the superficial layer of temporalis fascia with careful dissection to the zygoma may aid in minimizing this unsightly consequence. Incising the deep temporal fascia closer to the arch is associated with less temporal hollowing but a higher incidence of frontal branch injury, so care should be taken to make the incision on the superior aspect of the arch. The temporal branch of the facial nerve should be contained within the temporoparietal fascia, which is contained within the coronal flap.

To access the orbits and nasal region, the supraorbital neurovascular bundle must be released. If a bony foramen exists, an osteotome may be used to remove a bony ridge just inferior to the bundle. A subperiosteal dissection is then undertaken along the internal orbits. When dissecting the medial orbit, careful attention should be paid to avoid stripping the medial canthal tendon from the anterior and posterior lacrimal crests, which appear as dense fibrous attachments in the nasolacrimal fossa. As medial orbital wall dissection proceeds, the anterior and posterior ethmoidal arteries are found approximately 25 mm and 35 mm anterior to the anterior lacrimal crest,

respectively.[76] These vessels may be cauterized with bipolar electrocautery and transected with further posterior subperiosteal elevation. If necessary, the orbits may be dissected to their apices.

ACQUIRED ORBITOZYGOMATIC DEFORMITIES

Optimal reconstruction of orbitozygomaticomaxillary complex (OZMC) deformities remains controversial. The goal of zygoma reconstruction following trauma and ablative surgery should be based on reconstructing the buttresses of the facial skeleton.[77,78] Although there is general agreement that patients do not consistently require 3-point or 4-point fixation, as has been advocated by investigators in the past, there is still much confusion as to what approach offers adequate access for successful open reduction and internal fixation and minimal complications (**Fig. 13**). In addition, no consensus has been reached regarding objective criteria for exploration and/or repair of the orbital floor.

The author's approach to most OZMC fractures is a progressive technique that generally begins with an intraoral vestibular incision (Keen incision)

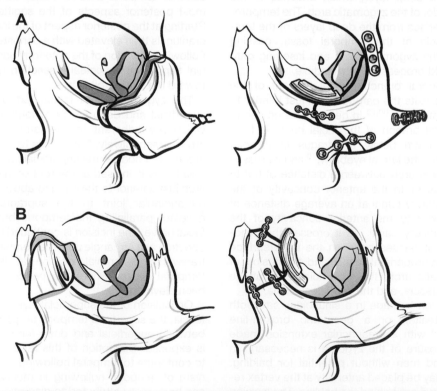

Fig. 13. Zygoma fracture with orbital rim and floor component and 4-point fixation was used (*A*). Medial orbital wall and nasoorbitoethmoid complex fracture and reduction and fixation (*B*). (*From* Manson PN. Fractures of the zygoma. In: Booth PW, Schendel SA, Hausamen JE, editors. Maxillofacial surgery. 2nd edition. St Louis: Churchill Livingstone; 2006; with permission.)

to approach the maxillary buttress. Many zygoma deformities are minimally displaced and do not require repair. Low-velocity OZMC fractures that are minimally to moderately displaced can often be managed with simple 1-point fixation at the maxillary buttress providing that no significant intraorbital component exists. More commonly, moderately displaced fractures of both low and high velocity can be managed with simple 2-point fixation provided at the maxillary buttress via a Keen incision and the frontozygomatic suture (FZ suture) approached via an upper lid blepharoplasty incision (**Fig. 14**). If the rotation of the OZMC complex is not adequately reduced following

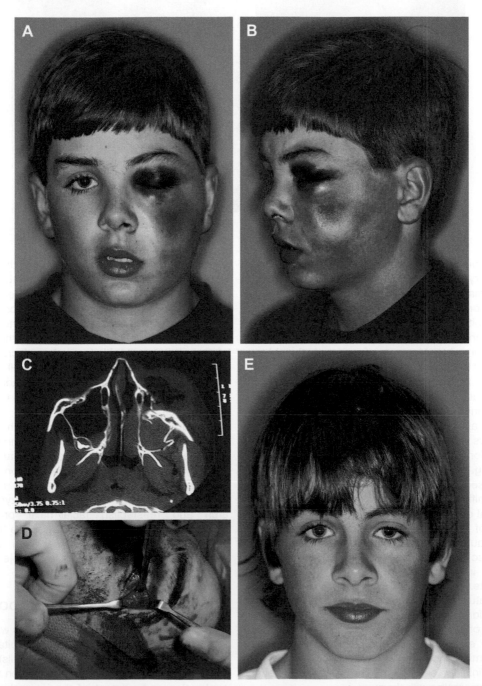

Fig. 14. Twelve-year-old boy with medially displaced left zygoma fracture and significant malar flattening (*A–C*). Blepharoplasty approach used to access the FZ suture (*D*). Frontal (*E*) and worm's-eye view (*F*) of patient 1 year after reconstruction. Frontal (*G*) and worm's-eye view (*H*) of patient 6 years after reconstruction.

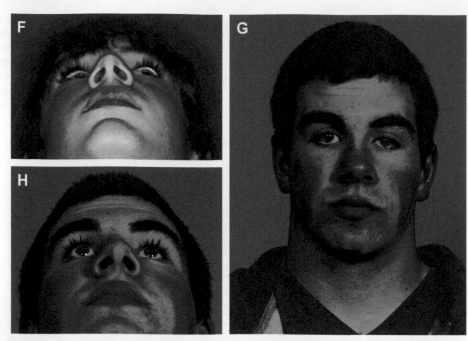

Fig. 14. (*continued*)

reduction and stabilization with 2 points at the maxillary buttress and FZ suture, or the infraorbital rim remains displaced, the transverse component of the orbital frame can then be stabilized at the infraorbital rim via a transconjunctival incision. Skeletonization of the infraorbital rim is avoided if at all possible. However, if adequate height or width of the inferior orbital rim cannot be achieved, then a 1.2-mm or 1.3-mm miniplate is placed along the infraorbital rim via either a transconjunctival or midlid incision.

Ellis and Kittidumkerng[17] analyzed a series of patients with OZMC fractures with regard to the need for repair of the orbital floor or infraorbital rim (**Fig. 15**). Their indications for repair included increased orbital volume or comminution as well as significant soft tissue prolapse.[17] The need for internal orbital reconstruction was only present in 44% of their series of patients. In patients who did require repair of the infraorbital rim or orbital floor, scleral show was associated with a lower eyelid incision in approximately 20% of the patients. In another study by Ellis and Reddy,[79] the status of the internal orbit was analyzed after reduction of a series of patients who underwent repair of OZMC fractures who did not undergo orbital exploration. Of these 65 patients, only 8 had minor increases in orbital volume that were not clinically significant. The residual defects became smaller with time.

The author therefore prefers an approach similar to that of Shumrick and colleagues,[80] which provides for selective management of the orbital rim and orbital floor in OZMC fractures based on clinical and radiographic findings. These findings include persistent diplopia, enophthalmos, significant comminution at the orbital rim, and/or displacement or comminution of greater than 50% of the orbital wall with herniation of orbital fat, combined orbital floor and medial wall defects with soft tissue displacement, and radiological evidence of fracture or comminution of the body of the zygoma.

Fractures that are the result of a high-velocity injury with severe fragmentation or comminution, or those associated with panfacial fractures, are typically repaired with 4-point stabilization. Unless there are large facial lacerations, this includes a coronal approach to expose the zygomatic arch and reestablish facial/malar projection (**Fig. 16**). Care must be taken to restore the arch to its normal flat contour rather than creating a rounded arch that will result in deprojection of the zygoma and widening of the face.

MANAGEMENT OF THE ORBITAL FLOOR

In the authors' experience, most patients with low-velocity injuries involving the external orbital frame (eg, bare-fisted assault or ground-level falls) can be adequately restored to form and function without exploration or treatment of the internal orbit. In contrast, most high-velocity injuries, such as those occurring in motor vehicle collisions, result in

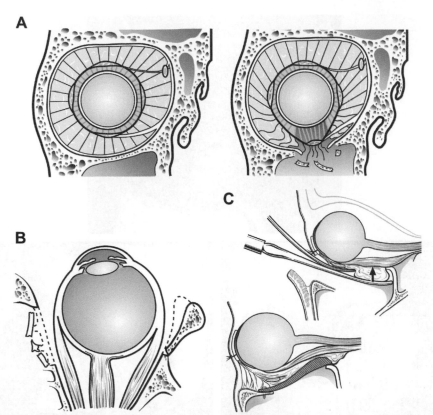

Fig. 15. Zygoma fractures with a significant orbital component may have orbital content herniation into the maxillary sinus antrum and associated increased orbital volume (*A*). The increase in orbital volume may not be seen until lateral reduction of the zygoma, which may create diastasis at the infraorbital rim. Severe zygoma fractures may be associated with medial orbital wall or nasoorbitoethmoid fractures, or lateral orbital wall fractures primarily at the SZ suture and may display additional associated increased orbital volume (*B*). Adequate reduction of the orbital floor will be crucial in restoring orbital volume and associated globe position (*C*). (*From* Manson PN. Fractures of the zygoma. In: Booth PW, Schendel SA, Hausamen JE, editors. Maxillofacial surgery. 2nd edition. St Louis: Churchill Livingstone; 2006; with permission.)

a displacement of energy that causes significant internal orbital disruption and necessitates repair of the internal orbit regardless of the level of displacement seen on CT. This selective approach to repair of the internal orbit takes into consideration the patient's subjective symptoms (eg, blurred vision, diplopia), physical findings (eg, entrapment of the inferior rectus muscle), limitation of extraocular muscle movement, radiographic findings (planar defect greater than 3.5 cm^2 and volumetric displacement greater than 1.6 cm^3), and mechanism of injury (ie, low velocity vs high velocity).

Complex, combined orbital fractures are some of the most challenging craniofacial injuries to manage. High-velocity trauma typically produces defects that affect 2, 3, or all 4 walls of the orbit. Such shattered orbits produce large volumetric increases intraorbitally, with massive herniation of periorbital contents into the surrounding anatomic spaces and occasional cranial neuropathies. These defects typically extend into the orbital cone and may involve the optic canal. Their complex patterns and loss of posterior support from the posteromedial and posteroinferior bulges make restoration of normal orbital anatomy challenging. Although refinements in surgical approaches and the development of new biologic materials have improved the ability to predictably restore these patients' form and function, a significant number of these individuals still require revision surgery despite the best efforts of an experienced surgeon.[16,18]

Four-wall fractures that involve the anterior skull base may require transcranial approaches, occasionally with the assistance of a neurosurgeon, and they often require management of the frontal sinus and occasionally the orbital apex. As the frontotemporal components are repositioned, the orbital roof must be restored with either titanium mesh or calvarial bone grafts and the anterior skull base lined to prevent leakage of cerebrospinal fluid.

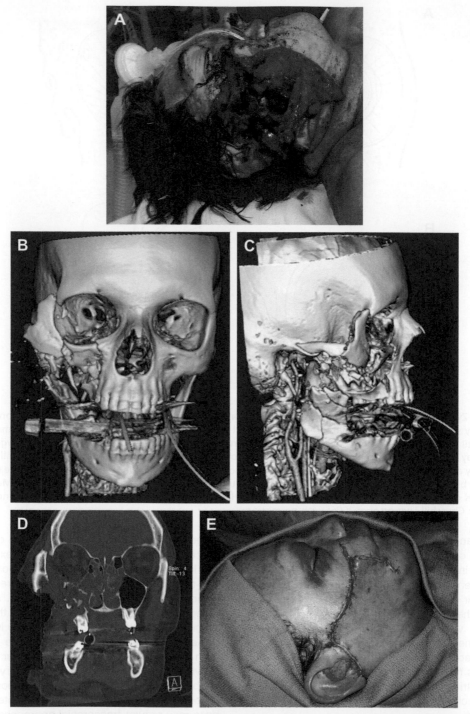

Fig. 16. A 55-year-old woman involved in motor vehicle accident with large facial laceration with cranial nerve VII transection, grossly displaced and comminuted left zygoma fracture involving all 4 sutures and significant infraorbital rim component, and comminuted mandible fracture (*A–D*). Patient underwent open reduction and internal fixation of her fractures with 4-point fixation and reduction and fixation of her medial orbital fracture, and comminuted right subcondylar fracture and primary closure of her facial laceration (*E*). Hardware CT showed 4-point fixation (*F*). Postoperative CT (*G–J*) showed restoration of vertical and anterior-posterior facial width with adequate projection from proper reduction of the zygomatic arch. Postoperative photographs showed adequate projection of facial width and projection; however, there was significant loss of right nasolabial fold and marginal mandibular nerve palsy (*K–M*). The patient will undergo facial reanimation surgery.

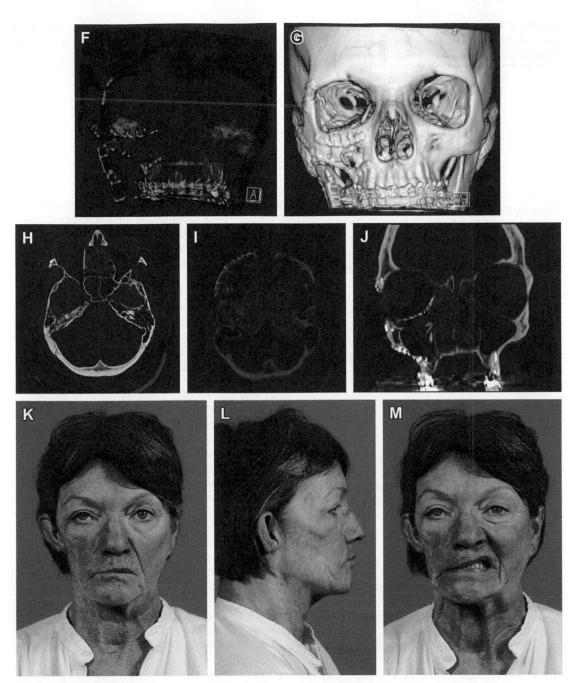

Fig. 16. (*continued*)

When the entire orbit is disrupted and there are no posterior landmarks to guide the reconstruction, accurate positioning of bone grafts or titanium mesh becomes problematic. It is difficult to establish proper orbital contour, volume, and medial bulge projection, and there is a risk of encroachment on the orbital apex and optic nerve. Presurgical computer planning to virtually reconstruct the affected orbit or orbits, stereolithographic models to establish proper plate contour, and the use of intraoperative navigation to ensure accurate and safe positioning of the plate in a poorly visualized anatomic region afford even experienced surgeons greater confidence and predictability in treating fractures of the deep orbit.[81]

COMPLICATIONS OF ZYGOMA TRAUMA AND TREATMENT
Orbital Complications

Superior orbital fissure syndrome

Superior orbital fissure syndrome involves damage to some or all of the contents that travel in the superior orbital fissure, which is a foramen of the skull lying between the lesser and greater wing of the sphenoid bones and including cranial nerves III, IV, VI, and the lacrimal, frontal, and nasociliary branches of the first division of cranial nerve V. Although there are multiple anatomic possibilities of the injury, most cases of superior orbital fissure syndrome can be divided into those that exhibit narrowing of the fissure and those that lack narrowing.[82] The ophthalmic vein and sympathetic branches from the cavernous sinus also travel through this foramen. Clinical symptoms include ptosis, anesthesia of the forehead, a fixed dilated pupil, and ophthalmoplegia. If suspected, immediate ophthalmologic consultation should be obtained. Management may include reduction of fractures, relief at the superior orbital fissure, possible exploration at the orbital apex, and systemic steroids.

Orbital apex syndrome

Signs of orbital apex syndrome or traumatic optic neuropathy may be seen on CT.[83] However, diagnosis is confirmed by clinical examination. Initial treatment of orbital apex syndrome includes ophthalmology consultation and usually systemic steroid administration and possible emergent decompression of the optic nerve by expansion of the optic canal and dural sheath incision of the optic nerve.

Retrobulbar hemorrhage

Retrobulbar hemorrhage may occur as a result of the initial injury or reparative surgery. Ischemic injury to the retinal vessel secondary to constriction of retinal blood flow may cause orbital compartment syndrome and irreversible blindness. Immediate identification for possible retrobulbar hemorrhage should be followed by lateral canthotomy and evacuation of the hematoma.[84–86] Occurring at a lesser incidence than retrobulbar hematoma is subperiosteal hematoma, which is more likely to occur with traumatic injury in the pediatric population.[87]

Diplopia

Ellis and colleagues[88] noted an incidence of diplopia of 5.4% to 74.5% in patients with zygoma fractures. Isolated zygoma and zygomatic arch fractures have a lower incidence than complex zygoma fractures. Diplopia may be binocular, which usually results from misalignment of the eyes relative to each other, such as a posttraumatic change in globe position; and monocular, which usually indicates a structural defect to the eye, such as dislocation of the lens, macula lesions, retinal detachment, and damage to the corneal surface or the visual cortex.

Contusion or entrapment of the extraocular muscles and their fascial attachments to the orbit may cause changes in visual acuity, ocular movement, and diplopia.[31] Neurogenic causes of diplopia, such as cranial nerve III, IV, and VI palsies, are uncommon following trauma and are caused by a false image in the affected eye in the same direction of movement produced by the unaffected eye. On examination, the eyes should be covered in sequence and the patient should be asked when the more peripheral image disappears. This technique allows identification of the muscles involved. In the cases in which rotational muscles such as the superior or inferior obliques are involved, tilting of horizontal and vertical lines (rotary diplopia) occurs.

Diplopia in orbital floor or medial orbital wall fractures usually results from edema, hematoma, or entrapment of the fibrous septa or extraocular muscles rather than a nerve palsy. Late posttraumatic diplopia may be caused by fat scarring or fibrosis between extraocular muscles and the periosteum of the globe. For example, vertical diplopia is caused by failure of the affected eye to be elevated and the false image is above or below the true image in the affected eye. The greatest separation of images occurs opposite the muscles involved. For example, with an entrapped inferior rectus muscle, the superior rectus and inferior oblique are hyperactive, making limitation of movement more prominent. Reversal of images indicates a mechanical restriction rather than a paresis. In addition, overactivity of the opposing superior rectus and inferior oblique muscles moves the upper pole of the globe backward and causes deepening of the supratarsal fold (retraction sign).

Soft tissue coronal CT views provide good visualization and can aid in determining whether muscle is entrapped. Diminished orbital volume following blowout fractures also contributes to diplopia because of alteration in globe position. Damage to the cornea intraoperatively and failure of the soft tissues of the periorbita and eyelids may contribute to change in globe position postoperatively. Vertical and horizontal dystopia results in not only esthetic deformity but often in diplopia, and can be prevented by the use of scleral shields, tarsorrhaphy sutures, and Frost sutures (sutures from the lower eyelid taped to the forehead aid in reestablishing preoperative eyelid and globe position).

Enophthalmos

Any subtle increase or decrease in orbital volume may cause enophthalmos or exophthalmos, respectively.[89] Fractures of the orbital floor encompassing an area of greater than 4.08 cm^2, or herniated tissue contents with a volume greater than 1.89 mL, are associated with enophthalmos of greater than 2 mm.[90] Enophthalmos or exophthalmos of more than 2 to 3 mm has been shown to be perceivable to the human eye.[91] Therefore, the orbital volume and soft tissue content of the orbits are integrally related and must be addressed by the surgeon. Restoration of normal orbital volume and globe projection following traumatic injury or ablative tumor surgery is often difficult. Improper implant placement may often lead to inadequate restoration of orbital volume resulting in residual enophthalmos.[92,93] Secondary repair of gross orbital deformities is difficult. Preoperative computer planning and intraoperative navigation have been shown to be useful adjuncts for secondary orbital reconstruction.[94,95]

Traumatic hyphema

Traumatic hyphema is the result of bleeding into the anterior chamber of the eye.[96,97] Immediate ophthalmology consultation is recommended if detected. Visual prognosis can be made from the percentage of hemorrhage obliterating the anterior chamber (microhyphema, I–IV). Complications include corneal staining, increased intraocular pressures, and rebleeding.[96] Treatment is directed at preventing rebleeding and maintaining normal intraocular pressure. Treatment includes elevating the head of the bed, wearing an eye patch, β-blockers, antifibrinolytics, osmotic agents, carbonic anhydrase inhibitors, and topical cycloplegics. Surgical intervention is rarely needed.

Trismus

Trismus associated with zygoma fractures occurs for 2 reasons. The cause is secondary to restriction in mandibular range of motion from inferior or posterior displacement of the zygoma impeding the coronoid process of the mandible. A medially displaced zygomatic arch secondary to edema of the muscles of mastication and soft tissues may also occur. This problem is usually corrected with proper reduction of the zygoma. The second and often longer lasting reason for trismus is fibro-osseous ankylosis of the coronoid process to the zygomatic arch, caused by medial depression of the zygomatic arch and interference with the coronoid process.

Facial Widening/Cheek Flattening

Gruss and colleagues[3] recognized the importance of the zygomatic arch in complex midfacial fracture repair and correction of posttraumatic orbitozygomatic deformities (**Fig. 17**). There is a reciprocal relationship between anterior-posterior projection

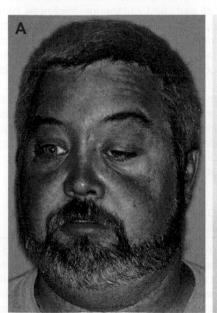
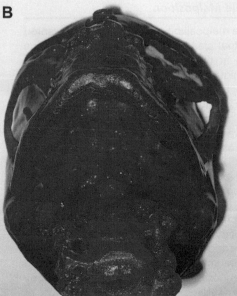

Fig. 17. Patient with left zygoma fracture with postoperative anterior-posterior deficiency and reciprocal facial widening from inadequate straightening of the zygomatic arch (A, B).

and facial width. As projection of the zygoma decreases, facial width increases. The zygoma is therefore key to restoring facial/orbital projection in severely displaced and comminuted fractures and should be returned to its natural flat contour. The most common error in reestablishing zygomatic projection is failure to reduce the segments out of a displaced arch into a flat zygoma. Failure to adequately flatten the zygomatic arch and achieve optimal rotation of the ZM complex results in flattening of the malar eminence and widening of the ipsilateral face. If a coronal incision is not performed, accurate rotation of the ZM complex can be assessed by inspecting the SZ suture region via an upper lid blepharoplasty approach.

Malar deficiency in the acute setting is almost always caused by failure to achieve adequate anterior-posterior projection of the zygomatic arch, resulting in a widened, more round face, or failing to reduce inferiorly and posteriorly displaced zygomatic body fractures. Long-term malar deficiency may be related to deficiency of the maxillofacial skeleton but may also be caused by ptosis of the malar fat pad, which usually results from failure to resuspend the soft tissues of the midface at the time of repair. Secondary malar deficiency and widening, both with hard and soft tissue causes, is extremely difficult to manage. Osteotomies[98,99] (Fig. 18) of the zygoma and alloplastic augmentation[100] (Fig. 19) may be needed in the case of bony deficiency. Dermal fillers[101] or autogenous fat grafting may be used in the case of soft tissue deficiency.

Soft Tissue Malposition

Soft tissue malposition may be partially prevented by periosteal closure, which prevents soft tissue spreading at the areas of fracture and incision. This technique includes closure of the periosteum of the orbit to the anterior layer of temporalis fascia over the FZ suture, closure of the deep temporal fascia on coronal incision, repositioning of the muscle over the zygomatic buttress, and suturing of the periosteum and subcutaneous tissue to the orbital rim. The facial tissue should also be fixated at several points over the bony skeleton. These tissue closures should be overcorrected to prevent facial soft tissue ptosis. For example, the periosteum over the malar surface should be fixated to the bone of the infraorbital rim, placing the zygomaticus major and minor in a more favorable position. The periosteum of the malar surface can be sutured to the temporal area similarly to rhytidectomy suspension sutures. In addition, a Frost stitch, or a stitch through the lower eyelid that is taped to the forehead, may be used to prevent ectropion.

Temporal Hollowing

In an MRI study, Lacey and colleagues[102] showed that diminution of the temporal fat pad, not the temporalis muscle, contributes to temporal hollowing following the coronal approach. Thus they recommended dissection immediately deep to the superficial layer of temporalis fascia to minimize dissection through the fat pad, rather than dissection over the superficial layer of the temporalis fascia or dissection within the substance of the superficial fat pad to prevent temporal hollowing. Matic and Kim[103] found that suprafascial dissection immediately over the superficial layer of the temporalis fascia with incision directly over the zygomatic arch was associated with less temporal hollowing and less damage to the ZT nerve and middle temporal artery (injured more in deep dissection) than deep dissection and dissection through the temporal fat pad.

Baek and colleagues[104] recommended a similar approach superficial to the superficial layer of the temporalis fascia for exposure of the zygomatic arch in patients undergoing facial fracture and craniosynostosis repair, noting avoidance of the frontal branch of the facial nerve and temporal artery, and subsequently decreased incidence of temporal hollowing with this approach. There was a zero incidence of facial nerve damage in both groups. Steinbacher and colleagues[105] used three-dimensional CT planning software (Materialise, Leuven, Belgium) to compare along the frontal bandeau and from midline: temporal width, temporalis muscle, superficial temporal fat pad, and cutaneous thickness between the operated and nonoperated sides. Temporal hollowing was affected by boney constriction along the anterior frontal bandeau and decreased temporalis muscle thickness, and not change in superficial temporal fat pad thickness. However, these data can only be generalized to the unilateral craniosynostosis population because the investigators used a dissection deep to the deep layer of temporalis fascia, avoiding penetration of the superficial temporal pad and its septal attachments superiorly.

ONCOLOGIC RECONSTRUCTION
Basic Ablative Approaches

Reconstruction of maxillectomy and zygoma defects is similar to reconstruction after trauma: it is based on buttress reconstruction with a focus on reconstructing the ZM, pterygomaxillary, and nasomaxillary buttresses.[77] Surgical approaches for partial or complete zygomatic ablation are similar to those discussed previously. Anterior

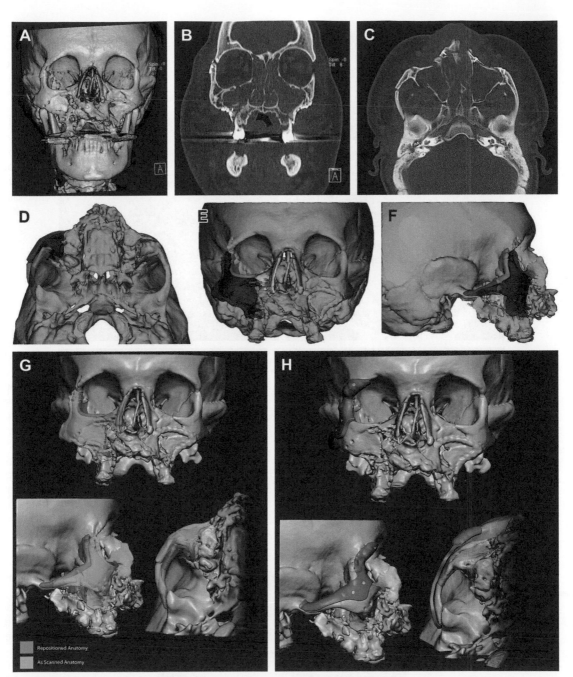

Fig. 18. Patient seen on referral after repair of multiple facial injuries including a right zygoma fracture (*A*, *B*). Inadequate anterior projection of the zygomatic arch resulted in residual reciprocal facial widening (*C*). Preoperative computer planning was used to virtually mirror the contralateral face to the right side for optimal zygoma positioning (red, true position; blue, goal mirrored position) (*D–F*). Based on the ideal position (*G*), a mounting gig was fabricated using computer-aided design/computer-aided monitoring (CAD/CAM) processes to guide the osteotomized segments into ideal position at the time of surgery (*H*). Frontal (*I*) and bird's-eye view (*J*) of patient before reconstruction. Stereolithographic model and mounting gig fabricated using CT data and CAD/CAM techniques (*K–M*). Coronal flap reflected to access zygomatic arch (*N*). Fixed fiducial marker placed on the skull to facilitate intraoperative navigation (*O*). Mounting gig applied to osteotomized segments (*P*). Postoperative frontal (*Q*) and worm's-eye (*R*) view of patient showing adequate restoration of facial width and malar projection.

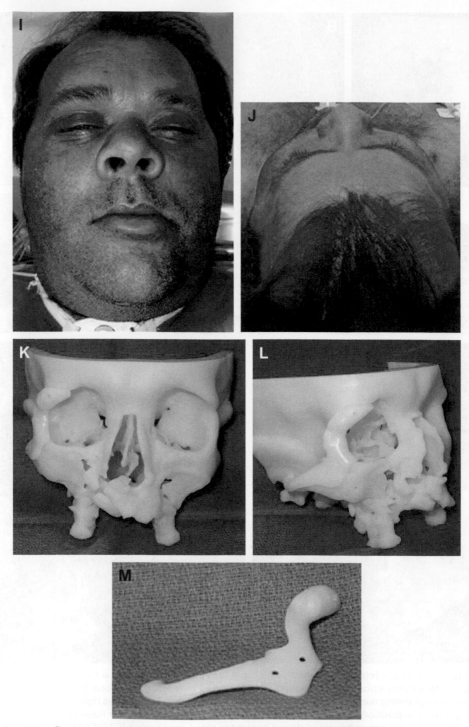

Fig. 18. (continued)

and infraorbital approaches may be considered when the defect includes the maxilla and a portion of the zygoma, but spares the orbit. Posterior approaches are preferred when the ablation involves the orbit. Cases that require postablation radiation are complicated by compromised tissue bed vascularity, which limits reconstructive options. These cases must be taken on an individual basis, and discussion is beyond the scope of this article.

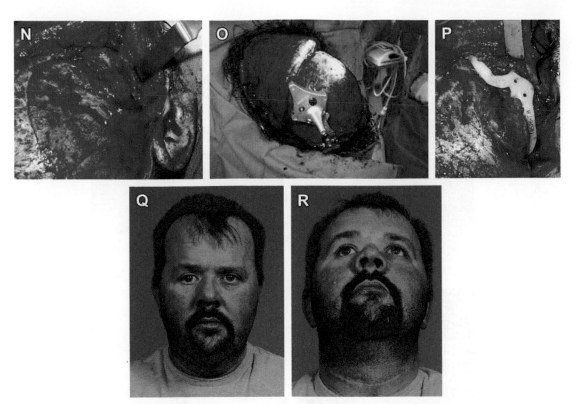

Fig. 18. (*continued*)

ALLOPLASTIC RECONSTRUCTION
Silastic (Silicone) Implants

Silastic silicone, an organosilicone polymer, is made of silicone, oxygen, and methyl-carbon groups. Once implanted into the face, silicone creates a fibrous capsule, which has the benefit of ease of removal if necessary. The main disadvantages of the implant relate to its instability and movement after placement. Metzinger and colleagues[106] reported an 85% success rate after 2 years for silicone malar implants, with only a 3.4% removal rate. Reported complications included undesirable esthetic results, malalignment requiring revision, displacement, and trigeminal hypesthesia. Potential complications included bony resorption, infection, seroma, hematoma, and facial nerve injury.

Medpor (Polyethylene Glycol) Implants

Polyethylene glycol implants are made of a high-density polyethylene material that is porous, thus allowing for vascular and fibrous ingrowth, but not bony ingrowth (**Fig. 20**).[107] This ingrowth may theoretically allow for more stability than Silastic implants, so polyethylene glycol implants may be stabilized with screw fixation, or left in place for soft tissue ingrowth, and fibrous capsule stabilization alone.

Polyetheretherketone Implants

Polyetheretherketone (PEEK) implants have become a popular method of orbitozygomatic reconstruction in recent years.[108] PEEK material is similar in density and strength to cortical bone, and can be used with traditional titanium plates and screws. CT imaging can be used to create custom implants for reconstruction of zygomatic defects.[109]

AUTOGENOUS RECONSTRUCTION
Calvarial Bone Grafts

The senior author has found the most success using cranial bone grafts, which typically are harvested in full-thickness fashion, split, and then used to reconstruct a zygoma/malar eminence (**Fig. 21**). Cranial bone grafts have an added benefit of being easily accessible, and can often be in the same operative field.[110] The curvature of the parietal eminence becomes the malar eminence, a strategy that is classically exploited in reconstruction of total zygomatic deformities, such as those seen in Treacher Collins syndrome.[111,112]

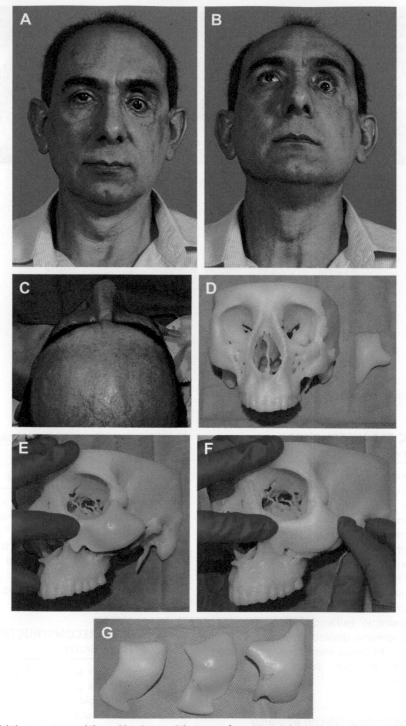

Fig. 19. Frontal (*A*), worm's-eye (*B*), and bird's-eye (*C*) views of a patient who was seen for secondary facial deformity with posttraumatic depressed and inferiorly positioned zygoma and globe rupture, enucleation, and placement of orbital prosthesis (*A–C*). Using preoperative planning and CAD/CAM techniques, a model of the patient's skull and a model of the patient's ideal alloplastic implant was fabricated using mirroring techniques (*D*). The stock implants were then tried on the skull (*E*), and the alloplastic implant was then shaped to match the CAD/CAM planned implant (*F, G*). Intraoperative navigation was used to compare the position on the implant of the implant with the preoperatively planned position (*H–L*). Postoperative frontal (*M*) and worm's-eye (*N*) views show significant restoration of midface projection and width, and favorable position of prosthesis.

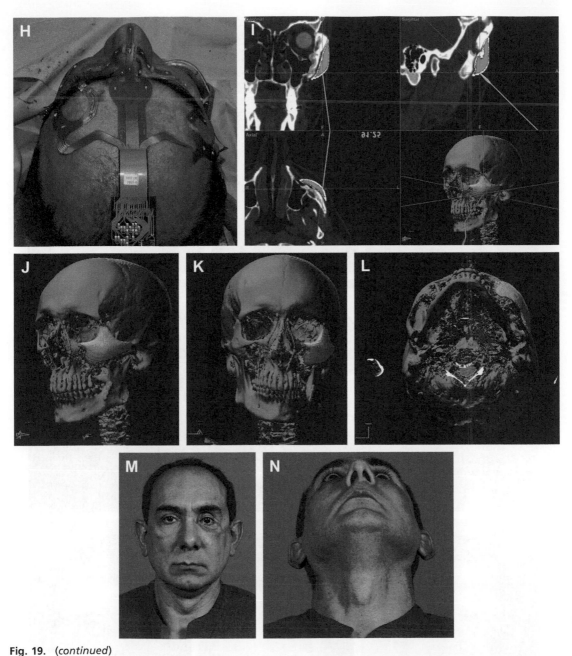

Fig. 19. (continued)

Costochondral Grafts

Autologous rib grafts are another option for free bone graft reconstruction of defects of the craniofacial skeleton.[113] The gentle curve of the rib, and the thick, bicortical bone, result in ipsilateral rib grafts being an acceptable reconstructive option for cases in which the zygomatic arch has been resected.[114]

Microvascular Free Tissue Transfer

Microvascular free flaps are becoming common for reconstruction of craniofacial cancer defects.[115] High maxillectomy defects are often restored with fibular myocutaneous flaps, because the fibula allows immediate or secondary dental implantation and prosthodontics rehabilitation.[116] Either vascularized or nonvascularized fibula

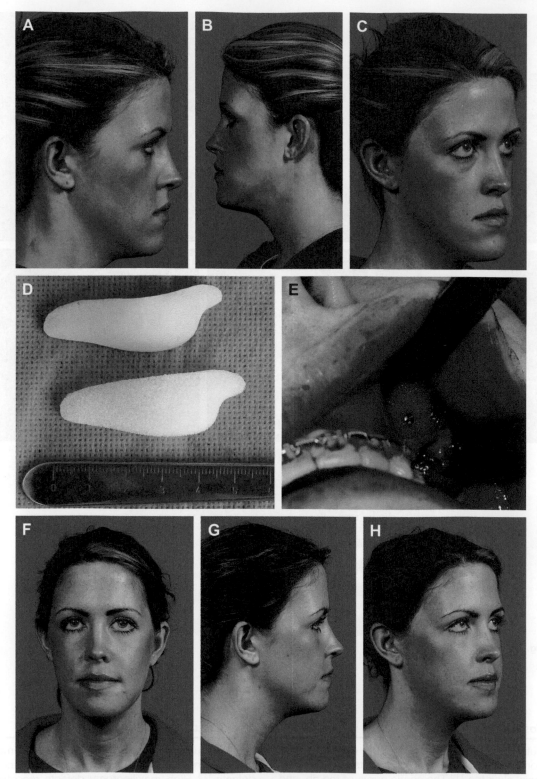

Fig. 20. Patient with class III occlusion and high midface deficiency (*A–C*). Patient underwent bilateral sagittal split osteotomy, reduction genioplasty, and bilateral alloplastic malar implantation. Trial (*top*) and actual malar (*bottom*) implants (*D*). Insertion and fixation of implant via a Keen approach (*E*). Postoperative frontal (*F*), side profile (*G*), and three-quarter-turn (*H*) views of patient.

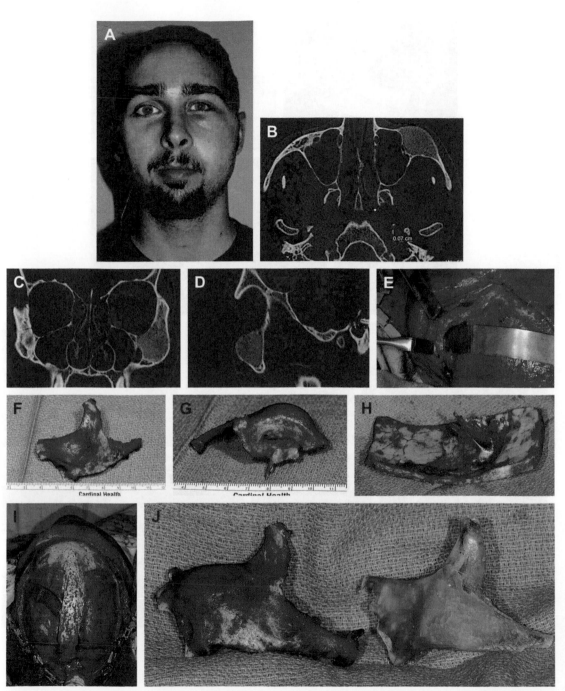

Fig. 21. Twenty-four-year-old man who presented with craniofacial fibrous dysplasia of the left zygoma (*A*). Axial (*B*), coronal (*C*), and sagittal (*D*) CT views of the patient. The zygoma was approached with a coronal incision (*E*). The tumor was resected (*F, G*). Biparietal calvarial bone grafts were harvested (*I*), with dimensions matching that of the resected zygoma (*H*). Using stereolithographic models (*J*), split-thickness calvarial bone grafts were adapted to restore previous orbitozygomatic dimensions (*K, L*). Split-thickness bone was then reapproximated and fixated to the skull (*M, N*). The adapted bone grafts were then applied and fixated to the patient's defect (*O*). Using the stereolithographic model, orbital mesh was adapted and applied to the lateral orbit and orbital floor defect (*P*). Immediate postoperative bird's-eye view (*Q*). Axial CT view showing restoration of zygomatic arch projection, width, and malar projection (*R*). Postoperative frontal (*S*) and worm's-eye (*T*) views of the patient 1 year after reconstruction.

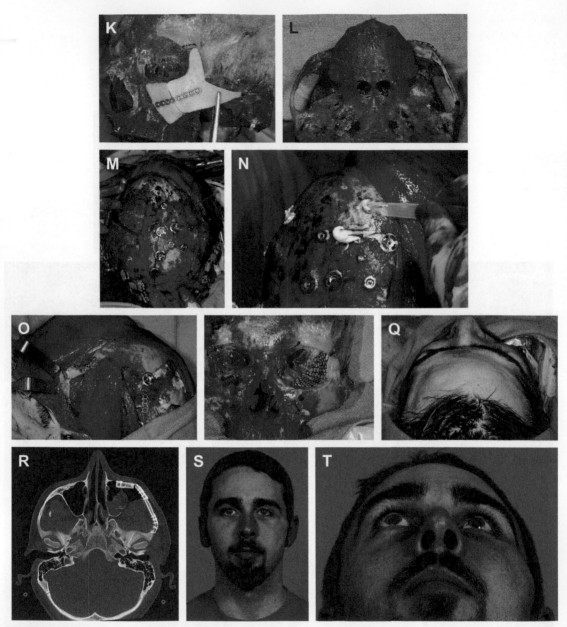

Fig. 21. (*continued*)

provides excellent length and may be fashioned to recreate the external orbit and zygoma when necessary.

COMPUTER-ASSISTED RECONSTRUCTION OF ACQUIRED ZYGOMATIC DEFORMITIES

Computer-aided, or virtual, surgery refers to the integration of three-dimensional data into the

surgical planning, treatment, and postoperative assessment of patients.

Virtual surgery generally consists of 4 phases: (1) the data acquisition phase, consisting of clinical and radiographic examinations; (2) the planning phase, in which CT scan data are imported into proprietary planning software and the ablation and reconstruction are planned; (3) the surgical phase, in which the virtual surgical plan is translated to the patient; and (4) the assessment phase, evaluating the accuracy of the virtual surgical plan using intraoperative or postoperative CT imaging.

Data Acquisition Phase

The data acquisition phase for all virtual surgical cases begins with a careful clinical examination. When planning for zygoma reconstruction, bony evaluation by CT scan must be balanced with evaluation of the soft tissue character and thickness. Zygoma reconstruction may include portions of the orbit and/or the maxilla and supporting dentition. If autogenous grafting is planned, CT scanning of the corresponding planned bony harvest site should be obtained (ie, cranial bone or fibula).

Planning Phase

The CT images are transferred to the proprietary surgical planning software in DICOM (Digital Imaging and Communications in Medicine) format using a process termed back conversion. The planning phase differs greatly depending on whether the orbit and/or the maxilla and dentition will be involved in the reconstruction. If the orbit will be involved, restoring orbital volume is a critical consideration in successful reconstruction. The normal, contralateral side is mirrored to the defective side for ideal orbital and zygomatic positioning (**Fig. 22**). For orbital reconstruction, stock implants can be prebent on the stereolithographic model, or custom plates may be constructed using the digital data alone. The virtual defect is reconstructed with a virtual bone graft, stents of which can be printed to serve as a cutting guide or template. Stereolithographic models of the unreconstructed and reconstructed skeletons are constructed, which then serve as a platform on which to try in the bone grafts and to prebend plates.

Surgical Phase

Intraoperative navigation is particularly useful in zygoma reconstruction as an aide to assess malar projection and orbital implant/bone graft positioning. Once the patient's position in space is registered to the CT dataset, the position of the surgical probe is tracked by a device called a localizer, and may be viewed in real time in the x, y, and z axes of the CT, as well as on the three-dimensional representation of the CT dataset.

Cutting guides allow reproduction of the ideal position and angle of osteotomy cuts created with the preoperative planning software, thus the assessment phase begins during the operation. In cases of full-thickness cranial bone grafting for malar reconstruction, cutting guides created with the planning software are used to cut the cranial bone to fit precisely into the defect left by the tumor resection.

Assessment Phase

A portable CT scanner is used to assess the accuracy of the reconstruction in the operating room before emergence from anesthesia, which allows immediate correction of discrepancies between the planned and actual treatment result. If intraoperative CT evaluation is not performed, postoperative CT imaging is used in the same way to evaluate planned versus actual outcomes. Postoperative CT is an invaluable tool to assess adequacy of reduction as well as assessing progress in

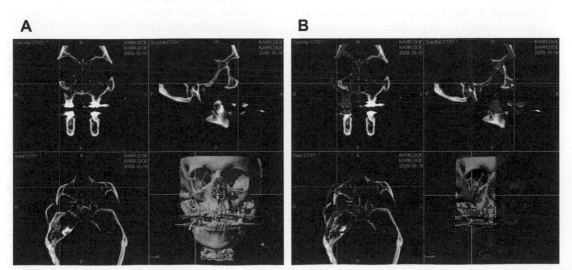

Fig. 22. Preoperative CT views of zygomatic deformity (*A*). Red represents the optimal mirrored side used as goal reconstruction (*B*).

surgical skill by allowing surgeons to evaluate their work.[16] However, the drawback of postoperative CT is the inability to readily fix inaccuracies in reduction. Intraoperative CT remediates this problem by allowing surgeons not only to evaluate their reduction and fixation, but to make immediate changes based on their assessments.[117,118] Additional details on computer-assisted zygoma reconstruction are given earlier in this article.

SUMMARY

The most common error in reconstruction of acquired deformities of the zygoma is inadequate restoration of malar projection. This error is typically caused by creating an outward curve of the zygomatic arch facilitated by medial rotation of the ZM complex. If a coronal incision is not performed, accurate rotation of the ZM complex can be assessed by inspecting the SZ suture region via an upper lid blepharoplasty approach. Failure to adequately flatten the zygomatic arch and achieve optimal rotation of the ZM complex results in flattening of the malar eminence and widening of the ipsilateral face. Modern digital technology may now be used to optimize treatment outcomes in patients with complex deformities. Intraoperative navigation is used to assess malar projection and orbital implant position, and stereolithographic models are used to fit bone grafts or flaps at the time of inset. In addition, modern mobile CT scanners are helpful to evaluate the accuracy of the reconstruction and the transfer of the virtual plan into reality.

REFERENCES

1. Bogusiak K, Arkuszewski P. Characteristics and epidemiology of zygomaticomaxillary complex fractures. J Craniofac Surg 2010;21:1018–23.
2. Knight JS, North JF. The classification of malar fractures: an analysis of displacement as a guide to treatment. Br J Plast Surg 1961;13:325–39.
3. Gruss JS, Van Wyck L, Phillips JH, et al. The importance of the zygomatic arch in complex midfacial fracture repair and correction of posttraumatic orbitozygomatic deformities. Plast Reconstr Surg 1990;85:878–90.
4. Manson PN, Hoopes JE, Su CT. Structural pillars of the facial skeleton: an approach to the management of Le Fort fractures. Plast Reconstr Surg 1980;66:54–62.
5. Majewski WT, Yu JC, Ewart C, et al. Posttraumatic craniofacial reconstruction using combined resorbable and nonresorbable fixation systems. Ann Plast Surg 2002;48:471–6.
6. Sicher H, Tandler J. Anatomie für Zahnärzte. Vienna (Austria): Springer; 1928.
7. Dingman OR, Native P. Surgery of the facial skeleton. Philadelphia: Saunders; 1964.
8. Rowe NL, Killey J. Fractures of the facial skeleton. Baltimore (MD): Williams & Wilkins; 1968.
9. Fujii N, Yamashiro M. Classification of malar complex fractures using computed tomography. J Oral Maxillofac Surg 1983;41:562–7.
10. Jackson IT. Classification and treatment of orbitozygomatic and orbitoethmoid fractures. The place of bone grafting and plate fixation. Clin Plast Surg 1989;16:77–91.
11. Rohrich RJ, Hollier LH, Watumull D. Optimizing the management of orbitozygomatic fractures. Clin Plast Surg 1992;19:149–65.
12. Stanley RB Jr. The zygomatic arch as a guide to reconstruction of comminuted malar fractures. Arch Otolaryngol Head Neck Surg 1989;115:1459–62.
13. Donat TL, Endress C, Mathog RH. Facial fracture classification according to skeletal support mechanisms. Arch Otolaryngol Head Neck Surg 1998;124:1306–14.
14. Bächli H, Leiggener H, Gawelin P, et al. Skull base and maxillofacial fractures: two centre study with correlation of clinical findings with a comprehensive craniofacial classification system. J Craniomaxillofac Surg 2009;37:305–11.
15. Ozyazgan I, Gunay GK, Eskitascioglu T, et al. A new proposal of classification of zygomatic arch fractures. J Oral Maxillofac Surg 2007;65:462–9.
16. Manson PN, Markowitz B, Mirvis S, et al. Toward CT-based facial fracture treatment. Plast Reconstr Surg 1990;85:202–12 [discussion: 213–4].
17. Ellis E 3rd, Kittidumkerng W. Analysis of treatment for isolated zygomaticomaxillary complex fractures. J Oral Maxillofac Surg 1996;54:386–400 [discussion: 400–1].
18. Makowski GJ, Van Sickels JE. Evaluation of results with three-point visualization of zygomaticomaxillary complex fractures. Oral Surg Oral Med Oral Pathol Oral Radiol Endod 1995;80:624–8.
19. Rohner D, Tay A, Meng CS, et al. The sphenozygomatic suture as a key site for osteosynthesis of the orbitozygomatic complex in panfacial fractures: a biomechanical study in human cadavers based on clinical practice. Plast Reconstr Surg 2002;110:1463–71 [discussion: 1472–5].
20. Rieger G. A rare cause of complete "spectacle hematoma". Ger J Ophthalmol 1996;5:415–6.
21. Altonen M, Kohonen A, Dickhoff K. Treatment of zygomatic fractures: internal wiring-antral-packing-reposition without fixation. J Maxillofac Surg 1976;4:107–15.
22. Bite U, Jackson IT, Forbes GS, et al. Orbital volume measurements in enophthalmos using

three-dimensional CT imaging. Plast Reconstr Surg 1985;75:502–8.

23. Hornby SJ, Ward SJ, Gilbert CE. Eye birth defects in humans may be caused by a recessively-inherited genetic predisposition to the effects of maternal vitamin A deficiency during pregnancy. Med Sci Monit 2003;9:HY23–6.

24. Karlan MS, Cassisi NJ. Fractures of the zygoma. A geometric, biomechanical, and surgical analysis. Arch Otolaryngol 1979;105:320–7.

25. Pearl RM. Surgical management of volumetric changes in the bony orbit. Ann Plast Surg 1987; 19:349–58.

26. Pearl RM, Vistnes LM. Orbital blowout fractures: an approach to management. Ann Plast Surg 1978;1: 267–70.

27. Zingg M, Chowdhury K, Ladrach K, et al. Treatment of 813 zygoma-lateral orbital complex fractures. New aspects. Arch Otolaryngol Head Neck Surg 1991;117:611–20 [discussion: 621–2].

28. Wiesenbaugh JM Jr. Diagnostic evaluation of zygomatic complex fractures. J Oral Surg 1970; 28:204–8.

29. Vriens JP, van der Glas HW, Moos KF, et al. Infraorbital nerve function following treatment of orbitozygomatic complex fractures. A multitest approach. Int J Oral Maxillofac Surg 1998;27:27–32.

30. Taicher S, Ardekian L, Samet N, et al. Recovery of the infraorbital nerve after zygomatic complex fractures: a preliminary study of different treatment methods. Int J Oral Maxillofac Surg 1993;22:339–41.

31. Koornneef L. New insights in the human orbital connective tissue. Result of a new anatomical approach. Arch Ophthalmol 1977;95:1269–73.

32. Manson PN, Clark N, Robertson B, et al. Subunit principles in midface fractures: the importance of sagittal buttresses, soft-tissue reductions, and sequencing treatment of segmental fractures. Plast Reconstr Surg 1999;103:1287–306 [quiz: 1307].

33. Kenn WW. Surgery: its principles and practice. Philadelphia: Saunders; 1909.

34. Manson PN, Ruas E, Iliff N, et al. Single eyelid incision for exposure of the zygomatic bone and orbital reconstruction. Plast Reconstr Surg 1987;79:120–6.

35. Wray RC, Holtmann B, Ribaudo JM, et al. A comparison of conjunctival and subciliary incisions for orbital fractures. Br J Plast Surg 1977; 30:142–5.

36. Baker TJ, Gordon HL, Mosienko P. Upper lid blepharoplasty. Plast Reconstr Surg 1977;60:692–8.

37. Eppley BL, Custer PL, Sadove AM. Cutaneous approaches to the orbital skeleton and periorbital structures. J Oral Maxillofac Surg 1990;48:842–54.

38. Haug RH, Van Sickels JE, Jenkins WS. Demographics and treatment options for orbital roof fractures. Oral Surg Oral Med Oral Pathol Oral Radiol Endod 2002;93:238–46.

39. Heckler FR, Songcharoen S, Sultani FA. Subciliary incision and skin-muscle eyelid flap for orbital fractures. Ann Plast Surg 1983;10:309–13.

40. Perman KI. Upper eyelid blepharoplasty. J Dermatol Surg Oncol 1992;18:1096–9.

41. Kung DS, Kaban LB. Supratarsal fold incision for approach to the superior lateral orbit. Oral Surg Oral Med Oral Pathol Oral Radiol Endod 1996;81: 522–5.

42. Ellis E, Zide MF. Surgical approaches to the facial skeleton. Philadelphia: Lippincott Williams & Wilkins; 2006. p. 251, xii.

43. Pozatek ZW, Kaban LB, Guralnick WC. Fractures of the zygomatic complex: an evaluation of surgical management with special emphasis on the eyebrow approach. J Oral Surg 1973;31:141–8.

44. Appling WD, Patrinely JR, Salzer TA. Transconjunctival approach vs subciliary skin-muscle flap approach for orbital fracture repair. Arch Otolaryngol Head Neck Surg 1993;119:1000–7.

45. Bahr W, Bagambisa FB, Schlegel G, et al. Comparison of transcutaneous incisions used for exposure of the infraorbital rim and orbital floor: a retrospective study. Plast Reconstr Surg 1992; 90:585–91.

46. Baumann A, Ewers R. Transcaruncular approach for reconstruction of medial orbital wall fracture. Int J Oral Maxillofac Surg 2000;29:264–7.

47. Holtmann B, Wray RC, Little AG. A randomized comparison of four incisions for orbital fractures. Plast Reconstr Surg 1981;67:731–7.

48. Kushner GM. Surgical approaches to the infraorbital rim and orbital floor: the case for the transconjunctival approach. J Oral Maxillofac Surg 2006; 64:108–10.

49. Lee CS, Yoon JS, Lee SY. Combined transconjunctival and transcaruncular approach for repair of large medial orbital wall fractures. Arch Ophthalmol 2009;127:291–6.

50. Netscher DT, Patrinely JR, Peltier M, et al. Transconjunctival versus transcutaneous lower eyelid blepharoplasty: a prospective study. Plast Reconstr Surg 1995;96:1053–60.

51. Rohrich RJ, Janis JE, Adams WP Jr. Subciliary versus subtarsal approaches to orbitozygomatic fractures. Plast Reconstr Surg 2003;111:1708–14.

52. Wilson S, Ellis E 3rd. Surgical approaches to the infraorbital rim and orbital floor: the case for the subtarsal approach. J Oral Maxillofac Surg 2006;64: 104–7.

53. De Riu G, Meloni SM, Gobbi R, et al. Subciliary versus swinging eyelid approach to the orbital floor. J Craniomaxillofac Surg 2008;36:439–42.

54. Ridgway EB, Chen C, Colakoglu S, et al. The incidence of lower eyelid malposition after facial fracture repair: a retrospective study and meta-analysis comparing subtarsal, subciliary, and

transconjunctival incisions. Plast Reconstr Surg 2009;124:1578–86.

55. Tenzel RR, Miller GR. Orbital blow-out fracture repair, conjunctival approach. Am J Ophthalmol 1971;71:1141–2.

56. Converse JM, Firmin F, Wood-Smith D, et al. The conjunctival approach in orbital fractures. Plast Reconstr Surg 1973;52:656–7.

57. Stoll W, Busse H, Kroll P. Transconjunctival incision and lateral canthotomy. A suitable approach for orbital floor and zygomatic bone correction. Laryngol Rhinol Otol (Stuttg) 1984;63:45–7 [in German].

58. Ciarallo RL, Ziccardi VB, Ochs MW. Combined transconjunctival lateral canthotomy approach for infraorbital nerve exploration: report of a case. J Oral Maxillofac Surg 1994;52:79–81.

59. Hadeed H, Ziccardi VB, Sotereanos GC, et al. Lateral canthotomy transconjunctival approach to the orbit. Oral Surg Oral Med Oral Pathol 1992;73:526–30.

60. Pospisil OA, Fernando TD. Review of the lower blepharoplasty incision as a surgical approach to zygomatic-orbital fractures. Br J Oral Maxillofac Surg 1984;22:261–8.

61. Feldman EM, Bruner TW, Sharabi SE, et al. The subtarsal incision: where should it be placed? J Oral Maxillofac Surg 2011;69:2419–23.

62. Goldthwaite RH. Plastic repair of depressed fracture of lower orbital rim. J Am Med Assoc 1924;82:628–9.

63. Carter TG, Bagheri S, Dierks EJ. Towel clip reduction of the depressed zygomatic arch fracture. J Oral Maxillofac Surg 2005;63:1244–6.

64. Gillies HD, Pomfret Kilner T, Stone D. Fractures of the malar-zygomatic compound: with a description of a new x-ray position. Br J Surg 1927;14:56.

65. Abubaker AO, Sotereanos G, Patterson GT. Use of the coronal surgical incision for reconstruction of severe craniomaxillofacial injuries. J Oral Maxillofac Surg 1990;48:579–86.

66. Matras H, Kuderna H. Combined cranio-facial fractures. J Maxillofac Surg 1980;8:52–9.

67. Luo W, Wang L, Jing W, et al. A new coronal scalp technique to treat craniofacial fracture: the supratemporalis approach. Oral Surg Oral Med Oral Pathol Oral Radiol Endod 2012;113:177–82.

68. Markiewicz MR, Bell RB. Traditional and contemporary surgical approaches to the orbit. Oral Maxillofac Surg Clin North Am 2012;24:573–607.

69. Al-Kayat A, Bramley P. A modified pre-auricular approach to the temporomandibular joint and malar arch. Br J Oral Surg 1979;17:91–103.

70. Furnas DW. Landmarks for the trunk and the temporofacial division of the facial nerve. Br J Surg 1965;52:694–6.

71. Stuzin JM, Wagstrom L, Kawamoto HK, et al. Anatomy of the frontal branch of the facial nerve: the significance of the temporal fat pad. Plast Reconstr Surg 1989;83:265–71.

72. Munro IR, Fearon JA. The coronal incision revisited. Plast Reconstr Surg 1994;93:185–7.

73. Fox AJ, Tatum SA. The coronal incision: sinusoidal, sawtooth, and postauricular techniques. Arch Facial Plast Surg 2003;5:259–62.

74. Hanasono MM, Utley DS, Goode RL. The temporalis muscle flap for reconstruction after head and neck oncologic surgery. Laryngoscope 2001;111:1719–25.

75. Kim S, Matic DB. The anatomy of temporal hollowing: the superficial temporal fat pad. J Craniofac Surg 2005;16:651–4.

76. Rontal E, Rontal M, Guilford FT. Surgical anatomy of the orbit. Ann Otol Rhinol Laryngol 1979;88:382–6.

77. Yamamoto Y, Kawashima K, Sugihara T, et al. Surgical management of maxillectomy defects based on the concept of buttress reconstruction. Head Neck 2004;26:247–56.

78. Gruss JS, Mackinnon SE. Complex maxillary fractures: role of buttress reconstruction and immediate bone grafts. Plast Reconstr Surg 1986;78:9–22.

79. Ellis E 3rd, Reddy L. Status of the internal orbit after reduction of zygomaticomaxillary complex fractures. J Oral Maxillofac Surg 2004;62:275–83.

80. Shumrick KA, Kersten RC, Kulwin DR, et al. Criteria for selective management of the orbital rim and floor in zygomatic complex and midface fractures. Arch Otolaryngol Head Neck Surg 1997;123:378–84.

81. Bell RB, Markiewicz MR. Computer-assisted planning, stereolithographic modeling, and intraoperative navigation for complex orbital reconstruction: a descriptive study in a preliminary cohort. J Oral Maxillofac Surg 2009;67:2559–70.

82. Reymond J, Kwiatkowski J, Wysocki J. Clinical anatomy of the superior orbital fissure and the orbital apex. J Craniomaxillofac Surg 2008;36:346–53.

83. Peter NM, Pearson AR. Orbital apex syndrome from blunt ocular trauma. Orbit 2010;29:42–4.

84. Oester AE Jr, Sahu P, Fowler B, et al. Radiographic predictors of visual outcome in orbital compartment syndrome. Ophthal Plast Reconstr Surg 2012;28:7–10.

85. Karabekir HS, Gocmen-Mas N, Emel E, et al. Ocular and periocular injuries associated with an isolated orbital fracture depending on a blunt cranial trauma: anatomical and surgical aspects. J Craniomaxillofac Surg 2011;40(7):e189–93.

86. Turko A, Talbot S, Pomahac B. Medial orbital wall fracture with associated medial rectus entrapment and retrobulbar hematoma. Plast Reconstr Surg 2009;123:108e–9e.

87. Yazici B, Gonen T. Posttraumatic subperiosteal hematomas of the orbit in children. Ophthal Plast Reconstr Surg 2011;27:33–7.

88. Ellis E 3rd, el-Attar A, Moos KF. An analysis of 2,067 cases of zygomatico-orbital fracture. J Oral Maxillofac Surg 1985;43:417–28.

89. Manson PN, Clifford CM, Su CT, et al. Mechanisms of global support and posttraumatic enophthalmos: I. The anatomy of the ligament sling and its relation to intramuscular cone orbital fat. Plast Reconstr Surg 1986;77:193–202.

90. Ploder O, Klug C, Voracek M, et al. Evaluation of computer-based area and volume measurement from coronal computed tomography scans in isolated blowout fractures of the orbital floor. J Oral Maxillofac Surg 2002;60:1267–72 [discussion: 1273–4].

91. Dolynchuk KN, Tadjalli HE, Manson PN. Orbital volumetric analysis: clinical application in orbitozygomatic complex injuries. J Craniomaxillofac Trauma 1996;2:56–63 [discussion: 64].

92. Manson PN, Grivas A, Rosenbaum A, et al. Studies on enophthalmos: II. The measurement of orbital injuries and their treatment by quantitative computed tomography. Plast Reconstr Surg 1986; 77:203–14.

93. Raskin EM, Millman AL, Lubkin V, et al. Prediction of late enophthalmos by volumetric analysis of orbital fractures. Ophthal Plast Reconstr Surg 1998;14:19–26.

94. Markiewicz MR, Dierks EJ, Bell RB. Does intraoperative navigation restore orbital dimensions in traumatic and post-ablative defects? J Craniomaxillofac Surg 2012;40:142–8.

95. Markiewicz MR, Dierks EJ, Potter BE, et al. Reliability of intraoperative navigation in restoring normal orbital dimensions. J Oral Maxillofac Surg 2011;69:2833–40.

96. Brandt MT, Haug RH. Traumatic hyphema: a comprehensive review. J Oral Maxillofac Surg 2001;59:1462–70.

97. Romano PE, Robinson JA. Traumatic hyphema: a comprehensive review of the past half century yields 8076 cases for which specific medical treatment reduces rebleeding 62%, from 13% to 5% (P<.0001). Binocul Vis Strabismus Q 2000;15:175–86.

98. Layoun W, Guyot L, Richard O, et al. Augmentation of cheek bone contour using malar osteotomy. Aesthetic Plast Surg 2003;27:269–74.

99. Mommaerts MY, Nadjmi N, Abeloos JV, et al. Six year's experience with the zygomatic "sandwich" osteotomy for correction of malar deficiency. J Oral Maxillofac Surg 1999;57:8–13 [discussion: 14–5].

100. Yaremchuk MJ, Doumit G, Thomas MA. Alloplastic augmentation of the facial skeleton: an occasional adjunct or alternative to orthognathic surgery. Plast Reconstr Surg 2011;127:2021–30.

101. Hilinski JM, Cohen SR. Soft tissue augmentation with ArteFill. Facial Plast Surg 2009;25:114–9.

102. Lacey M, Antonyshyn O, MacGregor JH. Temporal contour deformity after coronal flap elevation: an anatomical study. J Craniomaxillofac Surg 1994;5:223–7.

103. Matic DB, Kim S. Temporal hollowing following coronal incision: a prospective, randomized, controlled trial. Plast Reconstr Surg 2008;121: 379e–85e.

104. Baek RM, Heo CY, Lee SW. Temporal dissection technique that prevents temporal hollowing in coronal approach. J Craniofac Surg 2009;20:748–51.

105. Steinbacher DM, Wink J, Bartlett SP. Temporal hollowing following surgical correction of unicoronal synostosis. Plast Reconstr Surg 2011;128:231–40.

106. Metzinger SE, McCollough EG, Campbell JP, et al. Malar augmentation: a 5-year retrospective review of the Silastic midfacial malar implant. Arch Otolaryngol Head Neck Surg 1999;125:980–7.

107. Spector M, Harmon SL, Kreutner A. Characteristics of tissue growth into Proplast and porous polyethylene implants in bone. J Biomed Mater Res 1979;13:677–92.

108. Chambless LB, Mawn LA, Forbes JA, et al. Porous polyethylene implant reconstruction of the orbit after resection of spheno-orbital meningiomas: a novel technique. J Craniomaxillofac Surg 2012;40:e28–32.

109. Scolozzi P. Maxillofacial reconstruction using polyetheretherketone patient-specific implants by "mirroring" computational planning. Aesthetic Plast Surg 2012;36:660–5.

110. Maves MD, Matt BH. Calvarial bone grafting of facial defects. Otolaryngol Head Neck Surg 1986; 95:464–70.

111. Zhang Z, Niu F, Tang X, et al. Staged reconstruction for adult complete Treacher Collins syndrome. J Craniofac Surg 2009;20:1433–8.

112. Posnick JC, Goldstein JA, Waitzman AA. Surgical correction of the Treacher Collins malar deficiency: quantitative CT scan analysis of long-term results. Plast Reconstr Surg 1993;92:12–22.

113. Wang X, Chen J, Zhang Y, et al. Associated balancing surgical treatments of hemifacial microsomia. J Craniofac Surg 2010;21:1456–9.

114. Ladehinde AL, Ogunlewe MO, Thomas MO. Zygomatic arch reconstruction with autogenous rib bone graft in a post irradiated patient – a case report. Niger Postgrad Med J 2005;12:61–4.

115. Fisher M, Dorafshar A, Bojovic B, et al. The evolution of critical concepts in aesthetic craniofacial microsurgical reconstruction. Plast Reconstr Surg 2012;130:389–98.

116. Sun J, Shen Y, Li J, et al. Reconstruction of high maxillectomy defects with the fibula osteomyocutaneous flap in combination with titanium mesh or a zygomatic implant. Plast Reconstr Surg 2011; 127:150–60.

117. Collyer J. Stereotactic navigation in oral and maxillofacial surgery. Br J Oral Maxillofac Surg 2010;48: 79–83.

118. Pham AM, Rafii AA, Metzger MC, et al. Computer modeling and intraoperative navigation in maxillofacial surgery. Otolaryngol Head Neck Surg 2007; 137:624–31.

Lip Reconstruction

Joshua E. Lubek, DDS, MD, FACS[a,b,*],
Robert A. Ord, DDS, MD, FRCS, FACS, MS[a]

KEYWORDS

- Lip reconstruction • Full-thickness lip defect • Microvascular flap reconstruction
- Oncologic ablation

KEY POINTS

- Defects covering less than one-third of the lip may be closed primarily.
- Innervated local flaps provide excellent cosmesis and function for defects from one-third to subtotal reconstruction.
- Subtotal or total defects, or involvement of other facial subunits will likely require microvascular flap reconstruction.
- A thorough knowledge of lip anatomy and various reconstructive local and distant flap techniques is required to reconstruct complex defects of the lips.

INTRODUCTION

This article discusses the reconstruction of full-thickness defects of the lower and upper lip. Although these may occur as a result of hereditary disorders (cleft lip) or trauma, reconstruction is described in relation to oncologic ablation for primary lip cancers. These defects will obviously be preplanned and of a regular shape, unlike injuries sustained from penetrating trauma. Therefore, precise elective planning of reconstruction techniques must be undertaken.

Anatomically the lips comprise 3 layers: skin, muscle, and mucosa. In an ideal functional reconstruction, all 3 will be replaced. A further subunit, the vermilion, will require consideration. The lips play an important role in speech, facial expression, swallowing, preservation of an oral seal, and facial cosmesis.

When considering lip reconstruction following tumor ablation, the "reconstruction ladder" starts with the simplest procedures, moving up to the most complex. Primary closure of the lip is the simplest technique for small defects. Local flaps are the next option, and these have the advantage of good color match, easy accessibility, simplicity in the surgical technique, and use of innervated muscle for function. Local flaps also have some disadvantages, including the need to make extra skin incisions on the face and the lack of sufficient tissue for major defects. Skin/mucosal grafts have little utility for lip reconstruction. Rarely are pedicled flaps used for massive defects, and microvascular free flaps are often used as the next option. Free flaps have the advantage of supplying large amounts of tissue that can be used to reconstruct the entire lip plus involved subunits such as the chin or mandible if needed. Many donor sites are available, and skin, fascia, muscle, tendon, and even bone can all be included within a particular flap. The disadvantages are poor color match, a longer operative time, the need to access the

[a] Oncology Program, Department of Oral & Maxillofacial Surgery, Greenebaum Cancer Center, University of Maryland, 650 West Baltimore Street Room 1401, Baltimore, MD 21201, USA; [b] Maxillofacial Oncology & Microvascular Surgery, Department of Oral & Maxillofacial Surgery, University of Maryland, 650 West Baltimore Street, Room 1401, Baltimore, MD 21201, USA
* Corresponding author. Maxillofacial Oncology & Microvascular Surgery, Department of Oral & Maxillofacial Surgery, University of Maryland, 650 West Baltimore Street, Room 1401, Baltimore, MD 21201.
E-mail address: jlubek@umaryland.edu

Oral Maxillofacial Surg Clin N Am 25 (2013) 203–214
http://dx.doi.org/10.1016/j.coms.2013.01.001
1042-3699/13/$ – see front matter © 2013 Elsevier Inc. All rights reserved.

neck for donor vessels, and the need for specialized equipment and surgical expertise.

PRIMARY CLOSURE

The lips are generally lax with redundant soft tissue, especially in the elderly patient, and when defects constitute less than one-third of the lip, primary closure is usually possible without causing a "tight lip" or significant microstomia, so that eating or placing dentures is not problematic. Older patients who have a higher incidence of lip cancers have more lax tissue, and the repaired lip will stretch somewhat with function. The normal lower lip is 7 cm in width, allowing for defects of 2 to 2.5 cm to be closed primarily without difficulty.[1] To obtain the best cosmetic and functional results, the following points are of surgical importance.

- Align the skin/vermilion border. If the border is not well aligned there will be an obvious "step" appearance, which will draw the observer's eye to the wound. In sun-damaged lips the normal clearly defined skin/vermilion border may be blurred, and alignment may be difficult. When working under local anesthesia, the vasoconstriction may blanch the area and prevent proper identification of the skin/vermilion. To prevent this problem, the border can be tattooed temporarily using a small syringe needle and methylene blue.
- Undermine the skin and mucosal edges of the wound, thus allowing the skin and mucosal edges to be everted without tension, to give an aesthetic wound closure (**Fig. 1**).

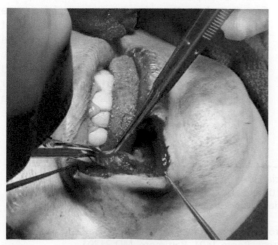

Fig. 1. Using sharp-pointed scissors to undermine skin and mucosal edges and define the orbicularis muscle following shield-shaped excision.

- Dissect out the orbicularis oris muscle. The muscle should be dissected free for a few millimeters to allow ease of deep-suture placement. Failure to close the 2 edges of muscle layer will give depressions and "whistle" deformities in function (**Fig. 2**).
- Use small 5-0 or 6-0 monofilament (nylon/prolene) sutures for skin closure.

When using W-shaped excisions for larger defects, it is important not to suture across the tip of the small inverted V-shaped flap at the inferior portion of the excision to avoid avascular necrosis of the tip (**Fig. 3**). In this circumstance a suture is passed through the skin of one edge of the defect, then passed through the subdermal layer of the tip of the V-shaped flap (see arrow in **Fig. 3**B) and out from deep through the skin on the opposite edge. This suture will secure the tip of the V-shaped flap in place without compressing the skin of the flap.

If the cancer is associated with dysplastic leukoplakia, the surrounding vermilion will need to be excised. It is best to excise the whole vermilion surface from wet line to skin vermilion border. If only part of the vermilion subunit is excised, the subsequent reconstruction looks very obvious. Simple undermining of the mucosa on the lingual side of the lip using sharp scissor dissection onto the vestibule followed by advancement of the mucosal flap is the simplest method of reconstruction (**Fig. 4**). This technique may cause thinning of the lip because of subsequent scar contracture, and care should be exercised in patients who do not have much vermilion showing preoperatively. However, it should be noted that in one study using anthropometric photography, all full-thickness reconstructions caused a tightening of the lip with retraction (**Fig. 5**), which caused thinning of the vermilion, leading to the impression of an aging face. The authors recommend that when using advancement flaps, it is important to introduce enough volume into the lip.[2]

In cases where vermilion replacement requires more bulk or the oral mucosa is not available, anterior-based tongue flaps are useful. Finally, when using W-shaped excisions in younger patients in whom it is more difficult to disguise scars, a design that places the W limbs in the submental fold can be considered (**Fig. 6**).

LOCAL FLAPS

Many local flaps have been described for lip reconstruction, and it is beyond the scope of this article to detail every type and variation.[3] These

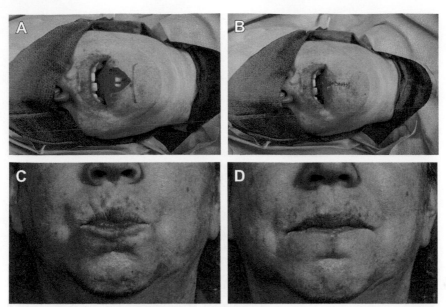

Fig. 2. (*A–D*) Wide local excision and primary closure of a lower lip squamous carcinoma. Good alignment of the lower vermillion and preservation of lip function.

local flaps work very well for patients with defects covering from one-third to two-thirds of the lip. Even though they may be used for total lip reconstructions, they often do not provide enough tissue for this purpose, resulting in a tight lower lip that tends to curl in beneath the upper lip. The authors prefer advancement flaps, which maintain the alignment of the orbicularis muscle fibers and are

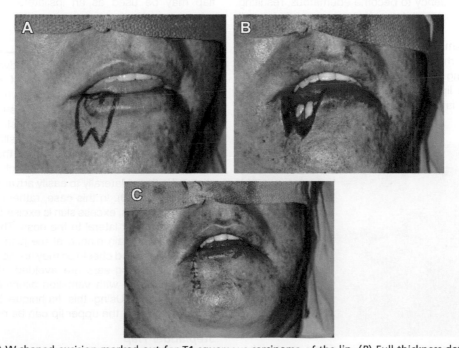

Fig. 3. (*A*) W-shaped excision marked out for T1 squamous carcinoma of the lip. (*B*) Full-thickness defect. Note pointed tip of inferior V-shaped flap. (*C*) Closure W to Y; sutures not placed across the tip of the inferior V-shaped flap.

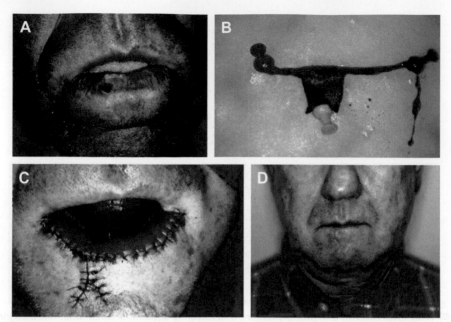

Fig. 4. (*A*) T1 squamous cell carcinoma of the lip with surrounding leukoplakia. (*B*) Surgical specimen pinned out to orient for the pathologist, showing W-shaped excision of the primary and vermilionectomy. (*C*) Surgical closure with mucosal advancement to replace the excised vermilion. (*D*) Postoperative result at 1 month. ([*C*] *Reproduced from* Amer Ord RA, Pazoki AE. Flap designs for lower lip reconstruction. Oral Maxillofac Surg Clin N 2003;15(4) 497–511.)

easy to design dimensionally. Although fan flaps work well, especially for cancers close to the commissure, they are often more difficult to design and have a tendency to become edematous, resulting in a "pincushion" deformity because of their small pedicle.

The simplest of the advancement flaps following a rhomboid excision is with a curved incision along the submental crease to release the adjacent lip and advance it into the defect. The incision is usually carried into the submental

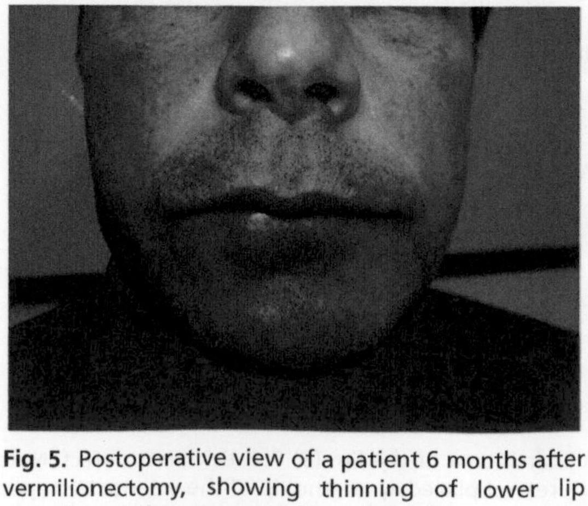

Fig. 5. Postoperative view of a patient 6 months after vermilionectomy, showing thinning of lower lip vermilion with some retraction of the lip.

region below the chin, where Burrows triangles can be removed in the skin to eliminate bunching or dog-ears as the flap is advanced (**Fig. 7**). This flap may be used as an ipsilateral or bilateral advancement.

Upper Lip Considerations

In the upper lip it is more difficult to advance flaps without causing distortion because of the central Cupid's bow, which can make any asymmetry obvious. The upper lip is released by a superior full-thickness incision through the lip just inferior to its junction with the nostril and nasal sill; this incision line is disguised by laying it at the junction of 2 facial subunits. The freely mobile cheek tissue allows the tissue laterally to easily advance toward the defect (**Fig. 8**). In this case, rather than using Burrows triangles, excess skin is excised as a perialar crescent just lateral to the nose. The excised tissue scar is again placed at the junction of the subunits (nose and cheek) so they are cosmetically pleasing and dog-ears are avoided. Closure is done in 3 layers with vermilion alignment as already detailed. Using this technique bilaterally, more than half of the upper lip can be replaced.

Stepladder Flap

In reconstruction of half to two-thirds of the lower lip, the stepladder technique has shown excellent

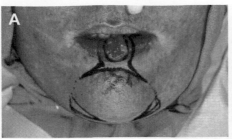 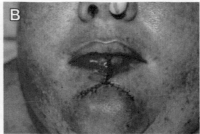

Fig. 6. (*A*) Modified W-shaped excision in a young woman with a large T1 of the central lower lip. Dotted lines indicate possible extension of incision if necessary, with submental Burrows triangles. (*B*) Final closure just as a modified W to T excision; no extension was required.

results.[4] This technique can be applied unilaterally, bilaterally (**Fig. 9**), or combined with vermilionectomy or other flaps (**Fig. 10**). The orbicularis remains aligned and the mouth opening is usually excellent. Placement of the incisions in the submental crease will give excellent cosmesis.

Fries Flap

When the commissure is involved, the stepladder flap can be combined with a Fries flap (**Fig. 11**).[5] The disadvantage of the Fries flap is the incision that extends from the commissure to the nasolabial fold, which can give a "Batman's Joker" appearance because of its location.

- When reconstructing defects at the commissure it is important to reconstruct the muscle

to prevent drooling. The orbicularis muscle of the upper lip is dissected free and sutured to the muscle in the lower lip flap with a large nonresorbable suture.
- When raising the Fries flap an excess of mucosa, which can then be folded over the flap and sutured to the skin edge of the flap to form the vermilion at the commissure, is taken.

Estlander Rotational Flap

Reconstruction of the commissure can also be achieved with the use of the Estlander rotational flap.[6] This technique involves a full-thickness (3-layer) lip-switch flap based on the labial artery. The flap is rotated 180° and sutured into the defect of the lower lip, allowing for restoration of perioral competence. Both upper and lower lip

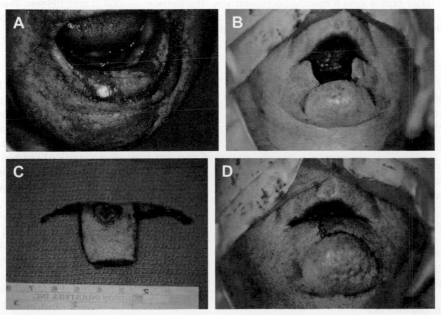

Fig. 7. (*A*) Squamous carcinoma of the lower lip with extensive premalignant changes in the vermilion. (*B*) Rhomboid excision with planned bilateral advancement flaps. (*C*) Surgical specimen with vermilionectomy. (*D*) Final closure needed only one flap advancement.

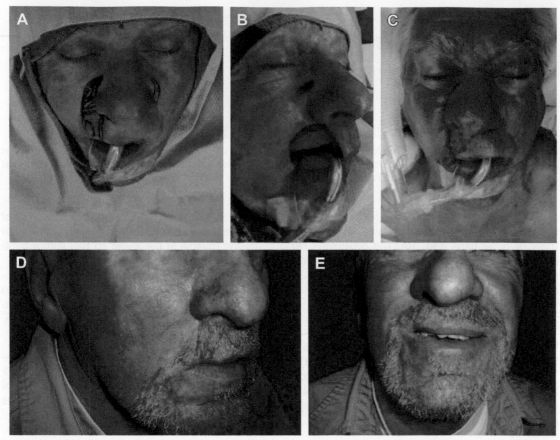

Fig. 8. (*A*) Adenoid cystic carcinoma of the right upper lip. In planning to resect the right lip, the blue arrow indicates area of perialar skin to be removed to allow advancement; the circle marks the tumor. (*B*) Excision of right upper lip. The edentulous alveolar ridge is visualized. (*C*) Following excision of perialar skin and advancement. (*D*) Three-quarter profile view 6 months postoperatively. The perialar incision is well hidden. There is a single vertical line in the upper lip. (*E*) Frontal view shows some rounding of the right commissure with some decrease in the width of the mouth. The patient was happy and does not wish revision commissurotomy.

commissure reconstruction can be performed using this technique. Often blunting of the commissure will result, and a secondary revision commissuroplasty will be necessary to improve aesthetics (**Fig. 12**).

- When designing the lip-switch rotational flap, the donor lip should be one-half the width of the defect to be reconstructed.
- Care must be taken to preserve the labial artery upon which the flap is pedicled.
- The flap can be divided and revision surgery can be performed at 3 to 4 weeks postoperatively, allowing for neovascularization and safe division of the pedicle.

Submental Island Flap

The submental island flap is a useful locoregional flap that can help in the reconstruction of lip defects. It provides the advantages of being a reliable flap with an axial-pattern blood supply, with excellent color match, tissue thickness, and ease of harvest.[7] It can be transferred either as a rotational flap or as free vascularized tissue (**Fig. 13**). Concerns regarding the risk of not being oncologically safe enough to perform a selective neck dissection (violation of lymph nodes within level I of the neck) have not been validated.

- A skin paddle measuring up to 15 × 7 cm can be harvested depending on the laxity of the cervical skin, allowing for primary closure of the donor-site defect.
- Preservation of the ipsilateral anterior belly of the digastric tendon can help to protect the submental pedicle, although this is not required for successful flap elevation and survival.

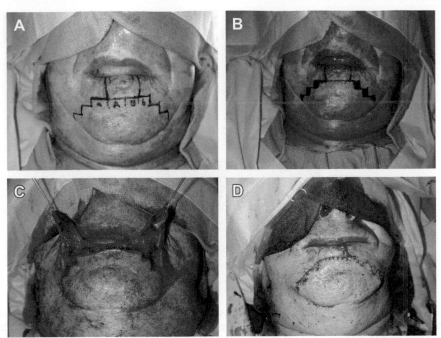

Fig. 9. (*A*) The cancer will be excised as a rectangle. The horizontal length of the excision is divided into 2 portions A + B. The flap lines a = A and b = B in length. The height of the steps is about 8 mm. (*B*) The areas of skin to be excised to allow advancement of the steps without bunching or dog-ears. Note that this skin removal is usually done as required after the flaps are raised and are being sutured. (*C*) The flaps are raised through skin and muscle; only the oral mucosa is left intact. (*D*) Following closure, the suture line approximates the line of the submental crease. (*Reproduced from* Amer Ord RA, Pazoki AE. Flap designs for lower lip reconstruction. Oral Maxillofac Surg Clin N 2003;15(4):497–511; with permission.)

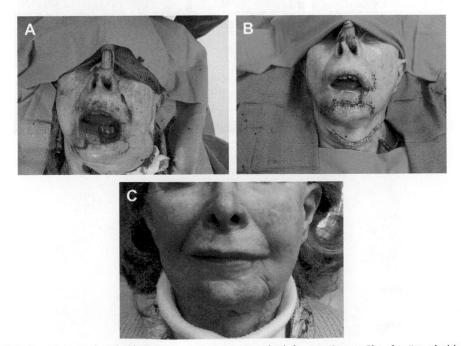

Fig. 10. (*A*) Defect of more than half of the lip, which involves the left commissure. Plan for "stepladder" flap on the right and Fries flap on the left. (*B*) Flaps sutured with commissurotomy on the left. An ipsilateral elective selective neck dissection has also been performed. (*C*) Final result after 6 months.

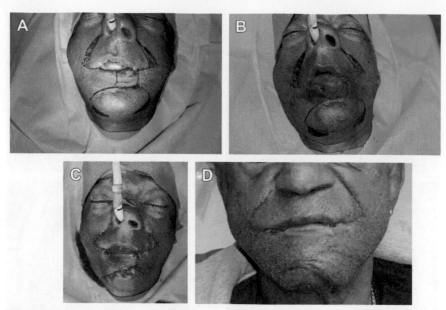

Fig. 11. (*A, B*) Reconstruction of half the lip with involvement of the commissure using bilateral Fries flaps. Note the Burrows triangles in the nasolabial folds and submental tissue. (*C*) Closure. Note that the horizontal excision at the commissure slopes cephalad toward the nasolabial fold. (*D*) Result after 1 month.

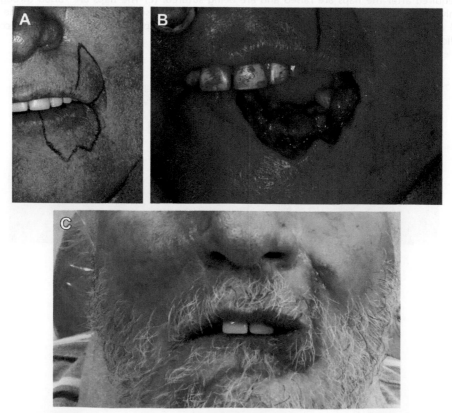

Fig. 12. (*A, B*) Estlander flap outlined for reconstruction of carcinoma involving the lower lip and commissure. (*C*) Estlander flap reconstruction of the lower lip with preservation of lip function. Note the blunting of the commissure.

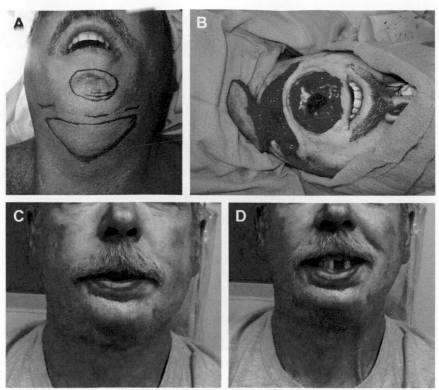

Fig. 13. (*A*) Recurrent basal cell carcinoma with involvement of the mentolabial fold. Anterior mandibular corticotomy and incisor tooth extraction was performed at initial surgery. (*B*) Submental island flap elevated to reconstruct the lip and chin defect. (*C, D*) After 18 months postoperative healing. A dental implant was placed into the incisor defect.

- One must ensure that there is no involvement of metastatic level I lymph nodes that could preclude the use of this flap.

Other Flaps

There are several techniques for using local flaps to reconstruct total/subtotal lip defects, including fan flaps, Fries flaps, and nasolabial flaps. The authors commonly use bilateral Fries flaps and even stepladder flaps, but usually the lip is tight and falls in below the upper lip, unless the patient has very lax tissues with redundant soft tissue in the cheeks. For these cases microvascular flaps should be discussed and considered, and this holds especially true if the tissues are already scarred or contracted locally (eg, after radiation) (**Fig. 14**).

- In flap reconstruction of the lip whereby vertical height is a problem leading to lip incompetence, as a result of extension of the defect to the commissure, excessive scarring, or inadequate tissue replacement by the flap reconstruction, the facial artery musculomucosal

(FAMM) flap is a readily available local flap (**Fig. 15**).[8]

The FAMM flap is also available bilaterally to replace vermilion if local mucosa is not available, although it is too bulky if only the vermilion is missing.

FREE-FLAP RECONSTRUCTION

Microvascular free tissue transfer is often required to reconstruct subtotal/total lip defects, especially when multiple facial subunits are to be included within the resection. Other reasons include previously irradiated tissue or previously reconstructed defects. Both the radial and ulnar forearm free flaps have been well described for use in reconstruction of total lip defects. The palmaris longus tendon can also be transferred with the flap to help provide support and suspend the lower lip.[9] In cases where the palmaris longus tendon is absent, a strip of flexor carpi radialis tendon can be used to help in the suspension of the lower lip (**Fig. 16**). The fibula osteocutaneous free flap can

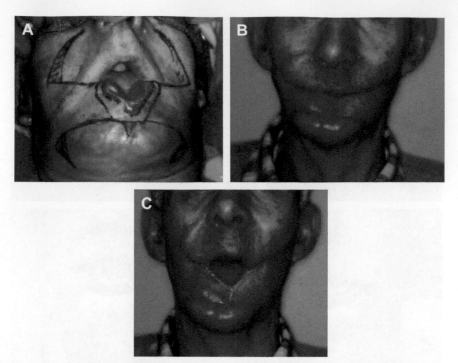

Fig. 14. (*A*) Recurrent lower lip cancer after radiation therapy. Intraoperative plan is for bilateral Fries flaps. (*B*) Lower lip retracted beneath upper lip. Note that this patient was medically unfit and therefore was not a candidate for a free flap. (*C*) Restricted opening and oral aperture as a result inadequate tissue, scar contracture, and lack of pliability of tissues after radiation.

be used to reconstruct defects from which bone and soft tissue have been removed (**Fig. 17**).

- Although microvascular tissue allows for coverage of tissue defect and partial perioral

competence, it fails to provide ideal aesthetics and true functional muscular support for the lip.

- Free flaps should be considered in situations where local flaps will cause significant

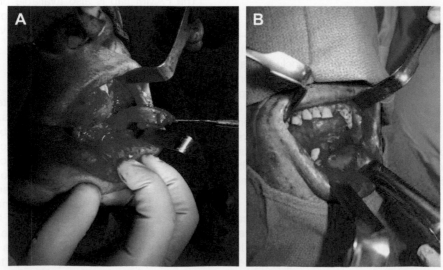

Fig. 15. (*A*) FAMM flap raised from left cheek to reconstruct the defect from alveolus extending into lower lip. (*B*) FAMM flap sutured to prevent retraction and loss of vertical height of the lip.

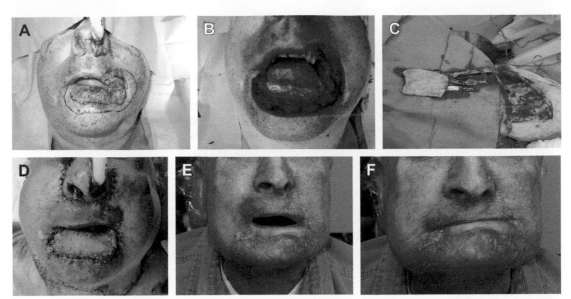

Fig. 16. (*A, B*) Squamous carcinoma involving 100% defect of the lower lip and 25% of the upper lip. (*C*) Ulnar forearm flap with flexor tendon transfer. (*D*) Lower lip reconstructed with ulnar flap with flexor tendon transfer. The upper lip was reconstructed with a sliding advancement flap with removal of perialar tissue. (*E, F*) The patient at 5 months postoperatively.

microstomia or in cases where there is a lack of locoregional tissue available for use in reconstruction.
- The suspended tendon should be attached to periosteum or via additional fascia lata

transfer to the temporalis tendon attachments or zygomatic arches.
- The forearm-flap donor-site defect is generally well tolerated, but closure will most often require a skin graft for tissue coverage.

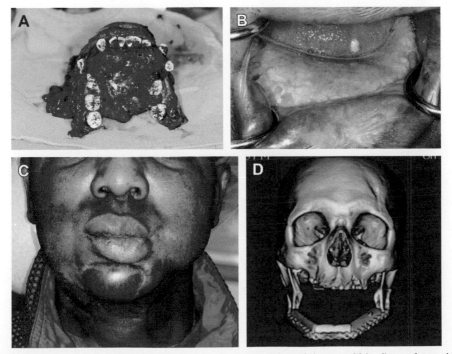

Fig. 17. (*A*) Squamous carcinoma composite defect requiring resection of the mandible, floor of mouth, and cutaneous chin. Vermillion was able to be preserved. (*B, C*) Reconstruction of the floor of mouth and cutaneous chin with de-epithelialized fibula osteocutaneous skin paddle. The patient 3.5 months after adjuvant chemoradiotherapy. (*D*) Postoperative 3-dimensional reconstruction scan demonstrating fibula reconstruction of the mandible.

REFERENCES

1. de Visscher JG, Gooris PJ, Vermy A, et al. Surgical margins for resection of squamous cell carcinoma of the lower lip. Int J Oral Maxillofac Surg 2002;31: 154–7.
2. Raschke GF, Rieger UM, Bader RD, et al. Lip reconstruction: an anthropometric and functional analysis of surgical outcomes. Int J Oral Maxillofac Surg 2012;41:744–50.
3. Karapandzic M. Reconstruction of lip defects by local arterial flaps. Br J Plast Surg 1983;36:40–7.
4. Johanson B, Aspelund E, Breine U, et al. Surgical treatment of nontraumatic lower lip lesions with special reference to the step technique: a follow up on 149 patients. Scand J Plast Reconstr Surg 1974; 8:232–47.
5. Fries R. Advantages of a basic concept in lip reconstruction after tumor resection. J Maxillofac Surg 1973;1:13–8.
6. Estlander JA. Eine Methode aus der einen Lippe Substanzverluster der andiron zu ersetzen. Arch Klin Chir 1872;14:622.
7. Chen WL, Li JS, Yang ZH, et al. Two submental island flaps for reconstructing oral and maxillofacial defects following cancer ablation. J Oral Maxillofac Surg 2008;66:1145–56.
8. Pribaz JJ, Meara JG, Wright S, et al. Lip and vermilion reconstruction with the facial artery musculomucosal flap. Plast Reconstr Surg 2000;105:864–72.
9. Sadove R, Luce E, McGarth P. Reconstruction of the lower lip and chin with the composite radial forearm-palmaris longus free flap. Plast Reconstr Surg 1991;88:209–14.

Maxillary Reconstruction

Nathan D. Lenox, DMD, MD[a], Dongsoo D. Kim, DMD, MD[b,c],*

KEYWORDS

- Maxilla/surgery • Head and neck neoplasms/surgery
- Reconstructive surgical procedures/methods • Surgical flaps

KEY POINTS

- The overall goals of maxillary reconstruction are to recreate facial form, anatomically partition the oral and nasal environments, and provide a stable framework for prosthetic dental rehabilitation.
- Complete understanding of the anatomic and functional requirements of maxillectomy defects, as appreciated by clinical examination and advanced imaging modalities, is an essential initial step in determining the most appropriate reconstructive plan.
- Anatomically based classification systems of maxillary defects offer a standardized, logical framework that allows accurate diagnosis, facilitates communication between surgeons, and offers guidance in selection of the most appropriate reconstructive options.
- Microvascular free-tissue techniques offer flexible reconstructive options for complex maxillary defects and offer many benefits to conventional obturator therapy.

INTRODUCTION

Functional and esthetic recreation of the maxilla presents many challenging opportunities to the reconstructive surgeon. Most patients requiring reconstruction of the maxilla suffer from defects resulting from the resection of malignant or locally aggressive disease. Reconstructive tumor surgery subjects the patient and family to a great deal of physical and emotional stress. Ablative defects of the maxilla commonly lead to facial disfigurement, loss of vision, compromised speech, difficulty swallowing, and diminished overall quality of life. Locally advanced disease often requires adjuvant chemoradiation, which further increases the psychological toll. However, with proper reconstruction, rehabilitation, and locoregional control, patients have the capability to return to premorbid functioning and maintain an overall good quality of life.

Ablative maxillary defects were traditionally managed almost exclusively with prosthetic obturators, but, over the past 20 years, with improved

refinements in microsurgical technique, vascularized free flaps have become increasingly integral to the overall reconstructive approach.[1] In the hands of an experienced prosthodontist, obturators provide a simple nonsurgical solution to fistula closure, allow improved speech and mastication, provide support to the facial tissue, and, when necessary, may restore missing structures such as the teeth, eyes, and nose. However, obturators also carry a negative psychosocial stigma; lead to painful areas of ulceration over time (especially during radiation therapy); develop foul odors and bad taste; and demand meticulous attention to oral hygiene.[2] Furthermore, dental obturators in patients after maxillectomy have not been shown to offer any significant advantage in esthetics or speech.[3] At one time, removable prosthetics were advocated for their ability to allow direct inspection of the tumor cavity and, over time, assess for recurrent local disease; however, with the widespread availability of advanced imaging modalities such as magnetic resonance imaging and positron

[a] Louisiana State University Health Sciences Center, 1501 Kings Highway, Shreveport, LA 71130, USA; [b] Department of Oral and Maxillofacial Surgery, Louisiana State University Health Sciences Center, 1501 Kings Highway, Shreveport, LA 71130, USA; [c] Department of Head and Neck Surgical Oncology and Microvascular Reconstruction, Louisiana State University Health Sciences Center, 1501 Kings Highway, Shreveport, LA 71130, USA
* Corresponding author.
E-mail address: dkim1@lsuhsc.edu

Oral Maxillofacial Surg Clin N Am 25 (2013) 215–222
http://dx.doi.org/10.1016/j.coms.2013.01.004
1042-3699/13/$ – see front matter © 2013 Elsevier Inc. All rights reserved.

emission tomography/computed tomography, this practice has a limited role in current clinical practice.

Nowadays, direct free-tissue transfer allows immediate single-stage reconstruction and obviates many of the day-to-day inconveniences of removable obturators. Tissue flaps offer a host of individually customizable reconstructive solutions for the spectrum of maxillary ablative defects. For example, simple local flaps such as the buccal fat pad flap (BFPF) offer straightforward solutions for small localized defects of the posterior maxilla and palate, whereas composite flaps such as the fibula free flap (FFF) offer skin, fascia, and high-quality vascularized bone. Microvascular free-tissue transfer allows primary healing in even the largest and most complex maxillofacial defects, improves support of the maxillary buttresses and overlying facial tissues, and offers a solid foundation for dental implant rehabilitation. Immediate single-stage microvascular reconstruction maximizes patient satisfaction and, when appropriate, should be the primary objective of the reconstructive surgeon.

CLASSIFICATION OF MAXILLARY DEFECTS

At the most fundamental level, successful maxillary reconstruction relies on an accurate assessment of the extent of the defect. Over the years, many classification schemes have attempted to standardize the description of maxillary defects, clarify communication between clinicians and researchers, and provide organized foundations for reconstructive treatment algorithms. In 1976, Lore[4] first introduced the terms partial and radical to depict ablative maxillary defects. Spiro and colleagues[5] later expanded the terminology to include limited, subtotal, and total for maxillectomies including 1, 2, or greater than 2 walls of the maxilla. This classification served to better detail the terms originally introduced by Lore[4]; however, the system still remained limited in its ability to reflect the intricacies of maxillary reconstruction.

Cordeiro and Chen[6,7] offered a graded system based on a simplified representation of the maxilla as a 6-walled geometric box. Postablative defects were classified according to the number of walls involved. The authors later modified this system and validated its reconstructive implications in a 15-year retrospective review of 100 flaps.[6,7] The Cordeiro classification is straightforward, easy to use, and offers a separate category for advanced defects exposing the intracranial contents.

Many oral and maxillofacial surgeons find the modified classification presented by Brown and colleagues[8] to be the most practical, clinically applicable, and widely recognized system available. In this classification scheme, independent evaluations of the vertical and horizontal components are combined to provide a three-dimensional description of the defect.[8] Defects are graded vertically from I to IV based on their extension from the maxillary alveolus toward the cranial base. Class I defects are limited to alveolus and palatal bone only. By definition, these defects do not involve the maxillary antrum. Also known as low maxillectomies, class II defects include alveolus and antral walls, but do not involve the orbital floor. Class III defects, or high maxillectomies, extend further superiorly to include the orbital floor; however, by definition the globe is not involved in the resection. Also known as radical maxillectomies, class IV defects are essentially the same as class III defects in terms of bony involvement, but orbital exenteration is included in the resection. Class V and VI were later added in the modified system to address isolated orbitomaxillary and nasomaxillary defects respectively.[9] Unlike the traditional class I to IV defects, these special categories do not involve the lower maxilla and alveolus.

Within the modified Brown classification, horizontal extent is graded separately as either a, b, c, or d. Isolated defects of the palate not including the alveolus are termed a. Defects involving 50% or less of the transverse width of the maxilla are termed b. Horizontal anterior defects of the maxilla are termed c. Large horizontal defects involving greater than 50% of the transverse width are termed d. Using the combined independent assessments of the vertical and horizontal dimensions, this 2-part classification system offers a straightforward method to accurately describe even the most seemingly complex maxillary defects (**Fig. 1**).

GOALS OF MAXILLARY RECONSTRUCTIVE SURGERY

Reconstruction of the maxilla is dictated by the overall objective to reestablish premorbid form and function. In this sense, the goals of maxillary reconstructive surgery are defined by the ability to maximize esthetic and functional outcomes while minimizing operative morbidity (**Box 1**). From a functional standpoint, surgery is intended to limit the deleterious effects on normal speech, swallowing, and velopharyngeal function. In certain situations, these effects are unavoidable, especially when striving to provide tumor-free margins; however, careful attention to flap selection, inset, and soft tissue suspension may limit undesirable outcomes. When faced with the prospect of long-term swallowing dysfunction and compromised

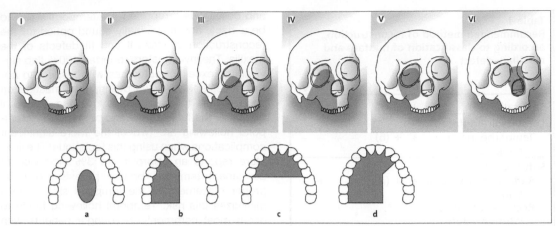

Fig. 1. Brown classification of maxillectomy defects. Vertical classification: I, maxillectomy not causing an oronasal fistula; II, not involving the orbit; III, involving the orbital adnexae with orbital retention; IV, with orbital enucleation or exenteration; V, orbitomaxillary defect; VI, nasomaxillary defect. Horizontal classification: a, palatal defect only, not involving the dental alveolus; b, less than or equal to one-half unilateral; c, less than or equal to one-half bilateral or transverse anterior; d, greater than one-half maxillectomy. (*From* Brown JS, Shaw RJ. Reconstruction of the maxilla and midface: introducing a new classification. Lancet Oncol 2010;11(10):1001–8; with permission.)

speech, early interventions such as parenteral enterogastric (PEG) tube support and speech therapy are recommended. Functional separation of the oral, nasal, and sinus cavities is important in preventing the negative sequela of chronic fistulae. In doing so, care must be taken not to obstruct normal patent airflow. The use of postoperative nasal trumpets assists in maintaining patency during early wound healing. From a structural standpoint, maxillary reconstructive surgery is intended to obliterate the dead space of large ablative defects and expedite the process of wound healing. This

---

Box 1
Goals of maxillary reconstructive surgery

Preservation of normal speech, swallowing, and velopharyngeal function

Close oral-antral and/or oral-nasal fistulae

Maintain nasal patency

Obliterate postoperative dead space

Expedite wound healing and transition to adjuvant therapy

Maximize mouth opening and masticatory function

Maintain functional lip competence

Provide vertical support to the globe and associated facial soft tissues

Create a stable preprosthetic framework for implant reconstruction and/or obturator fabrication

---

consideration becomes especially important when overall survival depends on the timely initiation of adjuvant chemoradiation therapy. Preservation of normal masticatory function and functional lip competence is important in maintaining nutrition and preventing sialorrhea. The senior author routinely offers coronoidectomy in advanced maxillary reconstructions to limit the late effects of trismus. Furthermore, adjunctive local tissue rearrangements such as the Abbe flap may be indicated to restore oral competence, depending on the extent of the reconstruction. For defects involving the orbital floor, reconstruction is intended to preserve support of the intact globe; if the globe is exenterated, attention should be given to preserving the lids and maintaining a functional cavity fit to ultimately receive an ocular prosthesis (**Table 1**).

Addressing individual patient desires and expectations openly (discussed within the context of general maxillary reconstructive goals) improves communication, facilitates trust, streamlines treatment planning, and ultimately improves satisfaction and tolerance of surgery.

RECONSTRUCTION OF MAXILLARY DEFECTS BY TYPE
Class I

Limited only to the resection of small amounts of alveolar and palatal bone, these defects do not classically include oral-antral fistulae. Brown and Shaw[9] reported the radial forearm fasciocutaneous flap (RFFF) to be the most common

Table 1
Recommended method of reconstruction, according to classification of midface and maxillary defect

	I	II	III	IV	V	VI
Obturation	+	+	–	–	–	–
Local pedicled flaps						
Temporoparietal, temporalis	+	+ (b)	–	–	–	–
Soft tissue free flaps						
Radial, anterolateral thigh	+	+ (a,b)	–	–	+	–
Rectus abdominis, latissimus dorsi	–	–	–	+	–	–
Hard tissue or composite flaps						
Radial	+	+ (b,c)	–	–	+	+
Fibula	–	+	–	–	–	–
DCIA/internal oblique	–	+	+	+	–	–
Scapula	–	+	+	+	–	–
TDAA (with scapula tip)	–	+	+	+	+	+

Letters (a,b,c) refer to the horizontal classification (see **Fig. 1**).
Abbreviations: +, recommended; –, not recommended; DCIA, deep circumflex iliac artery (supplies the iliac crest); TDAA, thoracodorsal angular artery (supplies the scapula tip).
From Brown JS, Shaw RJ. Reconstruction of the maxilla and midface: introducing a new classification. Lancet Oncol 2010;11(10):1001–8; with permission.

reconstructive solution for class I maxillary defects. In a series of 147 maxillary reconstructions, 8 class I defects were reported and all were reconstructed with the aforementioned flap.

Class II

When defects involve less than 50% of the transverse maxilla (class IIb), many potential reconstructive options exist. Depending on the experience of the surgeon, acceptable results may be achieved with prosthetic obturation, local tissue flaps, or microvascular free-tissue transfer. The temporalis flap and BFPF provide excellent local options for closure of select oral-antral and oral-nasal fistulae.[10–12]

The temporalis muscle flap was originally described by Lents in 1895 for condylar neck reconstruction in cases of temporomandibular joint ankylosis. Since that time, the temporalis flap has proved to be a versatile option for the reconstruction of palatal, floor of mouth, tongue, oropharyngeal, and retromolar defects. In a retrospective review of 39 postablative reconstructions, Djae

and colleagues[10] reported the temporalis flap to be a viable and functionally sound option for the reconstruction of class II and III defects of the maxilla. The investigators reported 100% flap survival and excellent outcomes with respect to appearance, speech, swallowing, and mastication on 2-month follow-up. Injury to the temporal branch of the facial nerve and postoperative temporal hollowing are two of the more significant complications when using this technique. The literature reports an approximate 3% incidence of permanent temporal branch paresis; however, proper placement of the temporal skin incision minimizes this risk. Temporal hollowing tends to occur most commonly in younger patients with minimal body fat and large ablative defects. To minimize this risk, the posterior portion of the temporalis muscle may be raised and rotated forward to supplement the deficiency at the anterior primary donor site.

Several additional options exist for the reconstruction of class IIb defects. First, depending on the status of the central incisors and ipsilateral canine, bony reconstruction may not be necessary to retain a final functional prosthesis. In addition, zygomatic implants may be used when other means of denture support are not available. The RFFF is the most commonly reported flap for the reconstruction of class II defects.[9] When vascularized bone is required, the FFF remains the most commonly used composite flap for the following reasons: the long vascular pedicle allows anastomosis with favorable vessels in the neck, the distant surgical site allows a comfortable and efficient 2-team approach, and the ample bone stock allows reliable placement of dental implants (**Figs. 2** and **3**).[13,14] In the isolated posterior class IIb defect, attention should instead focus on closure of the fistula, maintenance of vestibular depth, and preservation of the existing dentition. When using the FFF in reconstruction of oncologic defects, attention should also be paid to the location of the pterygomaxillary buttress. In advanced maxillary tumor ablation, the pterygoid plates are often included in the resection; however, when preserved, they may assist in alignment and provide posterior stabilization for the inset bone. Some investigators have disputed the usefulness of this concept, although failure to appreciate this relationship may lead to a misaligned bone flap, alterations in facial soft tissue support, and difficulties completing prosthetic dental rehabilitation (**Fig. 4**).[15] When adequate paranasal support remains, the FFF is an excellent option in the isolated posterior class IIb defect. In class IIc defects with paranasal collapse, the single-barrel fibula reconstruction may not provide adequate bony

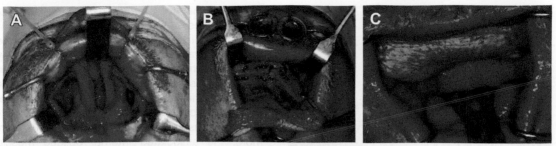

Fig. 2. (*A*) Class IId maxillary defect following resection of malignant variant of calcifying epithelial odontogenic tumor. (*B*) Reconstruction of the maxilla using composite free fibula flap. (*C*) Inset of skin paddle showing restored alveolar height and form.

support. Paranasal deficiencies must be evaluated on a case-by-case basis, but a simple solution is to inset paranasal strut grafts using the discarded segments of free fibula bone. An alternative is for surgeons to select an option such as the deep circumflex iliac artery (DCIA) flap, which provides a large supply of cortical bone and potential muscle. When fully mucosalized, free muscle flaps have the potential to recreate a more natural intraoral lining.

Flaps based on the scapular system are becoming more popular because of their versatility and ability to harvest multiple independent skin paddles, associated muscle, and bone from the lateral scapula.[16,17] These flaps were classically described as chimeric in nature and are ideal options for large-volume complex defects, especially those requiring only small amounts of

thin bone (class IIa, class IIb). Patients at risk of prolonged bed rest or postoperative gait disturbance may benefit from use of the scapula flap over iliac crest or fibula. In a retrospective review of 39 scapular system free flaps for maxillary reconstruction, Miles and Gilbert[17] found the scapular angle flap to be a reliable reconstructive option with minimal donor-site morbidity. The main limitations of this flap are its short vascular pedicle, poor overall bone quantity, need for intraoperative repositioning, and inability to perform a simultaneous 2-team approach. Modifications of the surgical technique have improved available pedicle length by raising the flap on a branch of the thoracodorsal artery instead of the circumflex scapular artery; however, for many microvascular surgeons, its other limitations often overshadow its use in routine clinical practice.

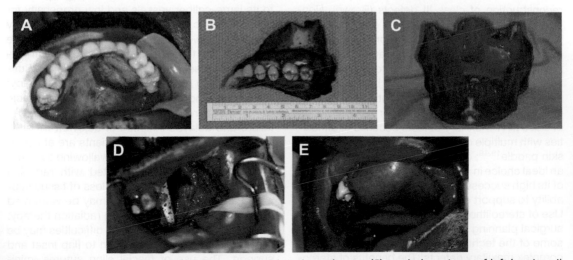

Fig. 3. (*A*) Preoperative view of left maxillary adenoid cystic carcinoma; (*B*) surgical specimen of left hemimaxillectomy; (*C*) stereolithographic model of postablative defect illustrating diagnostic wax-up of proposed bony reconstruction (patient was maintained with a dental obturator for tumor surveillance); (*D*) preparation of the defect for flap inset, Penrose drain marks tunnel for the pedicle into recipient vessels of the left neck; (*E*) postoperative view of skin paddle following flap inset.

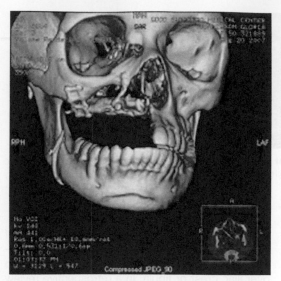

Fig. 4. Malalignment of the inset fibula with respect to the remaining pterygoid plates in oncologic hemimaxillary reconstruction.

Class III

The class III defect presents a moderate-volume to large-volume tissue requirement involving all 6 walls of the maxilla. Because of the extensive loss of facial soft tissue support and destruction of the orbital rim, class III defects are arguably some of the most difficult to treat. Providing adequate support to the globe and soft tissues of the cheek is paramount to any reconstructive endeavor. Fifty-eight percent of cases reported in the literature used only soft tissue flaps for the reconstruction of class III defects (Brown). Nonvascularized bone may be used in addition to provide bony reconstruction of the orbital floor, rim, and anterior maxillary wall; however, the risk of graft failure (especially when postoperative radiation therapy is indicated) must be considered. Some investigators have substantiated the claim that the FFF is less than ideal for reconstruction of class III/IV maxillary defects because of difficulties with multiple osteotomies and alignment of the skin paddle[18,19]; others have regarded the FFF as an ideal choice in maxillary reconstruction because of its high success rate, low complication rate, and ability to support osseointegrated dental implants. Use of stereolithographic modeling and predictive surgical planning software may assist in obviating some of the technical drawbacks of fibula inset in complex maxillary defects. The benefits of stereolithographic modeling have been well substantiated in mandibular reconstruction.[20,21] Use of planning software allows more efficient osteotomy design in the operating room, decreased overall

operative time, and more predictable reconstructive outcomes.

The DCIA is advocated as a more appropriate flap for advanced class III defects, especially those involving most of the remaining transverse maxilla (class IIId). The DCIA flap offers a large block of bone that can be contoured and inset to restore support to the missing zygomaticomaxillary and nasomaxillary buttresses.[22,23] Furthermore, the associated internal oblique muscle can be included to obliterate the dead space, close the fistulae, and provide a functional lining for the nose and oral cavity. The excellent bone stock supplied by the DCIA flap maintains the future option of using dental implants and, even if not used, mucosalized muscle from this flap has been used to support functional upper dentures.

Class IV

Advanced defects tend to portend a poorer long-term prognosis. In these situations, the focus becomes eradication of disease and preservation of life; certain functional and esthetic objectives may be sacrificed to optimize overall outcome. For example, reconstruction of the orbital floor is not a significant issue; instead, reconstructive efforts should be designed to eliminate dead space, separate the upper aerodigestive tract from areas of exposed dura, and prepare a mucosalized cavity for fabrication of an orbital prosthesis. The rectus abdominis, DCIA, and latissimus dorsi flaps all offer excellent reconstructive options depending on the preferences of the surgeon (**Fig. 5**). Owing to its large-caliber vessels and low propensity for atherosclerotic disease, the rectus flap typically carries the lowest incidence of overall flap failure and vascular thrombosis. By virtue of their advanced disease, many patients with class IV defects go on to require adjuvant radiation therapy; in these instances, the rectus flap offers a reliable option that minimizes the added morbidity of flap failure and delayed initiation of adjuvant therapy. In large composite defects, patients are at risk to experience chronic long-term swallowing dysfunction (especially when confronted with radiation therapy), speech difficulty, and loss of tissue support. Flap revision procedures may be warranted if excess bulk remains following radiation therapy; in the short term, some of these difficulties may be prevented with special attention to flap inset and support. The use of fascial sling sutures, miniplates, titanium mesh, or other implantable devices may be indicated to prevent prolapse within the oral cavity and excess sag of the facial skin.

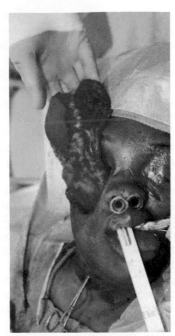

Fig. 5. Application of the latissimus dorsi myofascio-cutaneous flap for reconstruction of a large class IV maxillary defect.

Class V

Isolated orbitomaxillary defects typically require a more straightforward approach to the previous classifications. These defects do not involve the lower maxilla and alveolus and, therefore, bone is generally not required. Following orbital exenteration, the main objective of reconstructive surgery is to provide sufficient space for fabrication of an orbital prosthesis. Whenever possible, the anatomy of the lids must be preserved. In smaller defects, temporalis flaps may be appropriate; more commonly, radial forearm free flaps are preferred for their thin, pliable skin. Bulkier flaps are generally avoided and may prohibit optimal prosthesis fabrication.

Class VI

Class VI represents an uncommon subset of maxillary defects. In certain reports, these defects make up as little as 0.5% of all reconstructed defects.[9] By definition, class VI represents isolated nasomaxillary defects and these defects often do not require extensive reconstruction if the nasal bones, overlying skin, and palate remain undisturbed. Dural involvement and associated cerebrospinal fluid leak are possibilities in high-riding nasoethmoid tumors; however, for the most part, reconstructive challenges involve reconstruction of the nose. Depending on the experience of the surgeon and the available resources, acceptable reconstruction may be achieved with local tissue transfer, microvascular tissue transfer, or maxillo-facial prosthetics. Although these cases are limited, the osteocutaneous radial forearm free flap has been reported to provide excellent functional and esthetic outcomes when resection necessitates reconstruction of the bony nasal dorsum and overlying skin.[6,7]

SUMMARY

Postablative maxillary defects present the reconstructive surgeon with a wide range of functional and esthetic challenges. Over the years, several classification schemes have succeeded in adding clarity to the subject but, irrespective of the system adopted, the surgeon must maintain a clear vision of the defect at hand and appreciate its reconstructive implications throughout the spectrum of deformity. Local tissue flaps such as the temporalis and BFPF remain valuable tools in the reconstruction of small isolated defects of the posterior maxilla and palate; however, with advancements in modern technology and surgical technique, microvascular free flaps have eclipsed prosthetic obturators as the mainstay of therapy in advanced postablative defects of the maxilla. Depending on the skill and training of the surgeon, many excellent microvascular options exist and, regardless of the specific tools used, the overall objectives remain the same: recreate facial form, preserve oral function, and, most importantly, do so in accordance with the individual needs and desires of the patient.

REFERENCES

1. Andrades P, Militsakh O, Hanasono MM, et al. Current strategies in reconstruction of maxillectomy defects. Arch Otolaryngol Head Neck Surg 2011; 137:806–12.
2. Rogers SN, Lowe D, McNally D, et al. Health-related quality of life after maxillectomy: a comparison between obturation and free flap. J Oral Maxillofac Surg 2003;61:174–81.
3. Rieger JM, Tang JA, Wolfaardt J. Comparison of speech and esthetic outcomes in patients with maxillary reconstruction versus maxillary obturators after maxillectomy. J Otolaryngol Head Neck Surg 2011;40:40–7.
4. Lore JM. Partial and radical maxillectomy. Otolaryngol Clin North Am 1976;9:255–67.
5. Spiro RH, Strong EW, Shah JP. Maxillectomy and its classification. Head Neck 1997;19:309–14.

6. Cordeiro PG, Chen CM. A 15-year review of midface reconstruction after total and subtotal maxillectomy: part I. Algorithm and outcomes. Plast Reconstr Surg 2011;129:124–36.

7. Cordeiro PG, Chen CM. A 15-year review of midface reconstruction after total and subtotal maxillectomy: part II. Technical modifications to maximize aesthetic and functional outcomes. Plast Reconstr Surg 2011;129:139–47.

8. Brown JS, Rogers SN, McNally DN, et al. A modified classification for maxillectomy defect. Head Neck 2000;22:17–26.

9. Brown JS, Shaw RJ. Reconstruction of the maxilla and midface: introducing a new classification. Lancet Oncol 2010;11:1001–8.

10. Djae AK, Li Z, Li ZB. Temporalis muscle flap for immediate reconstruction of maxillary defects: review of 39 cases. Int J Oral Maxillofac Surg 2011;40:715–21.

11. Amin MA, Bailey BM, Swinson B, et al. Use of the buccal fat pad in reconstruction and prosthetic rehabilitation of oncological maxillary defects. Br J Oral Maxillofac Surg 2005;43:148–54.

12. Vuillemin T, Raveh J, Ramon Y. Reconstruction of the maxilla with bone grafts supported by the buccal fat pad. J Oral Maxillofac Surg 1988;46:100–5.

13. Chang YM, Coskunfirat OK, Wei FC, et al. Maxillary reconstruction with a fibula osteoseptocutaneous free flap and simultaneous insertion of osseointegrated dental implants. Plast Reconstr Surg 2004; 113:1140–5.

14. Kazaoka Y, Shinohara A, Yokou K, et al. Functional reconstruction after a total maxillectomy using a fibula osteocutaneous flap with osseointegrated implants. Plast Reconstr Surg 1999;103:1244–6.

15. Shipchandler TZ, Waters HH, Knott PD, et al. Orbito-maxillary reconstruction using the layered fibula osteocutaneous flap. Arch Facial Plast Surg 2012; 14(2):110–5.

16. Granick MS, Ramasastry SS, Newton ED, et al. Reconstruction of complex maxillectomy defects with the scapular-free flap. Head Neck Surg 1990; 12:377–85.

17. Miles BA, Gilbert RW. Maxillary reconstruction with the scapular angle osteomyogenous free flap. Arch Otolaryngol Head Neck Surg 2011;137: 1130–5.

18. Futran ND, Wadsworth JT, Villaret D, et al. Midface reconstruction with the fibula free flap. Arch Otolaryngol Head Neck Surg 2002;128:161–6.

19. Peng X, Mao C, Yu GY, et al. Maxillary reconstruction with the free fibula flap. Plast Reconstr Surg 2005; 115:1562–9.

20. Zheng GS, Su YX, Liao GQ, et al. Mandible reconstruction assisted by preoperative virtual surgical simulation. Oral Surg Oral Med Oral Pathol Oral Radiol 2012;113(5):604–11.

21. Antony AK, Chen WF, Kolokythas A, et al. Use of virtual surgery and stereolithography-guided osteotomy for mandibular reconstruction with the free fibula. Plast Reconstr Surg 2011;128(5): 1080–4.

22. Brown JS. Deep circumflex iliac artery free flap with internal oblique muscle as a new method of immediate reconstruction of maxillectomy defects. Head Neck Surg 1996;18:412–21.

23. Brown JS, Jones DC, Summerwill A. Vascularized iliac crest with internal oblique muscle for immediate reconstruction after maxillectomy. Br J Oral Maxillofac Surg 2002;40:183–90.

Zygoma Implant Reconstruction of Acquired Maxillary Bony Defects

Luis G. Vega, DDS[a,b,*], William Gielincki, DDS[c],
Rui P. Fernandes, DMD, MD[d,e]

KEYWORDS

- Zygoma implants • Maxillary defect • Maxillectomy

KEY POINTS

- Zygoma implant reconstruction of acquired maxillary defect is a safe, predictable and cost-effective treatment modality.
- The complexity of zygoma implant reconstruction of these defects calls for a prosthetically driven treatment plan in which a team approach between the surgeon and the restorative dentist is paramount for treatment success.
- The number, position, angulation, and length of the zygoma implants is going to depend on the size of the defect, residual bone, soft tissue coverage, and more important on the biomechanics of the prosthetic restoration.
- Closure of the oroantral/oronasal communication with placement of zygoma implants after or during closure facilitates the prosthetic reconstruction.

The reconstruction of acquired maxillary bony defects after pathologic ablation, infectious debridement, avulsive trauma, or previously failed reconstructions is among the most challenging areas in oral and maxillofacial reconstruction. The main goal of these reconstructive efforts is to maintain or improve the patient's quality of life by trying to restore the lost form and function. Multiple classifications, techniques and algorithms have tried to simplify the approach to these defects but the best reconstruction method remains controversial.[1–6] Traditionally, these defects have been reconstructed according to their size, residual anatomic structures, patient medical condition, and overall prognosis. Moreover, most of these techniques have the common denominator of long treatment time frames, multiple surgical procedures, donor site morbidity, high cost, and so forth. Maxillary obturators, with or without dental implant support, have been historically a great prosthetic option for selected patients.[7] Alternatively, microvascular tissue transfers in combination with dental implants have become a popular way to restore these defects (Fig. 1).[8,9]

Using the zygoma bone as anchorage, Brånemark, developed the zygomatic implant as

[a] Oral and Maxillofacial Residency Program, Health Science Center at Jacksonville, University of Florida, 653-1 West 8th Street, Jacksonville, FL 32209, USA; [b] Department of Oral and Maxillofacial Surgery, Health Science Center at Jacksonville, University of Florida, 653-1 West 8th Street, Jacksonville, FL 32209, USA; [c] Private Practice, Jacksonville Center for Prosthodontics and Implant Dentistry, 6855 Belfort Oaks Place, Jacksonville, FL 32216, USA; [d] Department of Oral and Maxillofacial Surgery, College of Medicine, University of Florida 653-1 West Eight Street, LRC 2nd Floor, Jacksonville, FL 32209, USA; [e] Department of Surgery, Division of Surgical Oncology, College of Medicine, University of Florida, 653-1 West Eight Street, LRC 2nd Floor, Jacksonville, FL 32209, USA
* Corresponding author. Department of Oral and Maxillofacial Surgery, Health Science Center at Jacksonville, University of Florida, 653-1 West 8th Street, Jacksonville, FL 32209.
E-mail address: luis.vega@jax.ufl.edu

Oral Maxillofacial Surg Clin N Am 25 (2013) 223–239
http://dx.doi.org/10.1016/j.coms.2013.02.007

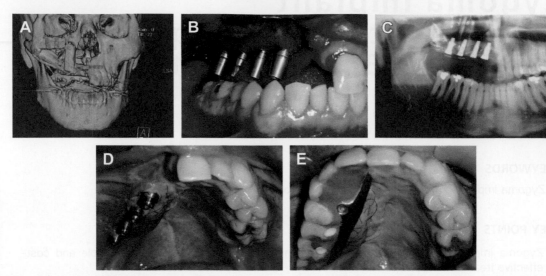

Fig. 1. Acquired right maxillary defect after myxoma resection reconstructed with a fibula free flap. (*A*) Postoperative three-dimensional computed tomographic reconstruction showing a right maxillary reconstruction with fibula free flap. (*B*) Intraoperative view of the placement of 4 dental implants. (*C*) Postoperative panoramic radiograph after implant placement. (*D*) Implants ready to be restored. (*E*) Fixed-hybrid prosthesis in place.

a solution to the lack of maxillary bony support for prosthetic rehabilitation.[10] Although they have become increasingly popular for the treatment of severely atrophic maxilla, several investigators have reported their use as a simple, predictable, and cost-effective solution to the reconstruction of acquired maxillary bony defects (**Box 1**).[11–17] The focus of this article is to review the surgical and prosthetic nuances to successfully reconstruct acquired maxillary bony defects with zygoma implants.

THE BASICS
Zygoma Bone

Several studies have described the anatomic characteristics of the zygoma bone with the purpose of implant placement.[10,18–21] These studies showed that mean dimensions of zygomatic bone range from 14.1 to 25.4 mm in the anteroposterior (AP) length and 7.6 to 9.5 mm in mediolateral (ML) thickness. In addition, when the length of the zygoma bone is measured along the potential implant axis, the measurements range from 14 to 16.5 mm. Clinically, Balshi and colleagues[22] found similar results. Their study of bone-to-implant contact (BIC), in 77 patients with 173 zygoma implants showed that the mean BIC was 15.3 mm (4.9–32.9 mm). This finding represented an average of 35.9% (12.2%–67.3%) of the implant that came into contact with the zygoma bone. A statistically significant difference was encountered between the BIC in males (16.5 mm ± 6 mm) and females (14.7 mm ±

5.4 mm). From a qualitative view, Nkenke and colleagues[19] indicated that the zygoma bone had poor trabecular bone density but a strong cortex. This finding led them to suggest that primary stability of the zygoma fixture could be achieved if it is inserted in zygomatic cortical bone. Furthermore in a microcomputed tomography study, Kato and colleagues[21] found that the trabecular bone at the end of the zygomatic fixture is thicker and wider than in other regions of the zygoma bone. These investigators suggested that after osseointegration, this thickening significantly assists the support of the zygoma fixture.

Zygoma Implant and Biomechanics

Worldwide, several manufactures have designed and commercialized zygomatic implants. The principal differences between them can be observed in **Table 1**. However, even in the presence of these differences, their main characteristic is being a long implant (30–62.5 mm) that obtains its main anchorage from the zygoma bone in presence or absence of maxillary alveolar bone. Several biomechanical three-dimensional finite elemental analyses have corroborated this distinctive feature.[23–25] Ujigawa and colleagues[23] compared functional stress distribution of zygoma implants with and without connected dental implants supporting a superstructure in a severely atrophic maxilla. These investigators found in the connected implant model that the stress was mostly concentrated in the zygoma bone and the middle of the implant. In contrast, the stress in the single implant model concentrated in zygoma bone, middle of the implant, maxillary alveolar bone and implant-abutment joint. These findings showed that a better distribution of forces occurs when all the implants are splinted with the prosthetic reconstruction. Romeed and colleagues[26] developed a model to study the effect of different amounts of zygoma bone support (10,15 and 20 mm) on the biomechanics of zygoma implants. These investigators found that 10 mm of zygoma bone support sustained double the stress of 15 and 20 mm. The stress within the fixture increased 3 times when the bone support decreased from 20 mm to 10 mm. Stresses within the fixture-abutment joint were not significantly different regardless of the level of bone support. Thus the investigators concluded that the abutment screw is not at risk of fracture and they suggested that the optimal amount of zygomatic bone support

should not be less than 15 mm. From a clinical perspective, these findings correlate with the average BIC from the study of Balshi and colleagues[22] described earlier.

Using different configurations in the number and position of implants, Miyamoto and colleagues[24] studied the biomechanics of an implant-retained prosthesis in hemimaxillectomy defects. Their results revealed that on the affected side, 2 zygoma implants instead of 1 allow for better stress distribution to the zygoma bone and the implant-abutment joint. In addition, in the unaffected side, the stress generated in the residual maxillary alveolus after the placement of 2 or 3 regular dental implants did not have a negative effect on their potential osseointegration. Using 1 zygoma implant in a unilateral maxillary defect, Korkmaz and colleagues[25] studied 4 different implant configurations to support a bar-retained obturator. These investigators concluded that an increase in the number of dental implants on the unaffected side did not decrease the maximum stress affecting the bone surrounding the implants. On the other hand, a marked decrease of the stress affecting the model was found when the dental implants on the unaffected side were substituted by a zygomatic fixture.

PREOPERATIVE EVALUATION

Multiple entities can be responsible for the creation of maxillary bony defects such as benign or malignant pathologic ablation (eg, ameloblastoma, myxoma, squamous cell carcinoma, mucoepidermoid carcinoma), infection debridement (eg, mucormycosis, actinomycosis), and avulsive trauma (eg, gunshot wound). The primary diagnosis, surgical management, and postoperative care of these conditions are not discussed because they are out of the scope of this review. However, because of the intricate nature of these causes, it is assumed during the rest of this article that the maxillary reconstruction with zygoma implants is performed as a secondary procedure in patients who are free of disease, with no contraindications for reconstruction. For immediate maxillary reconstruction with zygoma implants after oncology resection, readers are referred for further review to the protocol published in 2007 by Boyes-Varley and colleagues.[13]

History and Examination

The complexity of implant reconstruction of acquired maxillary bone defects calls for a prosthetically driven treatment plan, because surgical procedures might not always be as predictable as the prosthetic counterparts. Therefore the

Table 1

Zygoma implant differences according to the manufacture

Company	Headquarters	Implant Name	Length (mm)	Diameter (mm) (Apical [A]– Coronal [C])	Angulation (°)	Connection Type	Type of Surface	Type of Abutment
				Implant Size		**Platform**		
Brånemark Integration	Göteberg, Sweden	Z Fixture	5 (36, 40, 44, 48, 52)	4.0 (A)–5.3 (C)	0	External	Machined (smooth middle)	Standard
Conexão Sistemas de Protese	São Paulo, Brazil	Master Zigo	8 (30, 35, 40, 42.5, 45, 47.5, 50, 55)	4.0 (C)	45	External	Surface treated	Standard
		Zigo Max	8 (30, 35, 40, 42.5, 45, 47.5, 50, 55)	4.0 (C)	0	Internal	Surface treated	Angled 32° and 35°
Dentoflex	São Paulo, Brazil	TE (External Technique)	9 (35, 37.5, 40, 42.5, 45, 47.5, 50, 52.5, 55)		45	External	Machined (smooth middle)	
		TI (Intrasinus Technique)	9 (35, 37.5, 40, 42.5, 45, 47.5, 50, 52.5, 55)		45	External	Machined	
Neodent	Curitiba, Brazil	Zigomático Cone Morse	7 (30, 35, 40, 45, 47.5, 50, 52.5)	3.9 (A)–4.4 (C)	45	Internal	Machined	Standard
		Zigomático Hexágono Externo	7 (30, 35, 40, 45, 47.5, 50, 52.5)	3.9 (A)–4.4 (C)	45	External	Machined	Standard

Nobel Biocare	Göteberg, Sweden	Zygoma Machined	8 (30, 35, 40, 42.5, 45, 47.5, 50, 52.5)	4.0 (A)–5.0 (C)	45	External	Machined	Standard and angled 17°
		Zygoma TiUnite	8 (30, 35, 40, 42.5, 45, 47.5, 50, 52.5)	4.0 (A)–5.0 (C)	45	External	Surface treated	Standard
SIN (Sistema de Implante Nacional)	São Paulo, Brazil	Zygomatic	13 (32.5, 35, 37.5, 40, 42.5, 45, 47.5, 50, 52.5, 55, 57.5, 60, 62.5)	4.1 (C)	45	External	Machined	Standard
Southern Implants	Irene, South Africa	Zygomatic	8 (35, 37.5, 40, 42.5, 45, 47.5, 50, 52.5)	4.0 (A)–4.3 (C)	55	External	Machined	Standard and angled 17° and 30°
		Oncologic	3 (27, 32, 37)	4.0 (A)–4.3 (C)	55	External	Machined (7, 12, 17 mm smooth coronal)	Standard and angled 17° and 30°
Tecom Implantology	Lallio, Italy	Zygomatic	4 (35, 45, 50, 52.5)	4.0 (C)	45	External	Machined	Standard and angled 17°
Titanium Fix	São José dos Campos, Brazil	Z-Fix	11 (30, 32.5, 35, 37.5, 40, 42.5, 45, 47.5, 50, 52.5, 55)	3.75 (A)–4.5 (C)	0	Internal	Surface treated	Standard and angled 30°

single most important factor for treatment success is a team approach between the surgeon and the restorative dentist. Thus, treatment goals and potential limitations are determined after the patient's chief complaint, perceptions, expectations, cooperation, past surgical and medical history, clinical and radiographic evaluation are thoroughly reviewed and discussed by the reconstructive team. Special consideration should be given to patients with previous history of radiation because the literature on zygoma implants reports lower success rates in this population.[11,14,27]

Physical and radiographic examination is focused on the identification of residual areas in which sufficient bone is present for implant placement. It is important to evaluate the overall size of the defect, the presence of residual anatomic structures in affected and unaffected sides (eg, teeth, tuberosities, pterygoid plates), the existence of oroantral or oronasal communications, or the presence of previous reconstructive efforts (eg, local, regional flaps, or microvascular tissue transfers). The radiographic gold standard for the evaluation of acquired maxillary bone defects is computed tomography (CT) with three-dimensional reconstructions. These images help to establish the involvement of the zygoma bone into the defect, its AP and ML dimensions as well as its secondary topography such as curvature of the anterior maxillary wall. The images can also be used to determine the maxillary sinus health status and amount of residual maxillary bone

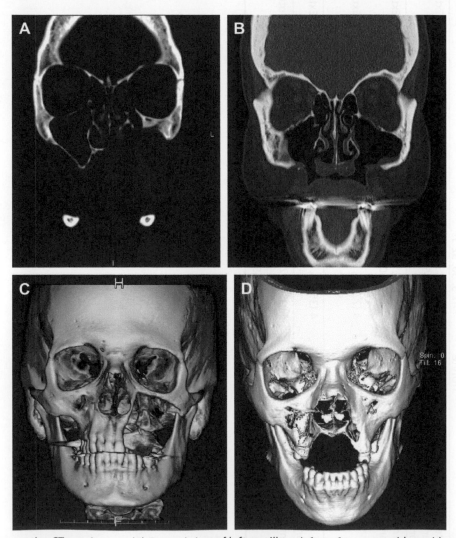

Fig. 2. Preoperative CT scan images. (*A*) Coronal view of left maxillary defect after mucoepidermoid resection. (*B*) Coronal view of bilateral maxillary defects after mucormycosis infection debridement. (*C*) Three-dimensional CT reconstruction of left maxillary defect after myxoma resection. (*D*) Three-dimensional CT reconstruction of anterior maxillary defect after ameloblastoma resection.

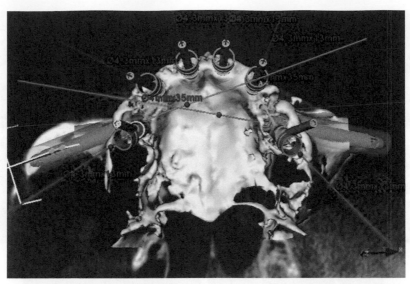

Fig. 3. Zygoma implant virtual planning surgery.

(**Fig. 2**). CT scan images can be used in virtual surgical planning (**Fig. 3**) and preliminary reports of computer-guided zygoma implant placement have been described in the literature.[20,28,29] Alternatively, stereolithographic models can be constructed to help in the establishment of the treatment plan by offering a better understanding of the defect, improving the communication within the team and allowing for model surgery (**Fig. 4**).

TREATMENT PLANNING
Prosthetic Considerations

When reconstructing acquired maxillary bony defects with zygomatic implants, the first step in the treatment plan is to choose between 1-stage or 2-stage functional rehabilitation:

1. One-stage approach: implants are placed and immediately loaded. This type approach

requires good coordination between the surgeon, restorative dentist, and laboratory personnel. It has the advantage that the patient functions immediately without further delay. Usually, this result is achieved with a fixed provisional prosthesis (modified existing denture or obturator); alternatively, the implants can be splinted with a stabilization bar loaded with a provisional prosthesis (**Fig. 5**). In the presence of an oroantral/oronasal communication, a more sophisticated reconstruction is needed such as fixed provisional prosthesis with a separate temporary obturator. Some investigators have suggested that a 1-stage approach allows for a better soft tissue–implant interface, because it decreases the amount of tissue manipulation.[30] This approach is especially important in defects with thin soft tissue coverage. In these cases, lack of residual

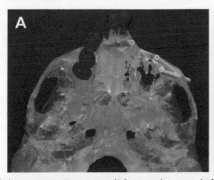

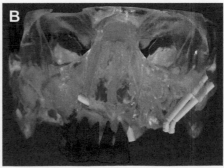

Fig. 4. Model surgery using stereolithography on a left maxillary defect after a myxoma resection. (*A, B*) Bottom and frontal view showing the placement of 3 zygoma implants on a left maxillary defect after a myxoma resection. Note how the presence of the residual dentition does not allow cross-arch stabilization. To circumvent this problem, a palatally placed anterior zygoma implant was planned.

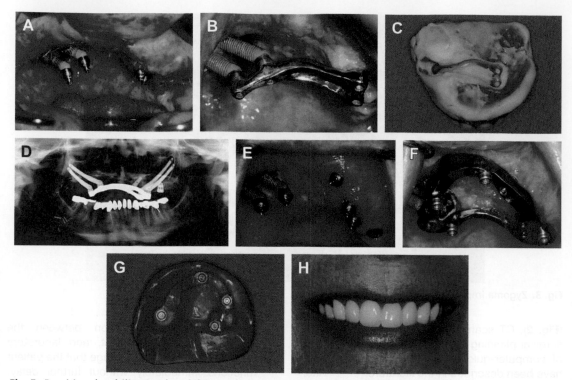

Fig. 5. Provisional stabilization bar. (*A*) Immediate postoperative view after the placement of 4 zygoma implants on a 68-year-old woman with a right maxillary defect after resection of a squamous cell carcinoma. Note how the implants on the affected side are protruding excessively in the oral cavity. Ideally, these implants should have been placed with the platform closer to the soft tissues. (*B*) A temporary stabilization bar was constructed while the implants osseointegrated. (*C*) Modified obturator. (*D*) Postoperative panoramic radiograph showing the provisional stabilization bar and 2 additional dental implants in the unaffected side. (*E*) Implants ready to be restored. Note the lack of AP spread of the zygoma implants in the affected side. (*F*) A circular superstructure was designed to better distribute functional forces. Note the 4 locator attachments within the superstructure. (*G*) View of the final removable prosthesis. Two attachments were blocked after delivery because of excessive retention of the prosthesis. (*H*) Result.

maxillary bone is encountered in the coronal portion of the zygomatic fixture, and excessive manipulation of these tissues could create soft tissue dehiscence, with potential oroantral communication (**Fig. 6**). Once osseointegration

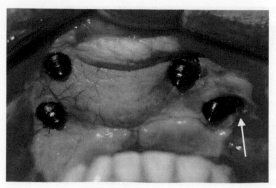

Fig. 6. Small oroantral communication caused by the lack of maxillary bone around the implant platform and thin soft tissue coverage (*arrow*).

has been achieved, after 4 to 6 months, the final prosthesis can be delivered.

2. Two-stage approach: implant placement and delayed loading. This is the traditional approach in which the implants are placed, and after 4 to 6 months of osseointegration, they are uncovered for further restoration. This approach has the disadvantage that it requires a second surgical procedure, and often, the patient's ability to function is delayed. On certain occasions, during the healing period, the patient is allowed to use a tissue-supported prosthesis. Once the implants are uncovered, ideally, they should be splinted as soon as possible, either with the provisional or final restoration.

The second step in the prosthetic treatment plan is the design of the prosthesis. The prosthesis should follow a physiologic approach that halts bone resorption and maintains the residual anatomic structures. Hence, the number and position of the implants depend on the biomechanics of the prosthetic restoration.

Several elements must be taken into consideration when designing the prosthetic restoration, as discussed in the following sections.

Zygoma implant biomechanics

As described earlier, zygoma implants are less resistant to rotational forces. It has been suggested that for better distribution of these forces, zygoma implants should be placed to allow the greatest AP spread. In addition, cantilevers in the prosthetic reconstruction should be avoided; cross-arch stabilization by splinting of all the implants is also recomended.[31] Few investigators treating acquired maxillary bony defects have reported prosthetic reconstruction success, even when some of these biomechanical principles could not be adhered to.[14,16,32,33] As an example, Landes and colleagues[14] reported an 89% cumulative 8-year zygoma implant survival rate using modified telescope prosthetic reconstructions. However, as a general guide, the necessary support for prosthetic restoration of bilateral maxillary defects can be obtained with the placement of 2 zygoma implants bilaterally. Unilateral defects without dentition in the unaffected side could be restored with 1 or 2 zygoma implants (preferably 2) in the affected side and 2 or 3 regular dental implants with long AP spread in the unaffected side (1 or 2 zygoma implants can be used if there is not enough bone for regular implants) (**Fig. 7**). These biomechanical principles are more difficult to follow in unilateral cases with residual dentition in the unaffected maxilla. Cross-arch stabilization in these cases could be achieved with more sophisticated designs, like using an anterior zygoma implant as a tilted implant (see **Fig. 3**).

Size of the defect/missing tissue

The size of the defect allows for the identification of tissues that have to be replaced. Acquired maxillary defects in which the residual structures allow fabrication of implant-retained crowns and bridges are unlikely to be encountered. Composite defects in which teeth, gingiva, alveolar bone, and maxillary bone is missing are more likely to be found. The best prosthetic option to replace these missing tissues is using a fixed-hybrid or a bar-retained prosthesis. As described earlier, in the presence of an oroantral/oronasal communication, a combination fixed-hybrid prosthesis and obturator or bar-retained prosthesis can be used. The size of the defect is also important in the determination of the zygoma implant angulation, length, and platform position. The ideal implant platform position (physiologically and biomechanically) should be at the level of the maxillary alveolar ridge, but this is rarely possible in the presence of maxillary

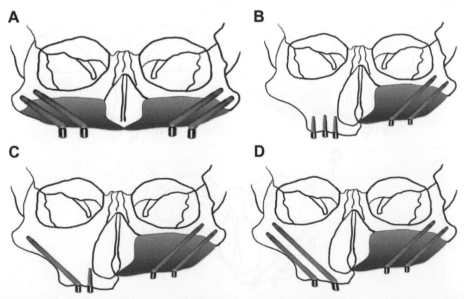

Fig. 7. Some possible scenarios of zygoma implant reconstruction of acquired maxillary defects. Note that the defects are covered with soft tissue and no oroantral or oronasal communication exists. (*A*) Four zygoma implants in a bilateral maxillary defect. (*B*) Two zygoma implants in the affected side in combination with regular implants in the unaffected side (adequate anterior and posterior bone). (*C*) Two zygoma implants in the affected side in combination with 1 zygoma and regular implants in the unaffected side (inadequate posterior bone). (*D*) Four zygoma implants (inadequate bone in the unaffected side).

defects. Instead, in these cases, the implant platform should be leveled as close as possible to the soft tissues of the residual defect. If the implant is too long, it protrudes too much into the oral cavity, making oral hygiene and prosthetic reconstruction difficult (**Fig. 8**). Large defects in which the residual zygoma bone is covered by a thin layer of soft tissue deserve special consideration because implant platforms might be placed too laterally and posterior to the original position of the missing maxillary alveolar ridge. Prosthetic reconstructions in these cases might require a vestibular flange to attach the implants.[13]

AP and ML cantilevers

The original description of the zygoma implant technique uses an intrasinus approach that has the potential to create ML cantilevers because of a more palatally position of the implant platform. The extrasinus technique, the zygoma anatomy guided approach (ZAGA) and implant design changes (55° platform) are modifications described in the literature to improve these cantilevers.[34–36] With regard to AP cantilevers, a greater AP spread of the implants provides better distribution of forces. When placing 2 zygoma implants in the same side of the maxilla, the position of the platform of the anterior zygoma implant is usually at the level of lateral incisor/canine. The platform

of the posterior zygoma is usually at the second premolar/first molar. AP cantilevers decrease by placing additional dental implants anterior or posterior to the zygoma fixtures. In the presence of maxillary defects, these principles are difficult to follow because the implant position is often dictated by the size of the defect, residual bone support, and implant position. Computer-aided design (CAD)–computer-aided manufacturing (CAM) technology is useful for the prosthetic design. This technology permits the study of these cantilevers and allows the design of complex superstructures in the presence of unfavorable cantilevers (**Fig. 9**). The unaffected side and opposing dentition require special attention. Cross-arch stabilization could be jeopardized if most of the teeth are present in the unaffected side. With regard to the opposing dentition, excessive forces can be avoided by eliminating cantilevers from the prosthetic design.

Hygiene

The ability to maintain good oral hygiene in this type of reconstruction is sometimes understated. Although a fixed restoration might be indicated, it is important to have the patient's feedback on their ability to maintain good oral hygiene. A bar-retained prosthesis should be considered whenever compliance is in question. Oral hygiene is

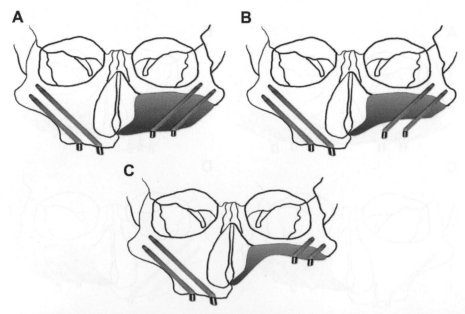

Fig. 8. Implant length, platform placement, and the relation to the defect soft tissue coverage. (*A*) Correct implant length, with implant platform placed at the level of the thick soft tissue coverage. (*B*) Incorrect implant length, with the implant platform placed in an overextended position in the oral cavity. This placement makes prosthetic reconstruction and oral hygiene more difficult. (*C*) Correct implant length, with implant platform placed at the level of thin soft tissue coverage. These implants are placed more laterally and posterior from the original maxillary alveolar ridge, but they can be restored by adding a flange to the prosthetic reconstruction.

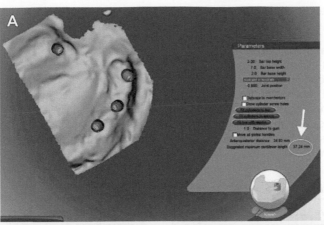

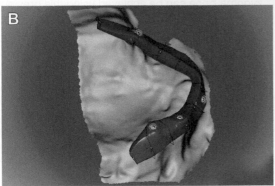

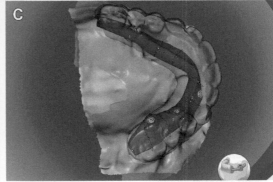

Fig. 9. CAD/CAM technology for the prosthetic design. (A, B) Study of the cantilevers and design of the superstructure. Note the suggested maximum cantilever length (arrow). (C) Design of the fixed-hybrid prosthesis.

especially important when the maxillary defect is covered with free soft tissue transfers, because the peri-implant tissues tend to become easily inflamed. This peri-implantitis is refractory to traditional methods of control and its management is difficult. These patients are better suited to a bar-retained prosthesis, which is easier to clean and maintain. If a fixed-hybrid design is selected, a great pearl is to place the shallow screw access channels of the prosthesis in metal. This strategy facilitates removal of the prosthesis because resin seals over the screws are not needed (Fig. 10).

Oroantral or oronasal communications

In the presence of communications, if no contraindications exist, an evaluation should be made to consider the possibility of a surgical closure with local, regional, or free tissue transfers. This topic is further discussed in the surgical considerations section. If closure cannot be achieved surgically, a prosthetic option is a bar-retained obturator. An additional option is a fixed-hybrid reconstruction, with an additional obturator. This obturator could be supported by using clasps or by adding extra locator attachments over the fixed-hybrid superstructure.

Lip support and aesthetics

Lip support and aesthetics are also closely related to the size and residual anatomy of the defect. Optimizing tooth position to create an ideal smile may increase the length of the cantilever. Sometimes, aesthetics must be compromised to adhere to sound biomechanical principles. The existent or the provisional prostheses are good

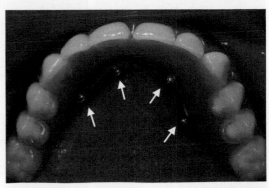

Fig. 10. Prosthesis shallow screw access channels placed in metal (arrows) for easier removal of the prosthesis.

indicators for the need to add or remove support (**Fig. 11**).

Patient preference and socioeconomics

Even when a fixed-hybrid is indicated, some patients (especially oncology patients) prefer to have a bar-retained reconstruction that allows easy access for cancer screening. These prosthetic reconstructions tend to be expensive, and sometimes, they must be tailored to the patient's socioeconomic means.

Surgical Considerations

For a comprehensive overview of the original zygoma implant technique, readers are referred to previously published articles by Sevetz[37] and Bedrossian[38] in *Oral and Maxillofacial Surgery Clinics of North America*. Several modifications to the original technique have been described in the literature, including:

1. Sinus slot technique by Stella and Warner[39] (2000)
2. Platform angulation changed from 45° to 55° to reduce the cantilevers by Boyes-Varley and colleagues[34] (2003)
3. Extrasinus implant placement by Maló and colleagues[35] (2008)
4. ZAGA by Aparicio[36] (2011)

During the surgical planning for the placement of zygoma implants in acquired maxillary defects,

the following factors should be taken into consideration.

Access

The patient's ability to open their mouth wide is important because of the implant placement angulation and the length of the burs. Heavy scarring or radiation usually compromises this capacity in patients with maxillary acquired defects. When mild to moderate trismus is encountered, the clinician should consider using a regular dental implant contra-angle instead of the zygoma implant handpiece because the former uses less space within the oral cavity. In patients with a preexisting Webber-Ferguson approach, access to the zygoma bone can be achieved using this previous approach.

Oroantral/oronasal communication/defect soft tissue coverage

The prosthetic reconstruction is facilitated in the absence of an oroantral/oronasal communication. When no contraindication exists, consideration must be given to creating a surgical closure using local, regional, or free tissue transfers. The surgeon may encounter 3 different scenarios for zygoma implant placement, described in the following sections.

1. Implant placement after closure: the advantage of this approach is that the soft tissues covering the defect are already conformed to the oral cavity. By knowing the amount of

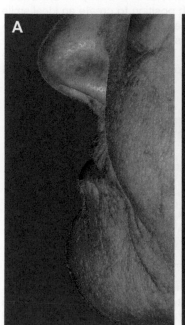 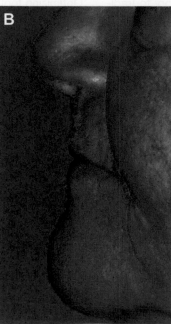

Fig. 11. Lip support. Because of the complexity of these defects, optimizing tooth position to create an ideal lip support and smile may increase the length of the cantilever. (*A*) Profile view without prosthesis. (*B*) Profile view with prosthesis.

soft tissue coverage, the surgeon is able to better determine the implant length, avoiding excessive extrusion in oral cavity. This approach also allows for the possibility of performing a 1-stage functional rehabilitation.

2. Implant placement at the same time of closure: this scenario usually requires a 2-stage rehabilitation, because once the implants are placed, they are covered completely by the soft tissue reconstruction. This approach avoids the possible overextension of the zygoma implant in the oral cavity (**Fig. 12**). During implant uncovering, care must be taken to avoid excessive soft tissue manipulation, because the lack of integration between these tissues and the implant surface has the potential to create a new communication.

3. Implants placed before closure: this scenario is the least favorable of the 3. Zygoma implants could potentially interfere with the soft tissue reconstruction and the communication could remain because of the lack of integration of the soft tissue and implant.

Implant length and angulation

Size of the defect, residual bone, and soft tissue coverage are factors that help determine the implant length and angulation. As an example, a bilateral maxillary defect requires shorter and more horizontal implants to avoid excessive protrusion in the oral cavity (see **Fig. 12**E). A duplicate of the patient's prosthesis or obturator can be used to help with the angulation of the implant and final platform position.

OUTCOMES

A recent systematic review[40] of the survival and complications of zygoma implants indicated that the overall success of these implants in the treatment of severely atrophic maxilla ranged from 90.3% to 100%. Higher survival rates (95.8%–100%) were found when the immediate function protocol was used in the same population. Few studies have focused on the outcomes of zygoma implant reconstructions in acquired maxillary defects. The success rate in these studies ranges from 78.6% to 91.7%.[11,14,27] Landes[27] identify 4 factors that could explain the lower success rates in this population: overloading leverage in extensive maxillectomies; overgrowth of local soft tissue, preventing abutment connection; recurrent infection; and tumor recurrence. However, Schmidt and colleagues[11] suggested a larger role of radiotherapy because all of their implant failures occurred at stage II, before loading.

COMPLICATIONS

The placement of zygoma implants is a safe and predictable technique. Complications are rare. Their incidence in zygoma implant reconstruction of acquired maxillary bony defects is unknown because only a few studies are available. Complications are more likely to develop in this population, because residual bone and soft tissues do not behave in the same manner as in the severely atrophic maxilla.

Common complications encountered in zygoma implant reconstruction of acquired maxillary defects are described in the following sections.

Sinusitis

Sinusitis is the most common complication reported in the literature of zygoma implants in severely atrophic maxilla (1.85%–18.42%).[30,40,41] It is uncertain if in acquired maxillary defects the development of sinusitis is caused by intrinsic factors of the sinus (eg, ostiomeatal obstruction after gunshot wound) or the presence of the zygoma implant. Davó and colleagues suggested 3 different etiopathogenic mechanisms:

1. Zygoma implant placement as invasive surgery for the sinus
2. Zygoma implant as intrasinus foreign body
3. Zygoma implant potentially creating an oroantral fistula

Regardless of the cause, antibiotics and decongestants are the first line of treatment. Refractory cases are better served with functional endoscopic sinus surgery (FESS) (**Fig. 13**).

Peri-implantitis

Peri-implantitis is commonly found when a free soft tissue flap was used to cover the defect. Even after debunking, keratinized tissue grafts, and multiple debridement, it remains difficult to control. Silver nitrate usually works well to control the peri-implant granulation tissue. These patients require close follow-up to ensure long-term success. In the absence of maxillary alveolar bone, this peri-implantitis does not compromise osseointegration, because the support of the implants is on the zygoma bone.

SUMMARY

Zygoma implant reconstruction of acquired maxillary defects is a safe, predictable, and cost-effective treatment modality. It should be part of the armamentarium of every clinician treating these complex defects. A team approach between

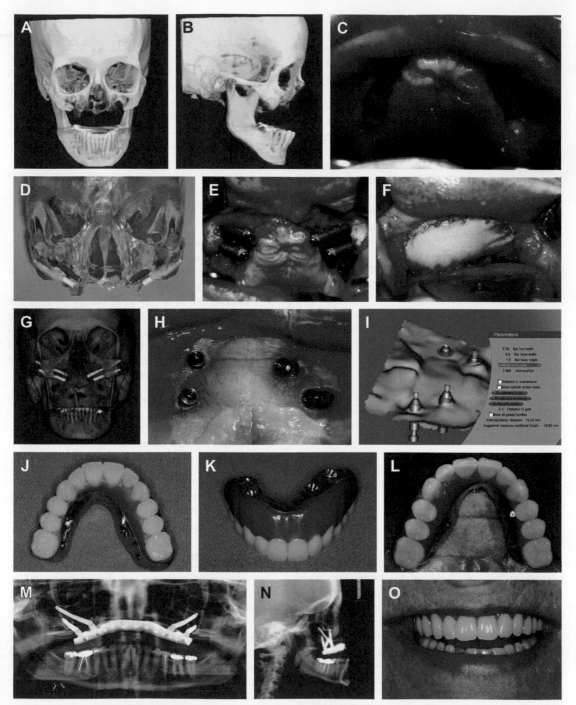

Fig. 12. Zygoma implant placement at the same time as the closure of bilateral oroantral communications. (*A, B*) Frontal and lateral views of a three-dimensional CT reconstruction of a 61-year-old woman with bilateral maxillary defects after surgical debridement of a mucormycosis infection. (*C*) Preoperative view of the oroantral communications. (*D*) Stereolithographic model surgery. (*E*) Intraoperative view of the placement of 4 zygoma implants. Note the lack of maxillary bony support and the implant platform placed at the level of the residual palatal tissue. (*F*) Intraoperative view of the closure of the oroantral communication with a radial forearm free flap. (*G*) Postoperative three-dimensional CT reconstruction showing the implants as planned in the model surgery. (*H*) Implants ready to be restored. (*I*) CAD/CAM study and prosthetic design. (*J–L*) Final prosthesis. (*M, N*) Final panoramic and cephalometric radiographs. Note the AP and vertical cantilevers. (*O*) Result.

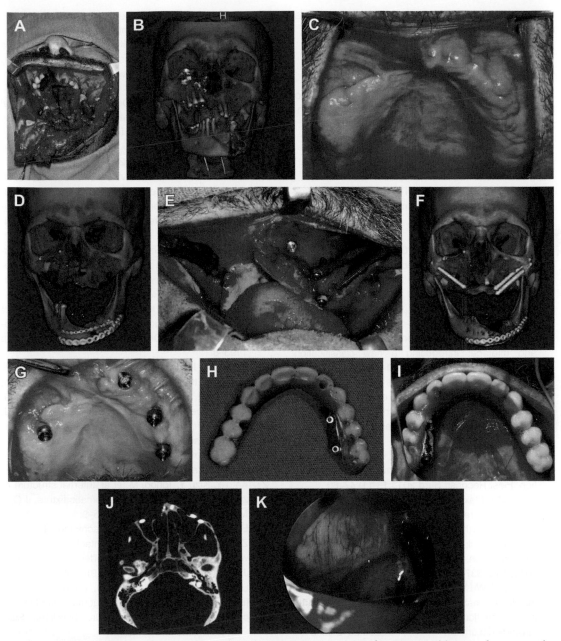

Fig. 13. Postoperative complications. Sinusitis. (*A*) Intraoperative view of a 57-year-old man after a gunshot wound to the face. (*B*) Preoperative three-dimensional CT reconstruction of the original injury. (*C*) Intraoral view of the maxillary defect 3 months after the original repair. (*D*) Postoperative three-dimensional CT reconstruction of the original repair. (*E*) Intraoperative view of the placement of 1 zygoma implant in the affect side in combination with 1 regular and 2 zygoma implants in the unaffected side. (*F*) Postoperative three-dimensional CT reconstruction after the zygoma implant placement. (*G*) Implants ready to be restored. (*H, I*) Final prosthesis. (*J*) Axial CT scan view showing right maxillary sinusitis, which developed 8 months after implant placement. Note the lack of involvement of the left maxillary sinus. This finding suggests that the development of the sinusitis in this case is probably caused by secondary effects of the gunshot wound in the permeability of the ostiomeatal complex. This sinusitis was refractory to antibiotics and decongestants and required FESS for resolution. (*K*) Intraoperative endoscopic view of the left maxillary sinus, which shows the zygoma implants in the sinus partially covered by healthy sinus membrane.

the surgeon and the restorative dentist is paramount for treatment success.

ACKNOWLEDGMENTS

The authors want to thank Dr Edward Sevetz for being instrumental in the establishment of the zygoma implant technique in our institution.

REFERENCES

1. Bidra AS, Jacob RF, Taylor TD. Classification of maxillectomy defects: a systematic review and criteria necessary for a universal description. J Prosthet Dent 2012;107(4):261–70.
2. McCarthy CM, Cordeiro PG. Microvascular reconstruction of oncologic defects of the midface. Plast Reconstr Surg 2010;126(6):1947–59.
3. O'Connell DA, Futran ND. Reconstruction of the midface and maxilla. Curr Opin Otolaryngol Head Neck Surg 2010;18(4):304–10.
4. Brown JS, Shaw RJ. Reconstruction of the maxilla and midface: introducing a new classification. Lancet Oncol 2010;11(10):1001–8.
5. González-García R, Naval-Gías L. Transport osteogenesis in the maxillofacial skeleton: outcomes of a versatile reconstruction method following tumor ablation. Arch Otolaryngol Head Neck Surg 2010; 136(3):243–50.
6. Hanasono MM, Silva AK, Yu P, et al. A comprehensive algorithm for oncologic maxillary reconstruction. Plast Reconstr Surg 2013;131(1):47–60.
7. Haug SP. Maxillofacial prosthetic management of the maxillary resection patient. Atlas Oral Maxillofac Surg Clin North Am 2007;15(1):51–68.
8. Kim DD, Ghali GE. Dental implants in oral cancer reconstruction. Oral Maxillofac Surg Clin North Am 2011;23(2):337–45, vii.
9. Huang W, Wu Y, Zou D, et al. Long-term results for maxillary rehabilitation with dental implants after tumor resection. Clin Implant Dent Relat Res 2012. http://dx.doi.org/10.1111/j.1708-8208.2012.00481.x.
10. Brånemark PI, Gröndahl K, Ohrnell LO, et al. Zygoma fixture in the management of advanced atrophy of the maxilla: technique and long-term results. Scand J Plast Reconstr Surg Hand Surg 2004;38(2):70–85.
11. Schmidt BL, Pogrel MA, Young CW, et al. Reconstruction of extensive maxillary defects using zygomaticus implants. J Oral Maxillofac Surg 2004; 62(Suppl 2):82–9.
12. Parel SM, Brånemark PI, Ohrnell LO, et al. Remote implant anchorage for the rehabilitation of maxillary defects. J Prosthet Dent 2001;86(4):377–81.
13. Boyes-Varley JG, Howes DG, Davidge-Pitts KD, et al. A protocol for maxillary reconstruction

following oncology resection using zygomatic implants. Int J Prosthodont 2007;20(5):521–31.
14. Landes CA, Paffrath C, Koehler C, et al. Zygoma implants for midfacial prosthetic rehabilitation using telescopes: 9-year follow-up. Int J Prosthodont 2009;22(1):20–32.
15. Zwahlen RA, Grätz KW, Oechslin CK, et al. Survival rate of zygomatic implants in atrophic or partially resected maxillae prior to functional loading: a retrospective clinical report. Int J Oral Maxillofac Implants 2006;21(3):413–20.
16. Hirsch DL, Howell KL, Levine JP. A novel approach to palatomaxillary reconstruction: use of radial forearm free tissue transfer combined with zygomaticus implants. J Oral Maxillofac Surg 2009;67(11): 2466–72.
17. Örtorp A. Three tumor patients with total maxillectomy rehabilitated with implant-supported frameworks and maxillary obturators: a follow-up report. Clin Implant Dent Relat Res 2010;12(4):315–23.
18. Uchida Y, Goto M, Katsuki T, et al. Measurement of the maxilla and zygoma as an aid in installing zygomatic implants. J Oral Maxillofac Surg 2001;59(10): 1193–8.
19. Nkenke E, Hahn M, Lell M, et al. Anatomic site evaluation of the zygomatic bone for dental implant placement. Clin Oral Implants Res 2003;14(1):72–9.
20. van Steenberghe D, Malevez C, van Cleynenbreugel J, et al. Accuracy of drilling guides for transfer from three-dimensional CT-based planning to placement of zygoma implants in human cadavers. Clin Oral Implants Res 2003;14(1):131–6.
21. Kato Y, Kizu Y, Tonogi M, et al. Internal structure of zygomatic bone related to zygomatic fixture. J Oral Maxillofac Surg 2005;63(9):1325–9.
22. Balshi TJ, Wolfinger GJ, Shuscavage NJ, et al. Zygomatic bone-to-implant contact in 77 patients with partially or completely edentulous maxillas. J Oral Maxillofac Surg 2012;70(9):2065–9.
23. Ujigawa K, Kato Y, Kizu Y, et al. Three-dimensional finite elemental analysis of zygomatic implants in craniofacial structures. Int J Oral Maxillofac Surg 2007;36(7):620–5.
24. Miyamoto S, Ujigawa K, Kizu Y, et al. Biomechanical three-dimensional finite-element analysis of maxillary prostheses with implants. Design of number and position of implants for maxillary prostheses after hemimaxillectomy. Int J Oral Maxillofac Surg 2010;39(11):1120–6.
25. Korkmaz FM, Korkmaz YT, Yaluğ S, et al. Impact of dental and zygomatic implants on stress distribution in maxillary defects: a 3-dimensional finite element analysis study. J Oral Implantol 2012;38(5):557–67.
26. Romeed S, Malik R, Dunne S. Zygomatic implants: the impact of zygoma bone support on biomechanics. J Oral Implantol 2012. http://dx.doi.org/10.1563/AAID-JOI-D-11-00245.1.

27. Landes CA. Zygoma implant-supported midfacial prosthetic rehabilitation: a 4-year follow-up study including assessment of quality of life. Clin Oral Implants Res 2005;16(3):313–25.

28. Schiroli G, Angiero F, Silvestrini-Biavati A, et al. Zygomatic implant placement with flapless computer-guided surgery: a proposed clinical protocol. J Oral Maxillofac Surg 2011;69(12):2979–89.

29. Vrielinck L, Politis C, Schepers S, et al. Image-based planning and clinical validation of zygoma and pterygoid implant placement in patients with severe bone atrophy using customized drill guides. Preliminary results from a prospective clinical follow-up study. Int J Oral Maxillofac Surg 2003;32(1):7–14.

30. Davó R, Malevez C, López-Orellana C, et al. Sinus reactions to immediately loaded zygoma implants: a clinical and radiological study. Eur J Oral Implantol 2008;1(1):53–60.

31. Bedrossian E, Stumpel LJ. Immediate stabilization at stage II of zygomatic implants: rationale and technique. J Prosthet Dent 2001;86(1):10–4.

32. Kreissl ME, Heydecke G, Metzger MC, et al. Zygoma implant-supported prosthetic rehabilitation after partial maxillectomy using surgical navigation: a clinical report. J Prosthet Dent 2007;97(3):121–8.

33. Shirota T, Shimodaira O, Matsui Y, et al. Zygoma implant-supported prosthetic rehabilitation of a patient with a maxillary defect. Int J Oral Maxillofac Surg 2011;40(1):113–7.

34. Boyes-Varley JG, Howes DG, Lownie JF, et al. Surgical modifications to the Brånemark zygomaticus

35. Maló P, Nobre Mde A, Lopes I. A new approach to rehabilitate the severely atrophic maxilla using extra-maxillary anchored implants in immediate function: a pilot study. J Prosthet Dent 2008;100(5):354–66.

36. Aparicio C. A proposed classification for zygomatic implant patient based on the zygoma anatomy guided approach (ZAGA): a cross-sectional survey. Eur J Oral Implantol 2011;4(3):269–75.

37. Sevetz EB. Treatment of the severely atrophic fully edentulous maxilla: the zygoma implant option. Atlas Oral Maxillofac Surg Clin North Am 2006; 14(1):121–36.

38. Bedrossian E. Rescue implant concept: the expanded use of the zygoma implant in the graftless solutions. Oral Maxillofac Surg Clin North Am 2011; 23(2):257–76.

39. Stella JP, Warner MR. Sinus slot technique for simplification and improved orientation of zygomaticus dental implants: a technical note. Int J Oral Maxillofac Implants 2000;15(6):889–93.

40. Chrcanovic BR, Abreu MH. Survival and complications of zygomatic implants: a systematic review. Oral Maxillofac Surg 2012. http://dx.doi.org/10.1007/s10006-012-0331-z.

41. Candel-Martí E, Carrillo-García C, Peñarrocha-Oltra D, et al. Rehabilitation of atrophic posterior maxilla with zygomatic implants: review. J Oral Implantol 2012;38(5):653–7.

protocol in the treatment of the severely resorbed maxilla: a clinical report. Int J Oral Maxillofac Implants 2003;18(2):232–7.

Reconstruction of Acquired Oromandibular Defects

Rui P. Fernandes, DMD, MD[a,b,*], Jacob G. Yetzer, DDS, MD[a,c]

KEYWORDS

- Mandible • Defect • Reconstruction

KEY POINTS

- Familiarity with mandibular and cervical anatomy is crucial in achieving mandibular reconstruction.
- The surgeon must evaluate which components of the hard and soft tissue are missing in selecting a method of reconstruction.
- Complexity of mandibular reconstruction ranges from simple rigid internal fixation to microvascular free tissue transfer, depending on factors related to both defect and patient.
- Modern techniques for microvascular tissue transfer provide a wide array of reconstructive options that can be tailored to patients' specific needs.

INTRODUCTION

Acquired defects of the mandible result from trauma, infection, osteoradionecrosis, and, most commonly, ablative surgery of the oral cavity and lower face. These defects are particularly debilitating not only because of the profoundly negative effect they have on facial appearance but also because they create disabilities of mastication and swallowing along with poor speech and oral competence.

For these reasons, surgeons have historically sought new and better methods to reconstruct mandibular defects. Early efforts are described from the ancient Chinese and Etruscans to Hippocrates himself involving prosthetics of wood, terracotta, and metal bound to bone or teeth in attempts to restore mandibular continuity.[1] Since then, modern surgery has developed more effective techniques including nonvascularized bone grafting, improved alloplastic materials, locoregional flaps, and vascularized soft-tissue and composite flaps. These components of the reconstructive surgeon's armamentarium have become indispensable.

ANATOMY

Considering the complex anatomy of the mandible, it is easy to appreciate why restoration of its form and function is so vital to patients' quality of life. The mandible and its associated soft tissues form the majority of the lower one-third of the face. It provides appropriate facial height anteriorly from the lower lip to the chin, and forms the skeletal framework for normal facial width at the level of the gonial angles. The alveolar process also houses the mandibular dentition within its tooth-bearing area, overlying the basal bone of the body and symphysis.

Functionally the temporomandibular joints allow for the complex movements involved in speech, chewing, and swallowing. These bilateral joints at the proximal aspects of the mandible are

[a] Department of Oral and Maxillofacial Surgery, College of Medicine, University of Florida, 653-1 West Eight Street, LRC 2nd Floor, Jacksonville, FL 32209, USA; [b] Department of Surgery, Division of Surgical Oncology, College of Medicine, University of Florida, 653-1 West Eight Street, LRC 2nd Floor, Jacksonville, FL 32209, USA; [c] Department of Surgery, College of Medicine, University of Florida, 653-1 West Eight Street, LRC 2nd Floor, Jacksonville, FL 32209, USA
* Corresponding author.
E-mail address: rui.fernandes@jax.ufl.edu

Oral Maxillofacial Surg Clin N Am 25 (2013) 241–249
http://dx.doi.org/10.1016/j.coms.2013.02.003
1042-3699/13/$ – see front matter © 2013 Elsevier Inc. All rights reserved.

ginglymoarthrodial; that is, they allow for rotational and translational movement within the glenoid fossa and articular eminence where the mandibular condyles approximate the skull base. Articulating on a fibrocartilage surface and supported by the capsular, temporomandibular, stylomandibular, and sphenomandibular ligaments, these paired joints are some of the more complex in the human body.

Major muscular attachments include the masticatory group: paired temporalis, masseters, and medial and lateral pterygoids create the forces necessary for efficient chewing and speech. Smaller, but no less important, muscular attachments such as extrinsic tongue and digastric muscles attach at the symphysis, and play a role in effective speech and swallowing along with airway maintenance.

Surgical access when reconstructing this region is almost always transcervical. Not only does this allow significantly better access than a transoral route, but it allows for access to recipient vessels for free flap reconstruction as well as the ability to perform any necessary lymphadenectomy. The dissection to the mandible requires a dissection of multiple layers. Just deep to skin lies the superficial cervical fascia. This fascia is closely associated with the platysma muscle, which is just deep, and may not be recognized as a separate layer. Continuing deeper, the superficial layer of the deep cervical fascia (SLDCF) can be identified just below the platysma.

Also known as the investing layer, the SLDCF is an important fascial component for the surgeon to understand because of its close association with several structures encountered during mandibular reconstruction. This layer envelops the trapezius and sternocleidomastoid muscles, and forms the parotidomasseteric sheath and submandibular capsule. More germane to the submandibular approach, this layer also contains the marginal mandibular branch of the facial nerve. It is important to identify and preserve this branch, because it has been found in anatomic dissections to curve below the inferior border of the mandible up to 53% of the time to a distance of up to 1.2 cm below the mandible.[2,3] Conveniently, the facial vein can be identified just deep to the SLDCF and superficial to the digastric muscle. By retracting this vein superiorly in a Hayes-Martin maneuver, the surgeon is assured that the marginal mandibular branch is safely retracted as well.

Continuing deep to the SLDCF, the submandibular triangle is encountered. The inferior border of the mandible and the anterior and posterior bellies of the digastric muscle bound this anatomically rich region. The digastric muscle has been referred to as the "resident's friend" because all clinically significant vessels and other important structures are found deep to this muscle. The facial artery is usually the first branch of the external carotid to be encountered in this area of dissection as it courses across the antegonial notch. It is important that this structure is identified and preserved because it, along with the facial vein, provides an ideal recipient vessel for anastomosis. Also within the submandibular triangle lies the submandibular gland, with the deep and superficial lobes enveloping the posterior margin of the mylohyoid muscle.

Retraction of the mylohyoid anteriorly gives access to the sublingual space and reveals the submandibular duct coursing anteriorly from the superior aspect of the gland. By following this structure anteriorly, the lingual nerve is identified as it loops below the duct on its course toward the tongue. The hypoglossal nerve will also be seen here, running just adjacent to the hyoglossus muscle, which forms the medial boundary of the sublingual space. Knowledge of the anatomy of these perimandibular areas is paramount in identifying and protecting critical structures when preparing the recipient site for oromandibular reconstruction.

GOALS OF RECONSTRUCTION

As is the case with many facial reconstructive procedures, the goals of the operation are most concisely summed up as restoration of original form and function. With this under consideration, there are more specific considerations on which to base surgical planning. First, primary reconstruction is preferable to delayed procedures when permitted by the patient's health status and motivation. Primary reconstruction allows the patient to avoid a second operation as well as the interim period of functional deficit. Outcomes are also better with primary reconstruction because the surgeon does not face the increased challenges of soft-tissue contracture, scarring, bone loss, or avascular tissue often dealt with in delayed reconstruction.[4]

Other specific goals of the reconstruction are primary closure, and soft tissue that allows for good tongue mobility and adequacy of the stoma. The reconstruction should reestablish mandibular continuity and should provide normal contour. In addition, there must be sufficient bone to provide a foundation for dental rehabilitation. Normal mobility of the mandible through its range of motion is also desirable. All of this must be accomplished in a manner whereby the aesthetic outcome allows the patient to remain socially functional (**Table 1**).

Table 1
Advantages and disadvantages of reconstructive techniques

Reconstruction	Advantages	Disadvantages
Gap-bridging plate	Fast and simple No donor site	Hardware failure Dehiscence, fistula No dental rehabilitation
Nonvascularized bone graft	Less technique sensitive than free flaps Shorter operating time	Requires soft-tissue presence Unpredictable
Fibula free flap	Long bone segment Two-team approach Soft tissue available Low donor-site morbidity	Limited cross-sectional bone stock
Scapula free flap	Soft tissue independent of bone Unaffected by atherosclerosis Large quantity of soft tissue	Cannot perform 2-team approach Limited cross-sectional bone stock
Iliac crest free flap	Large bone volume Two-team approach Soft tissue available	Donor-site morbidity
Radial forearm free flap	Relatively simple Pliable soft tissue	Limited available bone Significant morbidity with radius fracture

CLASSIFICATION

A review of the literature offers several classification schemes for oromandibular defects. Early classifications focused on hard-tissue defects, designating them based on central or lateral location and involvement of particular mandibular components.[5,6] Others have included a soft-tissue component, and differentiate defects of skin, mucosa, or both from bone-only defects.[7,8]

The most comprehensive system to date is that devised by Urken and colleagues.[9] This system categorizes defects based first on bony region: condyle, ramus, body, and symphysis. A coding system of superscripts and subscripts indicates the nature of the defect. For instance, a body defect with marginal resection is designated as B^M. It also specifically details the location of mucosal and soft-tissue defects including subsites of the palate, pharynx, floor of mouth, and tongue, and cutaneous defects. Examples would be FOM^L for lateral floor of mouth or $T^B_{1/4}$ for one-quarter of the tongue base. Finally, unique to the Urken classification is the description of neurologic problems involving the inferior alveolar, lingual, hypoglossal, and facial nerves.

The point to be emphasized from any classification system chosen is that the reconstructive surgeon must be cognizant of the specific structures lost. Before beginning a reconstruction, the surgeon should ask the following. (1) Which portions of the mandible must be recreated? (2) Where is soft tissue missing? (3) What functional loss can be expected as a result of this patient's particular defect? Only when these questions have been answered can the surgeon select the appropriate reconstruction (**Fig. 1**).

RECONSTRUCTIVE OPTIONS
Rigid Fixation with Internal Plating

Fixation of mandibular segments with an intervening bony gap using titanium plates has been a well-described option in mandibular reconstruction since the 1980s. This method provides a simple way to prevent collapse of the lower face and provide a framework for soft tissues supported by the mandible. When applying this technique, locking plates and screws can be helpful in preventing bone resorption around the hardware and subsequent loosening and infection of the plate. In addition, careful, tension-free soft-tissue coverage over the implant is crucial. Adequate closure can be facilitated with the use of locoregional flaps.

Despite these precautions, plating of the mandible alone tends to be fraught with long-term complications[10] including fistulae, plate fracture, soft-tissue breakdown, infection, and eventual plate removal.[11] Hardware failure has been reported from 21% to 37% of the time, and is particularly common in anterior segmental defects.[8,11,12] In addition to these problems, alloplastic reconstruction of this type is limited for dental reconstruction, and also fails to address soft-tissue defects. Overall, gap-bridging plates should be

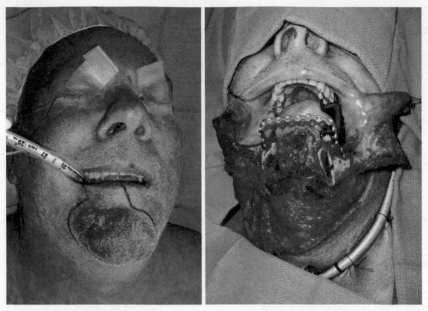

Fig. 1. Preoperative and completed composite resection for squamous cell carcinoma. Defect includes skin, anterior mandible, and floor of mouth. Thorough preoperative planning will direct and facilitate the reconstruction of oromandibular defects.

considered an option for patients who may not tolerate other means of reconstruction because of medical comorbidities or as a temporary measure before definitive reconstruction.

Nonvascularized Autogenous Bone Graft

Bone grafts can be harvested from any number of donor sites including rib, sternum, contralateral mandible, and calvarium. The most common option for mandibular reconstruction at present is the iliac crest graft from either an anterior or posterior approach (**Fig. 2**). The rationale is to transfer as many osteocompetent cells as possible to the recipient site. This action is best accomplished with cancellous bone chips, often with crib or scaffold that resorbs over time. Such a reconstruction can be a useful option for shorter segmental defects or marginal defects, especially those resulting from trauma or benign disease not requiring radiation.[13,14]

Because the survival of fragile osteoprogenitor cells determines the success or failure of these grafts, a specific set of circumstances must be

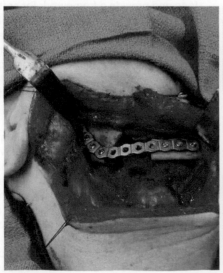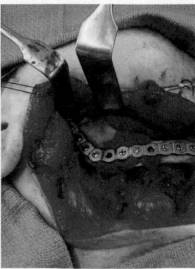

Fig. 2. Small segmental defect reconstructed using nonvascularized bone graft from the anterior iliac crest.

present, including stability of bone segments, adequate vascularity of surrounding tissue, and an uncontaminated donor site.[15] Owing to the nature of many oromandibular defects, the spectrum of uses for nonvascularized bone grafts is severely limited. Patients with cancer, for instance, generally have decreased vascularity of surrounding tissue resulting from their ablative surgery and radiation treatment. In addition, there are often coexisting soft-tissue defects, which prevent watertight closure of the site, which allows oral contamination and subsequent failure of the graft. These factors have led to an overall high failure rate of these techniques and a fall from favor for oromandibular reconstruction.[16,17]

Vascularized Free Tissue Transfer

The use of microvascular techniques for free tissue transfer has become the gold standard for oromandibular reconstruction. Since the 1980s this method has revolutionized maxillofacial reconstruction. These well-vascularized reconstructions are able to resist infection in the face of oral contamination, permit simultaneous hard-tissue and soft-tissue reconstruction, and allow rapid dental rehabilitation with endosseous implants. Their overall rate of success has been reported as greater than 95%.[18] For reconstruction of the oromandibular complex, 4 flaps are generally considered: fibula, iliac, scapula, and, in rare circumstances, radius (**Table 2**).

Although these flaps as a group have many favorable characteristics in comparison with other reconstructive methods, there are several considerations that must be understood by the surgeon preparing to perform such operations. First, the patient must be able to tolerate the longer operating time required for these technically demanding procedures. If medical comorbidities pose a barrier to prolonged anesthesia time, a simpler mode of reconstruction may be required. In addition, a degree of donor-site morbidity is to be expected, but can be minimized with appropriate foresight in selecting the harvest site. Handedness, lifestyle, occupation, and functional status should be recognized before proceeding to the operating room. Another necessary precaution when using free tissue transfer is ensuring adequate recipient vessels, which must be confirmed if previous surgeries have been performed near the planned anastomosis. A computed tomography angiogram (CTA) of the neck will generally suffice for this purpose. Finally, the procedure itself is relatively complex, and requires a surgeon be comfortable with the techniques needed to carry out harvest and anastomosis of the flap.

Fibula

The fibula flap was first described for mandibular reconstruction in 1989 by Hidalgo,[19] and remains a commonly used flap because of its versatility. Up to 25 cm of bone can be harvested for long segmental defects, and the flap can be used as either an osseous or osteocutaneous flap by including septocutaneous or musculocutaneous perforators to the skin. The skin paddle can be used to close several mucosal or cutaneous defects. The cross-sectional shape of the bone allows for bicortical placement of dental implants, thus allowing for immediate dental reconstruction because of the excellent primary stability.[20] The flap can also be made sensate by anastomosis to the lateral sural cutaneous nerve. In addition, the fibula can easily be harvested with a 2-team approach, saving time under anesthesia and in the operating room (**Fig. 3**).

Because the dominant pedicle to the fibula flap is the peroneal artery, preoperative assessment

Table 2
Defect-based reconstructive preferences

Defect	Favored Reconstruction
Short segment with no soft-tissue defect	Nonvascularized bone graft
Long segment	Fibula free flap
Condylar	Fibula free flap
Anterior mandible	Iliac crest free flap
Complex soft-tissue needs	Scapula
Patient with extensive vascular disease	Scapula
Palliative case	Spanning reconstruction plate

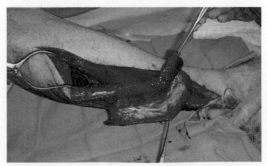

Fig. 3. Fibula flap osteotomized and configured for reconstruction of condyle-to-parasymphysis defect. The skin paddle can be used to reconstruct either mucosa or skin by reorienting the flap.

of the lower extremity vasculature is required to ensure adequate perfusion to the flap as well as to the foot by remaining tibial vessels. The method of this assessment depends on surgeon preference. Doppler ultrasonography, magnetic resonance angiography, CTA, and angiography are all reasonable as long as the peroneal artery is present and adequate blood supply to the foot can be confirmed. In vasculopathic patients this is not always possible, and other flaps must be considered.

Another potential challenge with the fibula is the height of the bone relative to the mandible. The fibula is only 1.5 cm thick compared with the 4- to 5-cm height of the mandible. Jones and colleagues[21] offered a solution to this problem with a "double-barrel" technique whereby the bone is osteotomized and stacked on itself. However, this must be done carefully to avoid insult to the pedicle or soft-tissue perforators, and its use may be limited in anterior defects for which multiple osteotomies are necessary. The fibula may also be fixated slightly above the inferior border of the mandible to reduce the crown-to-root ratio of dental implants. This action is also a compromise because to the extent that the fibula is elevated, a step will be created along the inferior mandibular border.

Donor-site morbidity is usually minor, but good hemostasis is essential before closure because of the potential for compartment syndrome. Other possible complications include infection, paresthesia, limited range of motion, and ankle instability.[22] Five days of splint wear followed by assisted ambulation and physical therapy is generally all that is required to have the patient functioning normally again by 4 to 5 weeks postoperatively.

Iliac

Taylor and colleagues[23,24] pioneered the use of the iliac crest flap as supplied by the deep circumflex iliac artery (DCIA), and its use in mandibular reconstruction. The increased bone height (2.5 vs 1.5 cm for fibula) and thickness of the bone that can be obtained makes it a useful alternative for mandibular reconstruction. It is particularly useful in areas requiring closer height match to the native mandible, such as in anterior defects. This closer match facilitates dental rehabilitation. Though not quite offering the length of the fibula, 14 cm of bone can still be harvested, which is adequate for most bony defects (**Fig. 4**).

This flap can also be harvested as an osteocutaneous or osteomyocutaneous flap for reconstruction of soft tissues. In general, inclusion of the internal oblique muscle allows for better closure of the mucosal side than does a skin paddle,[25] because the skin perforators travel along the inner table of the ilium and offer limited mobility, whereas the internal oblique is supplied by a separate ascending branch off of the DCIA that allows greater mobility and less chance of vascular compromise seen from difficult positioning of the skin paddle. Over time the denervated muscle will mucosalize, providing a thin mucosal lining. An additional benefit to this technique is that it leaves the separate skin paddle for closure of any skin defect that may exist, making this flap useful for through-and-through defects as well. Unlike the fibula, a DCIA flap is less likely to be compromised in patients with atherosclerosis, leaving this option available in the vasculopathic population.

The limitations of the DCIA flap come mostly from donor-site morbidity. Most commonly these relate to gait disturbance and pain. These deficits have been reported to affect around one-quarter of patients up to several months postoperatively.[26] These downsides have been debated. In fact, in 2003 Rogers and colleagues[27] reported that based on orthopedic and quality-of-life measures, the iliac

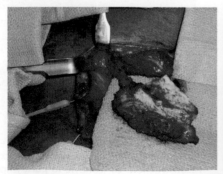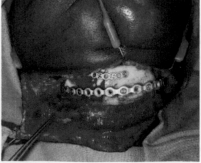

Fig. 4. Shown on the left is an iliac crest free flap elevated and ready for transfer. On right, the flap is shown inset at the recipient site for reconstruction of the anterior mandible.

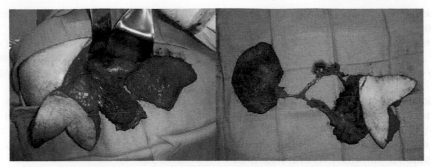

Fig. 5. Chimeric scapula flap demonstrates the flexibility of this flap, especially for geometrically complex defects.

crest flap was no different from the fibula in the long term. In any case, it remains important for patients to adhere to a physical-therapy protocol after surgery to minimize undesirable sequelae. Specific to this flap in comparison with others discussed here is the potential for hernia. Dissection of the abdominal musculature can weaken the rectus muscle as a result of denervation, and result in ventral hernia. Therefore a tight, layered closure is of critical importance.

Scapular flap

Another option for reconstruction of oromandibular defects is the scapular flap. Based on the subscapular system, specifically the circumflex scapular artery, a variety of composite flaps may be obtained. These flaps may contain skin, muscle, and bone, including separate soft-tissue paddles based on the transverse and descending cutaneous branches of the circumflex scapular artery, all of which makes the scapular flap versatile for complex reconstructions.[28] Further versatility is provided by the fact that the thoracodorsal system can be accessed simultaneously, allowing for harvest of latissimus dorsi or tip of scapula on a separate pedicle.[29]

Other advantages of the scapula flap include the large quantity of skin and its being independent of the bone. Also, because the subscapular artery is so rarely affected by atherosclerosis, this flap is a good choice in the face of peripheral vascular disease. Perhaps the biggest advantage of this option compared with those mentioned earlier is that the scapular flap has no associated disability with ambulation postoperatively. It is true that there may be some degree of shoulder pain after surgery, but by using the nondominant arm and providing physical therapy in the postoperative period, the morbidity is relatively limited (**Fig. 5**).

More problematic is that despite providing up to 14 cm of bone, the thickness is less predictable in comparison with the iliac crest and even the fibula

flap, which can create untoward challenges in dental-implant placement.[18] In addition, because of the need to turn the patient during surgery, a 2-team approach is essentially impossible, which prolongs the duration of the procedure and time under anesthesia.

Radial forearm

The radial forearm free flap is a fasciocutaneous flap that is useful in numerous ways for soft-tissue defects including components of the oral cavity, oropharynx, and skin. It provides a pliable skin paddle with good color match based on the radial artery and vena comitantes or cephalic vein (**Fig. 6**). Described initially by Yang and colleagues,[30] it was Soutar and colleagues[31] who introduced the osseous component by harvesting radius as part of the flap. Though it is worth mentioning as an option for mandibular reconstruction, the fact is that the bone stock is quite limited. Ten centimeters of length can be achieved, but only 40% of radius can be harvested.[32] Along with the significant risk of pathologic fracture,[33] this has relegated the radial forearm flap to a secondary role in oromandibular reconstruction.

Perhaps the radial forearm flap is best used in this setting when considering a second flap. Certain patients do require more tissue than can be provided using 1 flap. In these cases, 2 flaps can better fill the defect. Because of the excellent soft-tissue qualities of the forearm flap, in

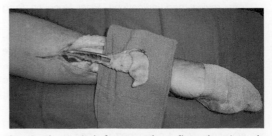

Fig. 6. The radial forearm free flap showing the pliable skin paddle, which can be used for soft-tissue coverage.

these situations it would provide additional tissue needed along with a primarily osseous flap using 2 separate sets of anastomoses.

SUMMARY

Overall, the long-term outcomes for patients undergoing reconstruction of the oromandibular complex can be good from an aesthetic and functional standpoint, including dietary and speech capabilities. Free tissue transfer with microvascular anastomosis has proved to be particularly useful in many of these patients whose defects result from cancer resection.[34] Although these are the clear choices much of the time, other reconstructive options such as alloplastic and grafting techniques continue to play an important role, based on the specific characteristics of patients and defects.

REFERENCES

1. Testelin S. History of microsurgical reconstruction of the mandible. Ann Chir Plast Esthet 1992; 37(3):241–5.
2. Dingmann RO, Grabb WC. Surgical anatomy of the mandibular ramus of the facial nerve based on the dissection of 100 facial halves. Plast Reconstr Surg 1962;29:266.
3. Ziarah HA, Atkinson MN. The surgical anatomy of the cervical distribution of the facial nerve. Br J Oral Maxillofac Surg 1981;19:159.
4. Farwell DG, Futran ND. Oromandibular reconstruction. Facial Plast Surg 2000;16(2):115–26.
5. David DJ, Tan E. Mandibular reconstruction with vascularized iliac crest: a 10-year experience. Plast Reconstr Surg 1998;82:792–803.
6. Jewer DD, Boyd JB. Orofacial and mandibular reconstruction with iliac crest free flap: a review of 60 cases and a new method of classification. Plast Reconstr Surg 1989;84:391–405.
7. Boyd JB, Gullane PJ, Brown DH. Classification of mandibular defects. Plast Reconstr Surg 1993; 92(7):1266–75.
8. Boyd JB, Mulholland RS, Davidson J, et al. The free flap and plate in oromandibular reconstruction: long-term review and indications. Plast Reconstr Surg 1995;95:1018–28.
9. Urken ML, Weinberg H, Vickery C, et al. Oromandibular reconstruction using microvascular composite free flaps. Report of 71 cases and a new classification scheme for bony, soft-tissue, and neurologic defects. Arch Otolaryngol Head Neck Surg 1991; 117:733–44.
10. Klotch DW, Prein J. Mandibular reconstruction using AO plates. Am J Surg 1987;154:384–8.
11. Gullane PJ. Primary mandibular reconstruction: analysis of 64 cases and evaluation of interface radiation dosimetry on bridging plates. Laryngoscope 1991;101:1–24.
12. Maurer P, Eckert AW, Kriwalsky MS, et al. Scope and limitations of methods of mandibular reconstruction: a long-term follow-up. Br J Oral Maxillofac Surg 2010;48:100–4.
13. Pogrel MA, Podlesh S, Anthony JP, et al. A comparison of vascularized and nonvascularized bone grafts for reconstruction of mandibular continuity defects. J Oral Maxillofac Surg 1997; 55:1200.
14. Anthony JP, Foster RD, Pogrel MA. The free fibula bone graft for salvaging failed mandibular reconstructions. J Oral Maxillofac Surg 1997;55:1417.
15. Turk JB, Vuillemin T, Raveh J. Revascularized bone grafts for craniofacial reconstruction. Otolaryngol Clin North Am 1994;27:955–82.
16. Adamo AK, Szal RL. Timing, results, and complications of mandibular reconstructive surgery: report of 32 cases. J Oral Surg 1979;37:755–63.
17. Hamaker RC. Irradiation of autogenous mandibular grafts in primary reconstructions. Laryngoscope 1981;91:1031–51.
18. Urken ML, Buchbinder D, Costantino PD, et al. Oromandibular reconstruction using microvascular composite flaps. Arch Otolaryngol Head Neck Surg 1998;124:46–55.
19. Hidalgo DA. Fibular free flap: a new method of mandible reconstruction. Plast Reconstr Surg 1989;84:71.
20. Chang YM, Santamaria E, Wei FC, et al. Primary insertion of osseointegrated dental implants into fibula osteoseptocutaneous free flap for mandible reconstruction. Plast Reconstr Surg 1998;102: 680–8.
21. Jones NF, Swartz WM, Mears DC, et al. The "double-barrel" free vascularized fibular bone graft. Plast Reconstr Surg 1988;81:378.
22. Fernandes RF. Fibula free flap in mandibular reconstruction. Atlas Oral Maxillofac Surg Clin North Am 2009;14:143–50.
23. Taylor GI, Townsend P, Corlett R. Superiority of the deep circumflex iliac vessels as the supply for free groin flap. Experimental work. Plast Reconstr Surg 1979;64:595.
24. Taylor GI. Reconstruction of the mandible with free composite iliac bone grafts. Ann Plast Surg 1982; 9:361.
25. Urken ML, Vickery C, Weinberg H, et al. The internal oblique-iliac crest osseomyocutaneous free flap in oromandibular reconstruction. Report of 20 cases. Arch Otolaryngol Head Neck Surg 1989;115:339–49.
26. Valentini V, Gennaro P. Iliac crest flap: donor site morbidity. J Craniofac Surg 2009;20(4):1052–5.
27. Rogers SN, Lakshmiah SR, Narayan B. A comparison of the long-term morbidity following deep

circumflex iliac and fibula free flaps for reconstruction following head and neck cancer. Plast Reconstr Surg 2003;112(6):1517–25; discussion 1526–7.

28. Swartz WM, Banis JC, Newton ED, et al. The osteocutaneous scapular free flap for mandibular and maxillary reconstruction. Plast Reconstr Surg 1986;77:530–45.

29. Coleman JJ, Sultan MR. The bipedicled osteocutaneous scapula flap: a new subscapular system free flap. Plast Reconstr Surg 1991;87:682–92.

30. Yang G, Chen B, Gao Y. Forearm free skin flap transplantation. Natl Med J China 1981;61:139–41.

31. Soutar DS, Scheker LR, Tanner NS, et al. The radial forearm flap: a versatile method for intra-oral reconstruction. Br J Plast Surg 1983;36:1–8.

32. Urken M, Cheney M, Sullivan M, et al. Atlas of regional and free flaps for head and neck reconstruction. 1st edition. Philadelphia: Lippincott Williams & Wilkins; 1995.

33. Bardsley AF, Soutar DS, Elliot D, et al. Reducing morbidity in the radial forearm flap donor site. Plast Reconstr Surg 1990;86:287–92.

34. Hidalgo DA, Pusic AL. Free-flap mandibular reconstruction: a 16-year follow-up study. Plast Reconstr Surg 2002;110:438–49.

Reconstruction of Acquired Temporomandibular Joint Defects

Luis G. Vega, DDS[a],*, Raúl González-García, MD, PhD[b],
Patrick J. Louis, DDS, MD[c]

KEYWORDS

- Temporomandibular joint defects • Temporomandibular joint reconstruction • Condylar defect
- Condylar reconstruction • Costochondral graft • Fibula free flap
- Total temporomandibular joint prosthesis

KEY POINTS

- Reconstruction of acquired temporomandibular joint (TMJ) defects represents a unique challenge because of the important role of the TMJ in daily activities such as mastication, deglutition, and phonation.
- Autogenous reconstructions such as costochondral or sternoclavicular joint graft continue to be the best option in children, owing to their ability to transfer a growth center.
- In adults, alloplastic reconstructions are a safe and predictable option.
- In regions of the world where prosthetic reconstruction is not available, is cost prohibitive, or is contraindicated because of patient-related factors such as allergy to materials or multiple previous infections associated with the prosthesis, autogenous reconstruction should be considered.
- Vascularized tissue transfers have also become a popular and reliable way to restore these defects, especially when larger amounts of tissue are missing or in the presence of an irradiated bed.

Temporomandibular joint (TMJ) ankylosis, ablation of benign or malignant pathology, loss of the condyle due to trauma, degenerative or inflammatory disorders, infection, idiopathic resorption, and previous failed reconstructions are some of the various conditions responsible for the development of acquired TMJ defects. The reconstruction of these defects represents a unique challenge, as the TMJ plays an important role in the function of the jaw including mastication, deglutition, and phonation. The condyle also serves as an important growth region of the mandible and lower face.[1] Hence the principles of reconstruction of acquired TMJ defects in the growing individual are different in comparison with the adult. However, even in the presence of these differences the main goal of these reconstructive efforts is to stop and restore the limitation of function, degeneration, growth disturbance, and pain.

Multiple surgical techniques using autogenous tissues and alloplastic materials have been described for the reconstruction of these defects. The indications of each technique vary depending on the severity of the problem, age of the patient, ability to perform postoperative physical therapy, surgeon's experience, and socioeconomic factors.[2,3]

ETIOLOGY AND INDICATIONS

Proper selection of the patient and type of reconstruction are crucial for long-term treatment success. General indications for reconstruction of

a Department of Oral & Maxillofacial Surgery, Health Science Center at Jacksonville, University of Florida, 653-1 West 8th Street, Jacksonville, FL 32209, USA; b Department of Oral and Maxillofacial-Head and Neck Surgery, University Infanta Cristina, C/Avda. De Elvas s/n, 06006, Badajoz, Spain; c Department of Oral & Maxillofacial Surgery, School of Dentistry, University of Alabama at Birmingham, 1919 Seventh Avenue South, SDB 419, Birmingham, AL 35294, USA
* Corresponding author.
E-mail address: luis.vega@jax.ufl.edu

Oral Maxillofacial Surg Clin N Am 25 (2013) 251–269
http://dx.doi.org/10.1016/j.coms.2013.02.008
1042-3699/13/$ – see front matter © 2013 Elsevier Inc. All rights reserved.

TMJ-acquired defects are shown in **Box 1**. Traditionally, classification schemes and treatment algorithms have been used to aid the clinician in the decision-making process. Although these protocols exist for the treatment of mandibular defects, very few have been described for the reconstruction of TMJ-acquired defects. Potter and Dierks[4] proposed a classification of TMJ defects and its respective treatment algorithm, based on reconstruction with microvascular free tissue transfers. When discussing TMJ reconstruction, a difference should be discerned among cases according to the etiology. Potter and Dierks suggested that autogenous bone grafting or alloplastic prosthetic replacement can usually be achieved in cases where the cause of the defect has created a residual tissue deficit that is relatively small, such as severe degenerative or inflammatory joint disease or bony ankylosis. Furthermore, microvascular free tissue transfers were recommended in cases of large tissue deficits or irradiated or soon to be irradiated defects, such as malignant pathology or avulsive trauma.[4]

Children with acquired TMJ defects will usually present with facial asymmetry secondary to growth disturbance. This condition also can be secondary to bony ankylosis, condylar resorption, hyperplasia, or previous tumor resection.[5] Of importance is that not all cases of asymmetry are treated, because some patients have a mild deformity that either does not require treatment or can be corrected with orthognathic surgery once growth is complete. In general, children are best managed with autogenous reconstruction that transfers a growth center that would parallel the growth of the mandibular condyle. Although the costochondral graft (CCG) is used most frequently, other options include sternoclavicular graft (SCG) and distraction osteogenesis (DO).[6–8] TMJ ankylosis is a particularly difficult problem that requires aggressive resection and physical therapy for proper management. Kaban and colleagues[9] published an elegant 7-step protocol for TMJ reconstruction in children with ankylosis, shown in **Box 2**.

In the adult, the need for TMJ reconstruction generally focuses on improving pain-free range of motion, establishing the best dental occlusion, and reducing the chances of ankylosis or reankylosis. Autogenous reconstruction can be used, but in cases of ankylosis it is usually not recommended, owing to the high risk of reankylosis.[10] Prosthetic reconstruction is often the preferred method of treatment, as it has a lower risk of reankylosis, is volumetrically stable, and allows for immediate physical therapy.[11,12] Custom and stock

---

Box 1
Indications for reconstruction of acquired TMJ defects

Children

Ankylosis

Posttraumatic TMJ deformity

TMJ tumors

TMJ defects after radiation therapy

Condylar resorption

Condylar hyperplasia

Juvenile rheumatoid arthritis

Osteomyelitis

Previous failed reconstructions

Adults

Ankylosis

Posttraumatic TMJ deformity

TMJ and mandibular tumors

Severe degenerative joint disease

Severe inflammatory joint disease

Condylar resorption

Condylar hyperplasia

Osteomyelitis

Previous failed reconstructions

Box 2
Protocol for surgical management of TMJ ankylosis in children

1. Aggressive excision of fibrous and/or bony mass

2. Coronoidectomy on affected side

3. Coronoidectomy on opposite side if steps 1 and 2 do not result in maximum interincisal opening of greater than 35 mm or to point of dislocation of opposite side

4. Lining of joint with temporalis fascia or the native disc

5. Condylar reconstruction with either DO or CCG with rigid fixation

6. Early mobilization; if DO used, mobilize day of surgery; if CCG used, early mobilization with minimal intermaxillary fixation (not >10 days)

7. Aggressive physiotherapy

From Kaban LB, Bouchard C, Troulis MJ. A protocol for management of temporomandibular joint ankylosis in children. J Oral Maxillofac Surg 2009;67:1966–78; with permission.

devices are available, which both have advantages and disadvantages when reconstructing the TMJ.[13,14] In regions of the world where prosthetic reconstruction is not available, is cost prohibitive, or is contraindicated because of patient-related factors such as allergy to materials or multiple previous infections associated with the prosthesis, autogenous reconstruction should be considered.

PREOPERATIVE EVALUATION

The evaluation of the patient with acquired TMJ defects begins with a detailed history and physical examination. The goal is to elicit the severity of limitation of function, degeneration, growth disturbance, and pain. Patients may have failed more conservative management, and many give a history of multiple failed surgical procedures. Previous history of irradiation is important, as this is likely to reduce the treatment options to vascularized tissue transfers.

Children will usually present with facial asymmetry secondary to growth disturbance.[15] In the adult the persistence of pain and decreased ability to open wide or chew are common features, but asymmetry can also be present.

Advanced imaging such as computed tomography (CT) with 3-dimensional reconstruction is needed to confirm the diagnosis and plan the reconstruction, as it shows the bony architecture well. Magnetic resonance imaging may be needed to aid in diagnosis and surgical resection in cases of neoplasm; however, CT/positron emission tomography has better specificity and sensitivity.[16] Finally, stereolithographic models are always helpful in understanding the deformity and establishing the treatment plan.

NONVASCULARIZED AUTOGENOUS RECONSTRUCTION

Historically, nonvascularized autogenous reconstruction with costochondral graft was considered the gold standard for TMJ reconstruction. However, other options include sternoclavicular graft (SCG), iliac crest bone graft, coronoid, and posterior border of the mandible (sliding osteotomy). In addition, cranial bone graft has been used in the rare cases of acquired glenoid fossa defects (trauma, abnormality, previous failed reconstructions).[17] A more complete list of autogenous grafts for condylar reconstruction is given in **Table 1**. With the advent of better materials and technology, autogenous reconstruction has largely been replaced by alloplastic prosthesis, except in the growing patient. As already described, in children autogenous reconstruction is indicated for the

treatment of TMJ growth disturbances and ankylosis. This type of reconstruction helps to correct the asymmetry and at the same time allows for potential growth. This option is also indicated in adults as an alternative to prosthetic reconstruction.

Distant Sites

Costochondral graft
The costochondral graft is used for replacement of the condyle because of its shape, ease of harvest with low risk of morbidity, and potential for growth.[6] Potential risks include reankylosis, overgrowth, undergrowth, nonunion, and donor-site morbidity. In the child who has mandibular asymmetry, preoperative planning must include a history and physical examination and CT. The surgeon must determine the ideal position to place the mandible to level the occlusal plane. A surgical guide must be fabricated to position the mandible at the time of surgery.

During surgery, the rib graft is usually harvested first, thus decreasing the risk of infection of the chest wound. The sixth or seventh rib on the right side is usually harvested to minimize injury to the myocardium.

An incision is made along the superior aspect of the rib medial to the midclavicular line. The incision is carried through the pectoralis minor muscle to the inferior border of the rib. The periosteum is then excised along the rib except at the costochondral junction, where the periosteum and perichondrium are left intact to avoid disruption of this junction. The dorsal periosteum is elevated with a Doyen elevator and the rib is cut with a rib cutter. The wound is checked for any pleural tears by asking the anesthetist to hold positive pressure and observe for any air bubbles from the wound. If a leak is present, it is repaired by placing a small catheter into the pleural tear, passing a purse-string suture along the defect and around the catheter. While the anesthetist holds positive pressure, the catheter is slowly removed and the suture is tightened and tied. The wound is then closed primarily. A postoperative chest radiograph is imperative to assure the absence of a pneumothorax.

The mandible is approached through a periauricular and submandibular or retromandibular approaches. The condyle, if present, is removed via the periauricular approach. Any scarring around the mandible must be freed to better mobilize it. While maintaining the sterility of the field, the splint is wired into position and the patient is placed in maxillomandibular fixation (MMF). The costochondral graft is then mortised into position, which usually requires the decortication of an area with a size similar to the width and length of the rib along the

Table 1
Advantages and limitations of autogenous grafts for reconstruction of TMJ-acquired defects

	Advantages	Limitations
Distant Sites		
Costochondral graft	Most widely used Has a cartilage cap, mimicking both the bone and cartilaginous components Has intrinsic growth potential Easy accessibility and adaptation Gross anatomic similarity to the mandibular condyle	Unpredictable growth Poor bone quality Possible separation of cartilage from bone Possible donor-site complications: pleural tear, pneumothorax, pleural effusion, atelectasis, empyema
Sternoclavicular joint graft	Similar anatomic and physiologic characteristics Contains a cartilaginous cap Has the potential for growth Probability of regeneration at donor site	Unacceptable location of surgical scar Donor-site complications: damage to the great vessels, instability of the shoulder, clavicle fracture
Cranial bone graft	Easy accessibility and adaptation Excellent for reconstruction of glenoid fossa	Mostly cortical bone Limited amount of bone Lack of growth Donor-site complications: alopecia, dural tear, superior sagittal sinus laceration, epidural hematoma
Iliac crest bone graft	Has a cartilage cap, mimicking both the bone and cartilaginous components Has potential for growth More suitable for large mandibular defects	Donor-site complications: altered gait, poor scar/bone contour, herniation of abdominal contents, ilium fracture, peritonitis, retroperitoneal hematoma
Local Sites		
Coronoid process	Avoidance of secondary surgical site and associated donor complications	Relatively pointed architecture No long-term studies
Mandibular condyle	Readily available as part of the normal anatomy Avoidance of secondary surgical site and associated donor complications	Possibility of resorption Requires enough bony surface for placement of at least 2 fixation screws
Ramus sliding osteotomy	Bone of a size and shape adequate for new condyle with similar histologic characteristics Is a pedicled graft	Damage to the contour of the mandibular angle Lack of growth Lack of long-term studies
Distraction osteogenesis	No need for interpositional material Patient can function during distraction osteogenesis Simultaneous correction of secondary deformities	Lengthy procedure Patient cooperation is a must
Vascularized Sites		
Fibular free flap	Tubular shape and densely cortical Vascularized graft has better survival rate More suitable for large mandibular defects	Lacks articular cartilage Donor-site complications: ankle stiffness, instability and weakness, numbness of the lateral side of the leg, pedal ischemia, foot edema
Metatarsophalangeal joint flap	Combination of articular cartilage and bone Fitting anatomy because of small size Has potential for growth	Donor-site complications: esthetic loss of a toe Simple hinge joint does not follow the same movements as the TMJ

Modified from Khadka A, Hu J. Autogenous graft for condylar reconstruction in treatment of TMJ ankylosis: current concepts and considerations for the future. Int J Oral Maxillofac Surg 2012;41:94–102; with permission.

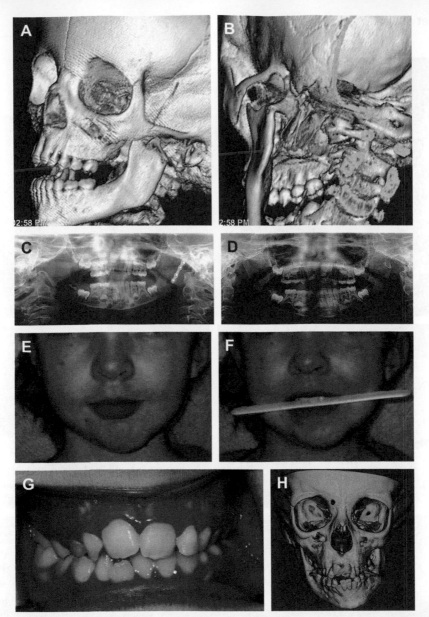

Fig. 1. Costochondral graft reconstruction of an acquired TMJ defect in a growing patient. A 5-year-old girl sustained a left subcondylar fracture when she tripped and fell, striking her chin. She initially had limited opening with persistent malocclusion, contacting only the left molars. She underwent open reduction and internal fixation (ORIF) of her mandible fracture. At approximately 1 year postoperatively, she had hardware removal. At the time of removal she was noted to have significant resorption of her condyle. Subsequently she had asymmetric facial growth with deviation of the chin to the left and a maxillary occlusal cant. At 10 years of age she underwent a left costochondral graft to the mandible and leveling of the mandible. The patient subsequently had an orthodontic occlusal appliance placed to maintain the mandibular position and encourage mandibular growth. (A) Lateral and (B) posterior 3-dimensional (3D) computed tomography (CT) views of reconstructions showing displaced left subcondylar fracture. (C) Postoperative panoramic radiograph after ORIF of the subcondylar fracture. (D) Postoperative panoramic radiograph approximately 1 year after ORIF of the subcondylar fracture. The hardware has been removed and there is marked resorption of the condyle. (E, F) Frontal photographs showing mandibular asymmetry and maxillary cant. (G) Intraoral occlusal view. (H) 3D CT scan of reconstructions showing the asymmetric mandibular growth and (I) resorbed left condyle. (J) Intraoperative view showing incision for harvest of the right sixth rib. (K) Exposure of the rib. (L) The lateral aspect of the rib has been cut. Note that the periosteum and perichondrium around the costochondral junction is intact. (M) The harvested rib. (N) Preauricular incision for exposure of the TMJ. (O) Intraoral view after the condyle has been removed. The teeth were not in the splint, so the left side of the mandible had to be mobilized to remove scar tissue along the TMJ. (P) Preauricular incision and (Q) retromandibular incision showing the rib graft in place. The lateral ramus has been decorticated and the costochondral graft has been secured with screws. (R) Frontal photograph after undergoing costochondral graft to reconstruct the left condyle. Note the improved symmetry. (S) Postoperative panoramic radiograph with costochondral graph. (T) Intraoral view with orthodontic appliance in place and leveling of the mandibular occlusal plane.

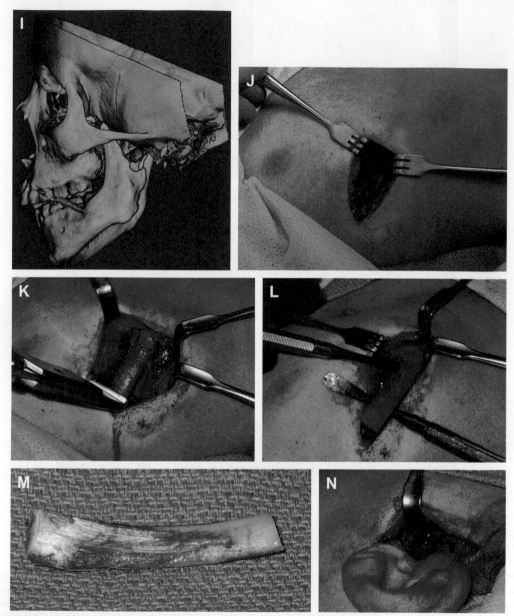

Fig. 1. (*continued*)

posterior ramus of the mandible. In addition, the rib should extend near the mandibular inferior border. The cartilage portion of the rib is trimmed, leaving 2 to 3 mm of cartilaginous cap in place. The rib is then inset along the mortised portion of the ramus and secured with bicortical screws. Larger-head screws are preferable because the cortex of the rib is easily compressed. The wound is irrigated with normal saline and closed in layers (**Fig. 1**).

Outcomes and complications Donor-site morbidity in CCG includes pneumothorax, hemothorax, pericardial and cardiac injury, seroma, hematoma, and neuritis.

As described earlier, overgrowth, undergrowth, nonunion, and reankylosis are some additional CCG complications (**Fig. 2**). In fact, a range of reankylosis of 5% to 39% has been described in the literature.[6] It must also be noted that recent publications in the management of ankylosis have suggested that patients who have undergone gap arthroplasty alone have significantly better postoperative maximal interincisal openings than those reconstructed with a costochondral graft.[3,18]

Sternoclavicular joint graft

The sternoclavicular joint (SCJ) is another potential choice for reconstruction of the mandibular

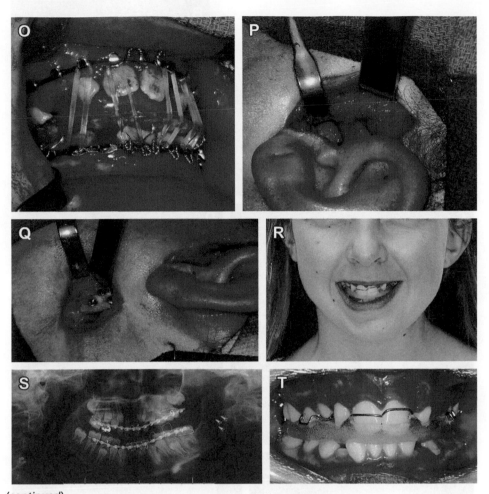

Fig. 1. (*continued*)

condyle. This graft has the advantage of being usable in the growing patient because there is transfer of a growth center. The main advantage of the superior portion of the sternal head of the clavicle is that it has microarchitecture similar to that of the mandibular condyle, and a similar growth pattern.[6] The harvest of the superior portion of the sternal head of the clavicle proceeds by making an incision over the proximal clavicle or 1 to 2 cm below the clavicle to help hide the incision. This incision is carried down through the periosteum, and a subperiosteal dissection is achieved to expose the superior half of the clavicle. The superior half of the proximal clavicle is harvested using a reciprocating saw. Only half of the width of the clavicle is needed for the reconstruction of the mandibular condyle, which offers several advantages: it allows for a better fit in the glenoid fossa, allows a better fit along the decorticated posterior ramus, and decreases the risk for fracture of the clavicle. Beveling the cut along the mid-shaft of the clavicle at the end of the graft

that is harvested can further reduce the risk of fracture. The length of the graft should be approximately the length of the ramus plus the needed height of the condyle it replaces. The superior portion of the clavicle is disarticulated from the sternum with a periosteal elevator while avoiding injury to the fibrocartilage on the head of the clavicle. The preparation of the mandible and the fixation of the graft are done in a fashion similar to that used for a rib graft, as already described. It is recommended that a figure-of-8 bandage supporting the shoulders and an arm sling to immobilize the arm be used for 3 months to reduce the risk of clavicular fracture.[6]

Outcomes and complications Donor-site morbidity in SCJ includes damage to the great vessels and clavicle fracture.

Few SCJ outcomes studies have been published. Although long-term studies comparing both grafts are lacking, reports suggest that SCJ is a viable alternative to CCG.[6,7]

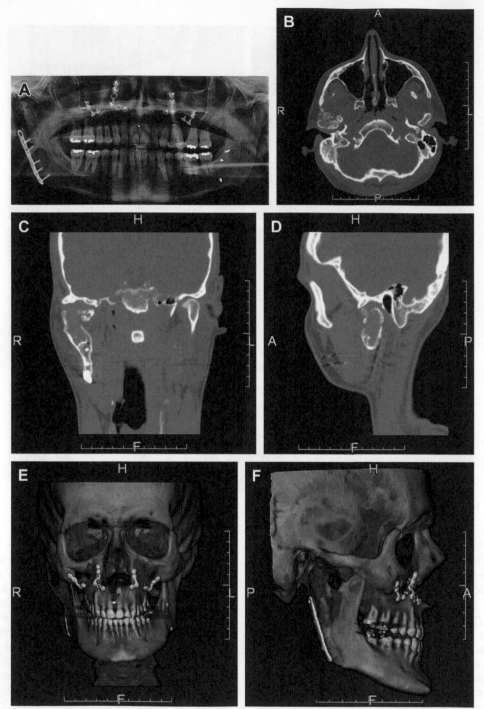

Fig. 2. Overgrown costochondral graft. A 28-year-old man underwent a right costochondral graft for TMJ reconstruction after the ablation of an osteochondroma. Ten years later, the patient presented to the authors' institution complaining of right TMJ pain and facial asymmetry. After clinical and radiographic evaluation, it was established that the patient had an overgrown costochondral graft that required removal and reconstruction with an alloplastic custom-made total TMJ replacement. (*A*) Panoramic radiograph showing deformed anatomy of the right costochondral graft. (*B*) Axial, (*C*) coronal, and (*D*) sagittal CT views showing an overgrown and deformed right costochondral graft. (*E*) Frontal and (*F*) lateral 3D CT reconstruction views. (*G*) Stereolithographic model showing the planned mandibular osteotomy and osteoplasty sites. (*H*) Right custom-made TMJ prosthesis. (*I*) Surgical specimen. (*J*) Preauricular and (*K*) retromandibular intraoperative views of the prosthetic fossa and mandibular components secured in place. (*L*) Frontal and (*M*) lateral postoperative 3D CT reconstruction views. (*N*) Postoperative maximum interincisal opening.

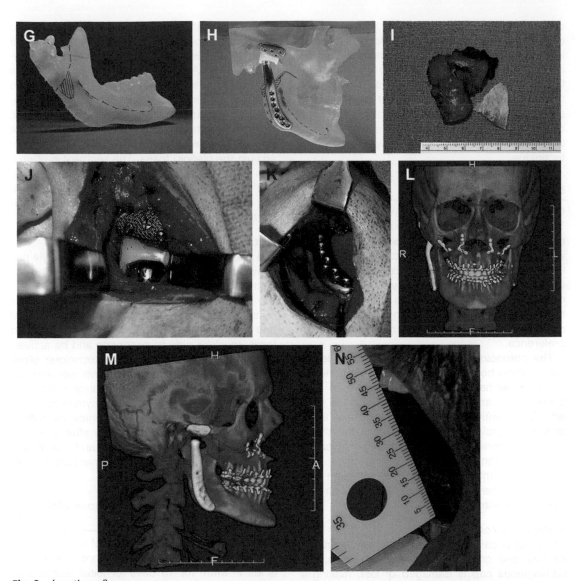

Fig. 2. (continued)

Other Distant Sites

Several other distant sites for reconstruction of the condyle have been described in the literature. With the exception of DO, these choices are not generally used in the child because of the limited growth potential. These sources can be used in the adult when growth is not needed.

Cranial bone graft

The calvarial bone graft has the advantage of being extremely dense, and thus resists resorption. It can be harvested in strops and lagged to the lateral aspect of the ramus of the mandible. Its main disadvantages are that it has no growth potential and is very thin. To form a broader articulation with the glenoid fossa, a "stacked" graft would be needed. In the region above the ramus,

2 or 3 1.5 × 2.0-cm pieces of calvarial bone are stacked together and secured with lag screws. The articulating surface is rounded to improve bony contact.

In addition, cranial bone graft can be used to reconstruct the glenoid fossa. An intracranial approach with the help of neurosurgery might sometimes be necessary, especially in cases of traumatic entrance of the condyle to the middle cranial fossa or pathologic ablation.[19]

Morbidity associated with calvarial bone graft harvest includes alopecia, dural tears, and intracranial hemorrhage.

Iliac crest bone graft

The iliac crest bone graft can be harvested with the associated cartilaginous cap.[6] This action would allow for some growth potential; however, sufficient long-term studies are lacking. Adequate length and width can easily be harvested, but the cortex is thin and may be prone to resorption. Donor-site morbidity associated with harvest from the iliac crest includes significant postoperative pain, gait disturbance, numbness along the lateral thigh, fracture, seroma, and hematoma. These complications can be minimized by good surgical technique.

Local Sites

Coronoid process

The coronoid process is usually resected in cases of condyle reconstruction, especially in patients with ankylosis. Coronoid resection is also indicated when patients suffer from an elongation of the coronoid process or ankylosis of the coronoid process to the surrounding structures. In patients with excellent range of motion of the TMJ, coronoid resection becomes a matter of surgeon preference.

The coronoid has been used for condyle reconstruction because it undergoes little bone resorption, but has several disadvantages.[20,21] The bone is thin and pointed, thus creating a poor articulation with the glenoid fossa. There is no cartilage or growth center, thus it lacks growth potential. The bone is often short, making it difficult to fixate to the ramus.

Donor-site morbidity is very low, although very few articles have reported experience with this type of reconstruction.[21–23]

Mandibular condyle

The condyle can be used as a graft, depending on its size and condition. In ankylosis cases, the cartilaginous cap is damaged or lost, making it a poor choice as a graft, because the risk of reankylosis and lack of growth would be high. The condyle can be of sufficient size, but fixation may be difficult because of the lack of overlap with the ramus. Plate fixation is generally required. Overall, the use of the condyle as a graft source is a poor choice for reconstruction, especially in the child.

Ramus sliding osteotomy

Reconstruction of the mandibular condyle using the mandibular ramus is an option that can be used in some situations when the condyle is resected for benign abnormality.[24] The segment contains no growth center and cannot be expected to have significant growth potential, so it is best used in nongrowing patients for small defects that involve the condyle only. After the condyle has been resected, a vertical osteotomy

is made from the posterior aspect of the sigmoid notch to the posterior aspect of the mandibular angle, thus preserving the prominence of the mandibular angle. A portion of the medial pterygoid is stripped from the inferior aspect of the ramus to slide the proximal segment superiorly.[24] The segment is stabilized in the fossa against the disc with 2 miniplates or a reconstruction plate. If the disc is not present, the segment is stabilized against the glenoid fossa. The segment is often a free graft, because it often must be freed and has little or no soft-tissue attachment. There is a risk of injury to the inferior nerve that can be minimized with proper osteotomy placement.

Distraction osteogenesis

The use of DO for lengthening of the condyle has shown some promise in selected cases.[8] The patient must have a large enough residual bone in the posterosuperior portion of the mandibular ramus to allow placement of 2 screws to control and transport the DO segment. The patient and family must be able to cooperate and be actively involved in the treatment. The technique eliminates the need for a separate donor site and can shorten hospitalization. The technique also has the advantage of correcting an asymmetric mandible but, because of lack of accuracy, the patient may require orthognathic surgery after growth is complete. Failure of the hardware and lack of consolidation of the transported segment are complications of this technique.[25]

Postoperative Care of Autogenous TMJ Reconstruction

Postoperative care for this kind of reconstruction is basically the same for all options. The patient is left in MMF for 10 days for initial stabilization of the graft, then physical therapy is started; this is done to prevent ankylosis of the graft. As mentioned earlier, when correcting asymmetry in a growing patient it is important to level the mandible at the time of surgery using a surgical splint. This splint is left in place during the initial healing phase and is changed to an appliance that facilitates the growth of the maxilla on the affected side. This changeover usually involves the orthodontist, and begins around 5 weeks.

VASCULARIZED AUTOGENOUS RECONSTRUCTION

Vascularized autogenous reconstruction has been mainly proposed for the reconstruction of large mandibular/TMJ defects following resection of tumor, debridement of osteoradionecrosis, osteomyelitis, and avulsive trauma. The fibula free flap

(FFF) is the most common vascularized reconstructive option, but the use of metatarsophalangeal joint transfer or a scapular tip flap have also been reported.[4,26,27]

Fibula Free Flap

The FFF is particularly well suited for condylar reconstruction because of its tubular shape and adaptability to the glenoid fossa. As a part of the primary or secondary reconstruction regimen following mandibular ablation, the FFF has become the first choice among vascularized bone grafts. Once the defect is created, the surgeon has to decide among 1 of 3 alternatives when using FFF: (1) to attach the resected condyle as a nonvascularized transplant to the pole of the graft, in cases where no direct tumoral extension is observed involving the condyle; (2) to insert a condylar prosthesis in addition to the graft; or (3) to place the distal pole of the graft into the glenoid fossa, with or without contouring.[26]

The technique for harvesting the FFF is performed according to the classic description by Taylor and colleagues[28] and Hidalgo.[29] If the tumor does not extend to the buccal cortex of the mandible, a template can be used to restore the normal mandibular curvature before its resection. This template can be used to place the osteotomies and replicate the original mandibular shape. Later on, the template is used to bend the mandibular reconstruction plate. The authors strongly recommend performing the osteotomies while the fibula is still attached to the pedicle at the donor site, to decrease the time of ischemia. Miniplates can be used to fix bone segments, although a mandibular reconstruction plate is more advisable because it accurately mimics the mandibular curvature. Locking-system reconstruction plates with screws that are placed monocortically are used to avoid damage to the vascularization of the periosteum on the inner side of the fibula. Alternatively, stereolithographic models of the mandible and fibula can be used to preoperatively design mandibular resection and fibula osteotomies, respectively.

Regarding condyle reconstruction, some specifications have to be considered. If a remnant of the condyle is left in place then the TMJ is not altered, and fixation of the condyle with the fibula is performed with the reconstruction plate, miniplates, or even wires. This approach is strongly recommended by Potter and Dierks,[4] who advocate

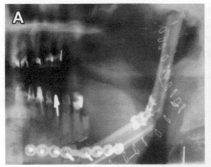
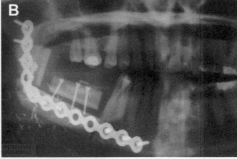
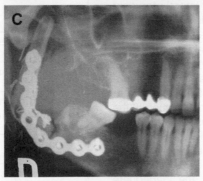

Fig. 3. TMJ reconstruction with fibula free flap. (*A*) Postoperative panoramic radiograph of a TMJ/mandibular reconstruction after cancer ablation. Note that the fibular pole is directly fitted into the glenoid fossa, as the native condyle was not preserved. (*B*) Postoperative panoramic radiograph of a TMJ/mandibular reconstruction after myxoma resection. Reconstruction was performed with a double-barreled vascularized free fibular flap attached to the remnant mandible and also to the remnant condyle with a mandibular reconstruction plate. (*C*) Postoperative panoramic radiograph of a TMJ/mandibular reconstruction after cancer ablation. Note that the fibular pole was incorrectly placed out of the glenoid fossa, anteriorly to the eminence.

leaving in place even small segments of the native condyle and attaching them to the fibular stump. However, this can be oncologically unsafe in certain cases where the tumor spreads largely into the mandibular ramus. For these cases, entire resection of the condyle has to be achieved. In the vast majority of such cases the TMJ disc can be preserved, thus allowing a more physiologic adaptation of the fibular pole into the glenoid fossa. The fibular pole can be smoothly contoured with a burr, although this is not mandatory, as remodeling will take place with neomandibular function. After positioning the fibula, the masseter muscle has to be sutured to the medial pterygoid muscle to actively seat the fibula into the glenoid fossa. Care should be taken to place the vascular pedicle in an anterior position by positioning the proximal stump of the fibula in contact with the remnant mandible. Last but not least, special attention must be paid to carefully tunnel the fibula through the soft tissue to avoid damage to the facial nerve.

Outcomes and complications

In a series of 6 cases regarding resection of the condyle and reconstruction with FFF, González-García and colleagues[26] found a maximal interincisal opening greater than 35 mm in all the cases but 1 that developed ankylosis of the neocondyle following a distraction procedure. The mean resorption rate of the neocondyle was almost 5% in the early postoperative period, with no further architectural changes in the longer term. Guyot and colleagues,[30] in a study of 11 patients undergoing condylar resection without disc removal and further reconstruction with FFF, found a tendency toward bone remodeling. Similarly to the first group, Thor and colleagues[31] stated that by preserving the TMJ disc, correctly securing the fibula in the fossa, and reattaching the lateral pterygoid muscle, it was possible to maintain normal rotation and translation, and to completely restore the mandibular function. Other investigators have reported the absence of translation in cases where the native condyle is removed, although a pseudarthrosis develops that is well tolerated and functional.[4] Nevertheless, although preservation of the disc has been proposed to be responsible for the good outcome in terms of function, this fact has not been studied in patients undergoing disc removal.

One possible complication is the inadequate positioning of the fibula into the glenoid fossa. It is more frequently observed in cases where severe fibrosis is present at the recipient site when reconstruction is performed at second look. Also, as stated by Potter and Dierks,[4] there exists a tendency for the neocondyle to "sag" regardless of whether the disc is preserved or not. Condylar suspension of the fibular pole to the zygomatic arc with sutures has been reported to better position the neocondyle into the temporal fossa.

Box 3
Indications and contraindications for alloplastic total TMJ reconstruction

Indications

Congenital and developmental disorders (condylar agenesis, condylar hyperplasia)

Neoplasia

Severe degenerative disease

Severe inflammatory disease

Posttraumatic deformities

Ankylosis

Previous failed autogenous reconstructions

Previous failed alloplastic reconstructions

Contraindications

Growing patients

Uncontrolled systemic disease

Psychiatric instability

Active infection

Allergy to prosthetic components

Uncontrolled parafunction

Table 2
Comparison between stock and custom-made total TMJ prostheses

Stock Prosthesis	Custom-Made Prosthesis
Make fit	Made to fit
Lower cost	Higher cost
Shorter treatment time frames	Longer treatment time frames
Removal of bone	No or minimal removal of bone
More difficult to obtained primary stability	Easier to obtain primary stability
Potential micromovement	No micromovement
Placement versatility	Less placement versatility
Potential for longer surgical time	Potential for less surgical time
Limited use for large or difficult anatomic defects	Excellent for large or difficult anatomic defects

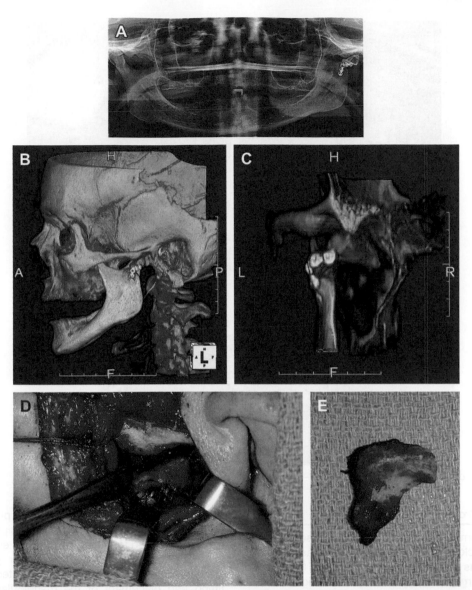

Fig. 4. TMJ reconstruction of posttraumatic deformity with stock prosthesis. A 41-year-old woman had a repair of a left subcondylar fracture 3 years before she presented to the authors' institution. Her complaints on presentation included left TMJ pain and facial asymmetry. After clinical and radiographic evaluation, it was established that the patient had poor fixation with hardware failure and subcondylar fracture malunion. Because of the limited size of the TMJ defect, a reconstruction with a stock prosthesis was indicated. (*A*) Panoramic radiographic showing a broken miniplate in the left subcondylar region. (*B*) Lateral 3D CT reconstruction. (*C*) Close-up view of the acquired left TMJ defect. (*D*) Intraoperative view of the broken miniplate and malposition condyle. (*E*) Surgical specimen. (*F, G*) Intraoperative views of the prosthetic fossa and mandibular components secured in place. (*H*) Postoperative panoramic radiographic.

Intermaxillary fixation before positioning the fibula can be a useful maneuver to avoid inadequate placement of the neocondyle (**Fig. 3**).

ALLOPLASTIC RECONSTRUCTION

Historically, alloplastic TMJ reconstruction has been surrounded by controversy; however, nowadays such reconstructions represent a safe and predictable way to restore TMJ-acquired defects.[14,32,33] Indications and contraindications of this type of reconstruction are listed in **Box 3**. Custom and stock prostheses are available (**Table 2**). At the time of writing, only 2 companies manufacture and distribute TMJ prostheses in the United States.

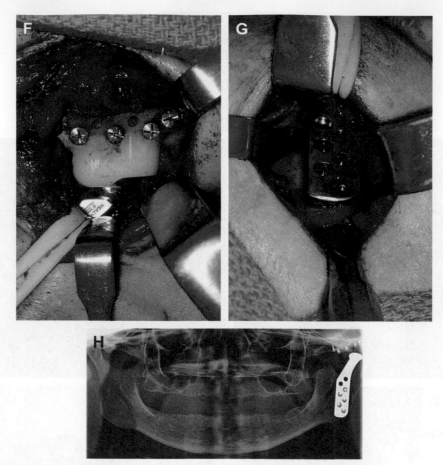

Fig. 4. (*continued*)

Stock Prosthesis

The Biomet prosthesis (Biomet, Jacksonville, FL) is a stock device, which the patient has to "make fit." It has a fossa component of 3 sizes (small, medium, large) made completely of ultrahigh molecular weight polyethylene. This component has the potential disadvantage that to be adapted it requires the removal of bone from the eminence and glenoid fossa. The mandibular ramus component is made of a cobalt-chrome alloy with a roughened titanium plasma coating on the host bone side. It comes in 3 different lengths: 45, 50, and 55 mm; and 2 different widths: standard and narrow.

Similar to previous descriptions, the standard surgical technique with this type of prosthesis requires periauricular and submandibular or retromandibular approaches. Alternatively a "facelift approach" can be used. Once exposure of the TMJ and mandibular ramus is achieved, a condylar osteotomy is done if necessary. Approximately between 2 and 2.5 mm of space are required between the articular surface and the residual mandible to be able to fit the prosthetic parts. A large-barreled burr or a reciprocating rasp is then used to flatten the articular eminence to adapt the fossa component. After properly sizing it, the fossa component is implanted before fitting and placement of the mandibular ramus component is performed. If indicated, fat grafts can be implanted around the condylar head. At this point MMF is released. (Depending on the case and surgeon preference, MMF is done either at the beginning or during the procedure.) Occlusion is checked and layer closure is done. A strict sterility protocol is recommended to avoid the potential risk of postoperative infection (**Fig. 4**).[34]

Outcomes and complications

Complications with this type of reconstruction include hardware failure, infection, and heterotopic bone formation. Nevertheless, outcomes studies with the Biomet stock prosthesis have shown that it is an efficacious option when alloplastic reconstruction is indicated.[33,35,36] However, patients with loss of a large portion of the

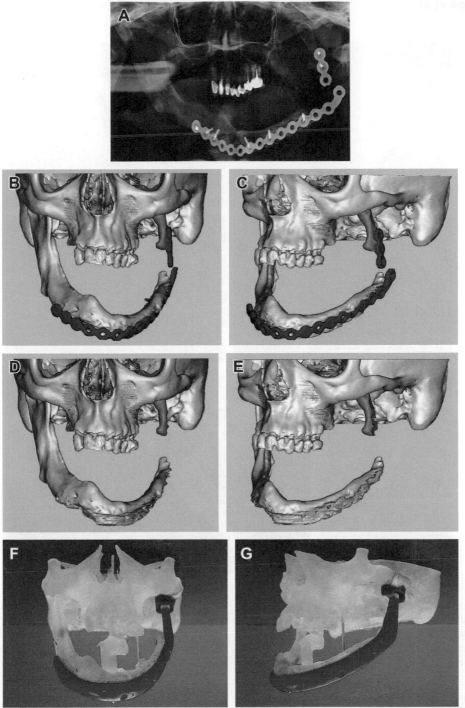

Fig. 5. TMJ reconstruction of postpathologic ablation deformity with custom-made prosthesis. A 53-year-old woman with a previous history of a large left mandibular vascular malformation underwent a mandibular resection and iliac crest bone graft reconstruction with preservation of her condyle. She presented to the authors' institution 15 years later complaining of pain and dysfunction. Clinical and radiographic evaluation showed that the patient had a broken reconstruction plate. Secondary to her complex medical history, a microvascular reconstruction was contraindicated, and a custom-made total TMJ prosthesis was selected because of the large size of the mandibular/TMJ defect. (*A*) Panoramic radiograph of a broken reconstruction plate. (*B, C*) 3D renderings showing the broken reconstruction plate and the residual malposition condyle. (*D, E*) Same 3D renderings after removal of the reconstruction plate digitally. (*F, G*) Prosthesis wax-up. Note the extension of the prosthesis all the way to native mandibular bone. (*H, I*) Actual total TMJ custom-made prosthesis. (*J*) Intraoperative view of the previous failed hardware. Note the extended surgical access and the bone growing over the reconstruction plate. (*K*) Surgical specimen. (*L, M*) Intraoperative views of the prosthetic fossa and mandibular components secured in place. (*N*) Postoperative 3D CT reconstruction (*O*) panoramic (*P*) and anteroposterior radiographs.

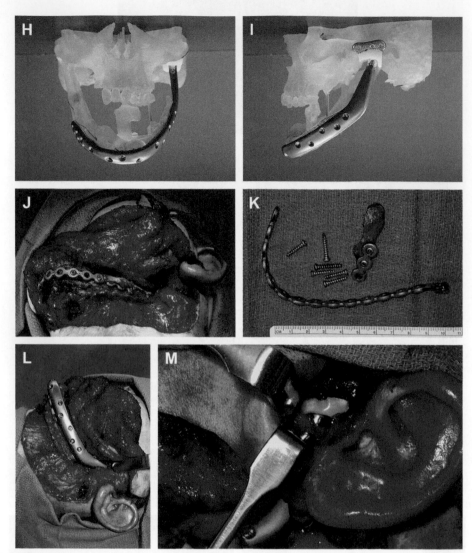

Fig. 5. (*continued*)

mandibular ramus or with a significant deformity of the mandibular ramus are usually not candidates for reconstruction with stock devices, and a custom-made device should be considered.

Custom-Made Prosthesis

The TMJ Concepts prosthesis (TMJ Concepts, Ventura, CA) has the distinct characteristic that it is a "made to fit" device, allowing for great versatility in the reconstruction of acquired TMJ defects (**Fig. 5**).

The process for construction of this type of device starts with a thin-cut maxillofacial CT scan that is used for the construction of a stereolithographic model. This model is then studied to determine if any osteotomies are to be made to achieve the necessary clearance for the placement of the prosthetic parts. The surgeon approves the prosthetic design after a wax-up is done in the stereolithographic model. The fossa component has a titanium mesh backing with an ultrahigh molecular weight polyethylene articulating surface. The mandibular component has a body made of machined alloyed titanium with a condylar head of chromecobalt-molybdenum alloy.

Similar to the surgical technique for the stock prosthesis, MMF is done at the beginning of the procedure or intraoperatively, depending on the case and surgeon's preference. Periauricular and submandibular or retromandibular approaches are also used to access the TMJ and the mandibular ramus. Modifications to these approaches are sometimes required, depending on the size of the acquired defect. Once these areas are exposed, the necessary planned osteotomies are

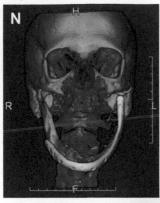

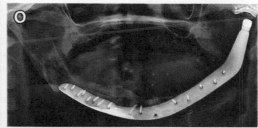

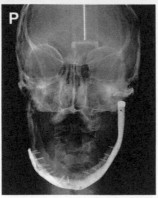

Fig. 5. (*continued*)

performed. The fossa component is placed and secured first, followed by the mandibular component. If indicated, fat grafts can be implanted around the condylar head. At this point MMF is released and occlusion is checked. In bilateral cases both joints are accessed and prepared before the placement of the prosthesis, as this will facilitate their placement. Sterility is paramount in avoiding contamination and potential infection of the prosthesis.[37]

Outcomes and complications

Complications with this type of reconstruction include hardware failure, infection, and heterotopic bone formation. Several protocols for the management of these complications have been reported in the literature.[38–42] At the same time, numerous outcomes studies with the TMJ Concepts prosthesis have shown that it is a safe and predictable option when alloplastic reconstruction is indicated.[35,43–46]

Postoperative Care of Alloplastic TMJ Reconstruction

Postoperative care should focus on avoiding dislocation. Head dressings or guiding elastics can be used for this purpose. Physical therapy must start as early as possible. One week of antibiotics is recommended, and diet is advanced as tolerated.[47]

SUMMARY

Reconstruction of acquired TMJ defects represents a unique challenge because of the important role of the TMJ in daily activities such as mastication, deglutition, and phonation. The clinician must be aware of the different autogenous and alloplastic reconstruction options. Autogenous reconstructions such as costochondral or SCJ graft continue to be the best option in children, owing to their ability to transfer a growth center.

In adults, alloplastic reconstructions are a safe and predictable option. However, in regions of the world where prosthetic reconstruction is not available, is cost prohibitive, or is contraindicated because of patient-related factors such as allergy to materials or multiple previous infections associated with the prosthesis, autogenous reconstruction should be considered.

Vascularized tissue transfers have also become a popular and reliable way to restore these defects, especially when larger amounts of tissue are missing or in the presence of an irradiated bed.

REFERENCES

1. Smartt JM, Low DW, Bartlett SP. The pediatric mandible: I. A primer on growth and development. Plast Reconstr Surg 2005;116(1):14e–23e.
2. Vesnaver A, Ahčan U, Rozman J. Evaluation of surgical treatment in mandibular condyle fractures. J Craniomaxillofac Surg 2012;40(8):647–53.
3. Katsnelson A, Markiewicz MR, Keith DA, et al. Operative management of temporomandibular joint ankylosis: a systematic review and meta-analysis. J Oral Maxillofac Surg 2011;70(3):531–6.
4. Potter JK, Dierks EJ. Vascularized options for reconstruction of the mandibular condyle. Semin Plast Surg 2008;22(3):156–60.
5. Kaban LB. Mandibular asymmetry and the fourth dimension. J Craniofac Surg 2009;20(Suppl 1): 622–31.
6. Khadka A, Hu J. Autogenous grafts for condylar reconstruction in treatment of TMJ ankylosis: current concepts and considerations for the future. Int J Oral Maxillofac Surg 2012;41(1):94–102.
7. Singh V, Dhingra R, Bhagol A. Prospective analysis of temporomandibular joint reconstruction in ankylosis with sternoclavicular graft and buccal fat pad lining. J Oral Maxillofac Surg 2012;70(4):997–1006.
8. Spagnoli DB, Gollehon SG. Distraction osteogenesis in reconstruction of the mandible and temporomandibular joint. Oral Maxillofac Surg Clin North Am 2006;18(3):383–98.
9. Kaban LB, Bouchard C, Troulis MJ. A protocol for management of temporomandibular joint ankylosis in children. J Oral Maxillofac Surg 2009;67(9): 1966–78.
10. Saeed NR, Kent JN. A retrospective study of the costochondral graft in TMJ reconstruction. Int J Oral Maxillofac Surg 2003;32(6):606–9.
11. Saeed N, Hensher R, Mcleod N, et al. Reconstruction of the temporomandibular joint autogenous compared with alloplastic. Br J Oral Maxillofac Surg 2002;40(4):296–9.
12. Mercuri LG. Total joint reconstruction—autologous or alloplastic. Oral Maxillofac Surg Clin North Am 2006;18(3):399–410.
13. Wolford LM, Dingwerth DJ, Talwar RM, et al. Comparison of 2 temporomandibular joint total joint prosthesis systems. J Oral Maxillofac Surg 2003;61(6): 685–90 [discussion: 690].
14. Mercuri LG. Alloplastic temporomandibular joint replacement: rationale for the use of custom devices. Int J Oral Maxillofac Surg 2012;41(9):1033–40.
15. Pedersen TK, Jensen JJ, Melsen B, et al. Resorption of the temporomandibular condylar bone according to subtypes of juvenile chronic arthritis. J Rheumatol 2001;28(9):2109–15.
16. Shintaku WH, Venturin JS, Langlais RP, et al. Imaging modalities to access bony tumors and hyperplasic reactions of the temporomandibular joint. J Oral Maxillofac Surg 2010;68(8):1911–21.
17. Lee JJ, Worthington P. Reconstruction of the temporomandibular joint using calvarial bone after a failed Teflon-Proplast implant. J Oral Maxillofac Surg 1999; 57(4):457–61.
18. Nitzan DW, Tair JA, Lehman H. Is entire removal of a post-traumatic temporomandibular joint ankylotic site necessary for an optimal outcome? J Oral Maxillofac Surg 2012;70(12):e683–99.
19. Li KK, Ung F, McKenna MJ, et al. Combined middle cranial fossa and preauricular approach to the temporomandibular joint: report of a case. J Oral Maxillofac Surg 1997;55(8):851–2.
20. Hong Y, Gu X, Feng X, et al. Modified coronoid process grafts combined with sagittal split osteotomy for treatment of bilateral temporomandibular joint ankylosis. J Oral Maxillofac Surg 2002;60(1):11–8 [discussion: 18–9].
21. Liu Y, Li J, Hu J, et al. Autogenous coronoid process pedicled on temporal muscle grafts for reconstruction of the mandible condylar in patients with temporomandibular joint ankylosis. Oral Surg Oral Med Oral Pathol Oral Radiol Endod 2010;109(2):203–10.
22. Zhu SS, Hu J, Li J, et al. Free grafting of autogenous coronoid process for condylar reconstruction in patients with temporomandibular joint ankylosis. Oral Surg Oral Med Oral Pathol Oral Radiol Endod 2008;106(5):662–7.
23. Yang X, Hu J, Yin G, et al. Computer-assisted condylar reconstruction in bilateral ankylosis of the temporomandibular joint using autogenous coronoid process. Br J Oral Maxillofac Surg 2011;49(8): 612–7.
24. Liu Y, Khadka A, Li J, et al. Sliding reconstruction of the condyle using posterior border of mandibular ramus in patients with temporomandibular joint ankylosis. Int J Oral Maxillofac Surg 2011;40(11): 1238–45.
25. Cheung LK, Lo J. The long-term effect of transport distraction in the management of temporomandibular joint ankylosis. Plast Reconstr Surg 2007; 119(3):1003–9.
26. González-García R, Naval-Gías L, Rodríguez-Campo FJ, et al. Vascularized fibular flap for reconstruction of the condyle after mandibular ablation. J Oral Maxillofac Surg 2008;66(6):1133–7.
27. Boahene KD, Owusu JA, Collar R, et al. Vascularized scapular tip flap in the reconstruction of the mandibular joint following ablative surgery. Arch Facial Plast Surg 2012;14(3):211–4.
28. Taylor GI, Miller GD, Ham FJ. The free vascularized bone graft. A clinical extension of microvascular techniques. Plast Reconstr Surg 1975;55(5):533–44.
29. Hidalgo DA. Fibula free flap: a new method of mandible reconstruction. Plast Reconstr Surg 1989;84(1):71–9.

30. Guyot L, Richard O, Layoun W, et al. Long-term radiological findings following reconstruction of the condyle with fibular free flaps. J Craniomaxillofac Surg 2004;32(2):98–102.

31. Thor A, Rojas RA, Hirsch JM. Functional reconstruction of the temporomandibular joint with a free fibular microvascular flap. Scand J Plast Reconstr Surg Hand Surg 2008;42(5):233–40.

32. Mercuri LG, Swift JQ. Considerations for the use of alloplastic temporomandibular joint replacement in the growing patient. J Oral Maxillofac Surg 2009; 67(9):1979–90.

33. Giannakopoulos HE, Sinn DP, Quinn PD. Biomet microfixation temporomandibular joint replacement system: a 3-year follow-up study of patients treated during 1995 to 2005. J Oral Maxillofac Surg 2012; 70(4):787–94.

34. Granquist EJ, Quinn PD. Total reconstruction of the temporomandibular joint with a stock prosthesis. Atlas Oral Maxillofac Surg Clin North Am 2011; 19(2):221–32.

35. Westermark A. Total reconstruction of the temporomandibular joint. Up to 8 years of follow-up of patients treated with Biomet(®) total joint prostheses. Int J Oral Maxillofac Surg 2010;39(10): 951–5.

36. Machon V, Hirjak D, Beno M, et al. Total alloplastic temporomandibular joint replacement: the Czech-Slovak initial experience. Int J Oral Maxillofac Surg 2012;41(4):514–7.

37. Mercuri LG. Patient-fitted ("custom") alloplastic temporomandibular joint replacement technique. Atlas Oral Maxillofac Surg Clin North Am 2011; 19(2):233–42.

38. Mercuri LG. Microbial biofilms: a potential source for alloplastic device failure. J Oral Maxillofac Surg 2006;64(8):1303–9.

39. Mercuri LG, Anspach WE. Principles for the revision of total alloplastic TMJ prostheses. Int J Oral Maxillofac Surg 2003;32(4):353–9.

40. Mercuri LG. Avoiding and managing temporomandibular joint total joint replacement surgical site infections. J Oral Maxillofac Surg 2012;70(10):2280–9.

41. Mercuri LG, Ali FA, Woolson R. Outcomes of total alloplastic replacement with periarticular autogenous fat grafting for management of reankylosis of the temporomandibular joint. J Oral Maxillofac Surg 2008;66(9):1794–803.

42. Wolford LM, Rodrigues DB, McPhillips A. Management of the infected temporomandibular joint total joint prosthesis. J Oral Maxillofac Surg 2010; 68(11):2810–23.

43. Mercuri LG, Wolford LM, Sanders B, et al. Custom CAD/CAM total temporomandibular joint reconstruction system: preliminary multicenter report. J Oral Maxillofac Surg 1995;53(2):106–15 [discussion: 115–6].

44. Wolford LM, Pitta MC, Reiche-Fischel O, et al. TMJ Concepts/Techmedica custom-made TMJ total joint prosthesis: 5-year follow-up study. Int J Oral Maxillofac Surg 2003;32(3):268–74.

45. Mercuri LG, Giobbie-Harder A. Long-term outcomes after total alloplastic temporomandibular joint reconstruction following exposure to failed materials. J Oral Maxillofac Surg 2004;62(9):1088–96.

46. Mercuri LG, Edibam NR, Giobbie-Harder A. Fourteen-year follow-up of a patient-fitted total temporomandibular joint reconstruction system. J Oral Maxillofac Surg 2007;65(6):1140–8.

47. Mercuri LG, Psutka D. Perioperative, postoperative, and prophylactic use of antibiotics in alloplastic total temporomandibular joint replacement surgery: a survey and preliminary guidelines. J Oral Maxillofac Surg 2011;69(8):2106–11.

Autogenous and Prosthetic Reconstruction of the Ear

Patrick J. Louis, DDS, MD[a,*],
Ruth A. Aponte-Wesson, DDS, MS[b,c],
Rui P. Fernandes, DMD, MD[d,e,f], Justin Clemow, DMD, MD[d,e]

KEYWORDS

- External ear injury • Acquired auricular defects • Prosthetic ear reconstruction
- Autogenous ear reconstruction • Facial implants • Microsurgery • Architecture of the ear
- Implant-retained prosthetic reconstruction

KEY POINTS

- Reconstruction of auricular defects must reproduce certain key dimensional measurements for optimal aesthetic and functional rehabilitation. These measurements include height, width, vertical axis, protrusion, and position.
- Initial evaluation of a patient for auricular reconstruction must include patient-related factors, patient's reconstructive goals, cause of the defect, type of tissue involved (partial thickness vs full thickness), size and location of the defect, and condition of surrounding local and regional tissues.
- Acquired auricular defects can be divided into cutaneous defects, involving only the auricular skin; composite defects, in which both cartilage and skin are lost; and total or near-total defects, in which the entirety of the auricle requires reconstruction.
- Autogenous reconstruction can be performed with local, regional, and, rarely, free-tissue transfer, based on the type of defect and condition of the surrounding tissue.
- Prosthetic reconstruction can be performed for nearly all acquired auricular defects, with ideal or poor condition of the surrounding tissue. The prosthesis can be implant or nonimplant retained.

Reconstruction of the ear brings about many challenges because of its three-dimensional anatomic complexity. There are multiple causes and multiple techniques that can be used in the reconstruction of the ear. This article presents the potential causes of complete or partial loss of the ear and the potential treatment options.

CAUSE

Causes of complete or partial loss of the ear include trauma, neoplasm, and infection. Because of the lateral position of the ear on the head, and high ratio of surface area to mass,[1] the ear is vulnerable to sharp and blunt trauma,

Funding Sources: None.
Conflict of Interest: None.
[a] Department of Oral and Maxillofacial Surgery, University of Alabama at Birmingham, 1919 7th Avenue South, SDB 419, Birmingham, AL 35294-0007, USA; [b] Department of General Dental Science, University of Alabama at Birmingham, 1919 7th Avenue South, SDB 330, Birmingham, AL 35294-0007, USA; [c] Maxillofacial Prosthodontics, School of Dentistry, University of Alabama at Birmingham, 1919 7th Avenue South, SDB 330, Birmingham, AL 35294-0007, USA; [d] Department of Oral and Maxillofacial Surgery, University of Florida – Jacksonville, 653-1 West Eight Street, LRC 2nd Floor, Jacksonville, FL 32209, USA; [e] Head and Neck Oncology and Microvascular Surgery, University of Florida – Jacksonville, Shands Jacksonville, 655 W 8th Street, Jacksonville, FL 32209, USA; [f] Section of Head and Neck Cancer, Shands Hospital, University of Florida – Jacksonville, Shands Jacksonville, 655 W 8th Street, Jacksonville, FL 32209, USA
* Corresponding author.
E-mail address: plouis@uab.edu

Oral Maxillofacial Surg Clin N Am 25 (2013) 271–286
http://dx.doi.org/10.1016/j.coms.2013.02.001
1042-3699/13/$ – see front matter © 2013 Elsevier Inc. All rights reserved.

burns, and exposure to the elements of nature, such as sun and extremes of temperature. In a study by Guo and colleagues,[2] the most common reasons for comlete prosthetic reconstruction of the external ear in a series of 46 patients were congenital deformities (65.2%), tumor resection (26.1%), trauma (4.3%), burns (2.2%), and infection (2.2%). In another study,[3] a literature review of trauma cases of the auricle was performed. There were 74 cases identified that had complete or partial amputation or extensive lacerations. The following causes were identified: motor vehicle accidents 33.8%, altercations 28.4%, work accidents 10.8%, home accidents 6.9%, sports 4%, and no information identified 14.9%. The number of injuries caused by bites was also reviewed, and 23% were human bites and 12.2% were dog bites.

EVALUATION AND TREATMENT OPTIONS

Options for reconstruction include autogenous reconstruction and prosthetic reconstruction. The clinical evaluation must include evaluation of the ear and the surrounding hard and soft tissue. The clinical evaluation of the residual ear and the periauricular tissue is the most critical part of the surgical planning. The information gathered allows the surgeon to determine which surgical option allows the best outcome. Some surgeons believe that prosthetic reconstruction should be reserved for patients with severe damage to the periauricular tissue or failed previous attempts at reconstruction.[3,4] Injury to the surrounding soft tissue alters the potential surgical options and may prevent local flaps for reconstruction. When planning implants for an anchored prosthetic device, a computed tomography (CT) scan is recommended to determine the amount and location of available bone.

Architecture of the Ear

In consideration of reconstruction of auricular defects, certain key dimensional measurements should be considered for the optimal aesthetic and functional rehabilitation. These measurements include, but are not limited to, the following:

- Height should approximate the distance between the lateral orbital rim and root of the helix at the level of the brow.
- Width of the pinna is roughly 55% of the height.
- The vertical axis has roughly 15° of inclination.
- The helical rim protrudes between 1 and 2.5 cm from the skull, creating an angle of 25° to 30°.
- The superiormost point is at the level of the lateral brow (**Fig. 1**).

Although these dimensions serve as generic standards, they provide only a framework for auricular reconstruction. In unilateral cases, strict adherence to these measurements should not trump the primary importance of using the contralateral ear as a template on which to base the reconstructive effort. As mentioned earlier, the topography of the ear is complex, and faithful recreation of this anatomy presents a considerable challenge to the reconstructive surgeon. Specific contour lines that have been identified as important include a helix, with its root beginning in the concha, tragus, antitragus, and conchal bowl.

Autogenous Reconstruction

Patient selection
In the initial evaluation of a patient for auricular reconstruction, several variables must be considered. These variables include:

- Patient-related factors, including medical health, medications, and smoking
- Patient's reconstructive goals

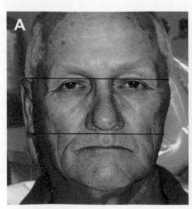
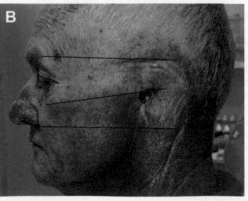

Fig. 1. (*A*) Frontal view of a patient after total resection of his left auricle caused by squamous cell carcinoma. (*B*) Lateral view of a patient after total resection or his left auricle caused by squamous cell carcinoma. The tragus is missing but the ear canal is present, which is useful in determining the position of the ear relative to the other ear.

- Cause of the defect
- Type of tissue involved: partial thickness versus full thickness
- Size and location of the defect
- Condition of surrounding local and regional tissues

Once these considerations have been assessed, the surgeon can begin to develop a treatment plan for reconstruction (**Fig. 2**); there are a variety of classifications in the literature for describing auricular defects, and all of them involve an evaluation of these factors.[5,6] In general, defects can be divided into cutaneous defects, involving only the auricular skin; composite defects, in which both cartilage and skin are lost; and total or near-total defects, in which the entirety of the auricle requires reconstruction. Composite defects can further be subdivided into marginal and nonmarginal defects, with specific reconstructive implications for each. Similarly, near-total and total auricular defects are further subdivided into those with healthy/intact surrounding tissues versus those in which the surrounding tissue is compromised or damaged.

Surgical technique

Cutaneous defects For auricular defects in which only soft tissue is missing, the first assessment in the reconstructive algorithm regards the integrity of the perichondrium. In cases in which skin and subcutaneous tissues are missing, but the perichondrium and cartilage are intact, these defects are best served with a full-thickness skin graft. The retroauricular skin provides the best color match and thickness for this purpose. For cutaneous defects with loss of perichondrium, the location of the defect becomes a consideration. If this defect occurs in an area

where the cartilage is not structure determining, such as the conchal bowl or scapha, removal of the cartilage followed by full-thickness skin graft is appropriate, relying on the posterior auricular skin as a donor site. With loss of perichondrium and skin and the helix or antihelix, consideration should be given to making the defect full thickness, followed by reconstruction in 1 of the ways described in the following sections.

Composite defects

Marginal defects With auricular defects involving skin and cartilage, consideration of the size and location of the defect is crucial. In general, smaller defects can usually be addressed by 1 of several types of reduction procedures. Composite defects measuring less than 15 mm of the helical rim or antihelix are generally amenable to full-thickness wedge excision and primary closure. For larger defects of the helical rim (no greater than 25 mm), the surgeon should consider the chondrocutaneous composite advancement flap as described by Antia and Buch in 1967.[7] The basic principle of this technique involves advancement of adjacent intact helical margin chondrocutaneous flaps based on a large postauricular pedicle. An incision in the helical sulcus through the skin and cartilage, leaving posterior perichondrium and postauricular skin intact, allows for advancement of the helix about the scapha. For inferior and middle marginal defects, most of the advancement is accomplished from the inferior segment at the expense of the lobule. Conversely, superior defects use advancement of both the inferior and superior segments, using a V-Y closure at the root of the helix (**Fig. 3**).[8]

As mentioned earlier, the Antia-Buch and other reduction and advancement techniques are best reserved for marginal defects less

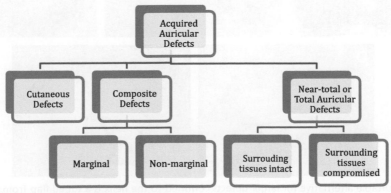

Fig. 2. Classification of acquired defects of the ear.

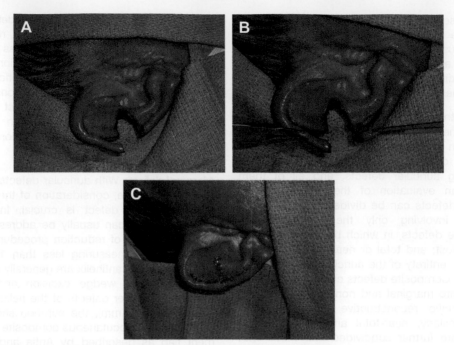

Fig. 3. (*A–C*) Superior defects use advancement of both the inferior and superior segments, using a V-Y closure at the root of the helix.

than 25 mm in length, or about one-third of the helical rim. With larger defects, the resulting microtia leads to a cosmetically unacceptable result. A suitable alternative for larger defects confined to the helix is a tubed flap from 1 of several periauricular areas (**Fig. 4**). Several variations of this concept have been described.

Masud and Tzafetta[9] described a 2-stage technique named a double-headed slug flap, which first reconstructs the superior half of a helical defect with an inferiorly based transposition interpolation flap, followed 3 weeks later by a second transposition flap to complete the reconstruction of the inferior half. The donor

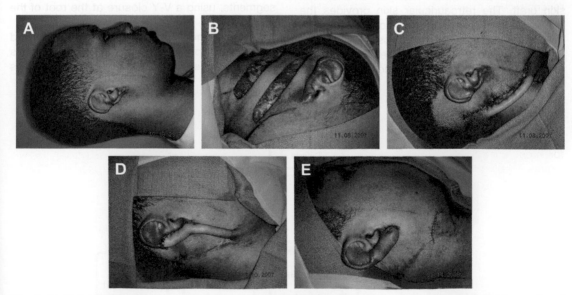

Fig. 4. (*A–E*) A suitable alternative for larger defects confined to the helix is a tubed flap from 1 of several periauricular areas.

site is closed primarily, resulting in a discrete posterior auricular scar.

Nonmarginal defects For nonmarginal defects, or defects involving the helix plus some combination of the conchal bowl, scapha, or triangular fossa, several adaptations of the original Antia-Buch technique have been described. An exhaustive summary of these modifications is beyond the scope of this text, but some of them include specifically placed anterior chondrocutaneous excisions at the borders of the advancement,[8,10] versus replacement of scaphal fossa tissue with a posterior auricular transpositional flap. Schonauer and colleagues[11] describe the varied uses of the posterior auricular soft tissues on either side of the auriculocephalic groove. The unusually rich arterial supply in this area, which supplies the auricular branch of the posterior auricular artery and the posterior branch of the superficial temporal artery, allows for great versatility for random-pattern flap design to reconstruct a variety of nonhelical full-thickness auricular defects.

For composite defects of up to 2 cm, a chondrocutaneous graft from the contralateral ear can be considered. The obvious consideration here is the degree of resultant microtia of the donor ear, and the difficulty of matching the outcome in the opposite ear.

Total or near-total defects For full-thickness auricular defects in which a significant amount of the structure-determining cartilage is lost, reconstruction depends on replacing the cartilaginous framework as well as the soft tissue coverage. This reconstruction presents a particular obstacle because the cartilaginous anatomy of the ear is intricate and the overlying auricular skin must be thin to adequately portray the cartilaginous topography.

The major tenants of reconstruction of acquired ear deformities are borrowed from the principles of congenital microtia surgery described by Tanzer's original 6-stage procedure.[12] Subsequent revisions by Brent[13] led to Nagata's[14] introduction of a 2-stage procedure, which provides the basis for most current auricular reconstruction techniques. The basic principle of this method involves a first stage in which costal cartilage is harvested, fashioned to recreate the acquired auricular defect and sutured to remaining native auricular cartilage if applicable, then buried in the postauricular soft tissue. This stage is followed 3 to 6 months later by a second stage, which involves elevating this cartilaginous construct from the mastoid skin by creating a posterior auricular sulcus and therefore accomplishing the desired projection from the mastoid region.

Hard tissue reconstruction Cartilaginous structure can be provided by autologous sources like conchal cartilage in the case of small defects or costal cartilage for larger defects. For helical defects, costal cartilage from the floating (eighth) rib may be sufficient. However, for total auricular reconstruction, a block of cartilage from the synchondrosis of the sixth and seventh ribs is also required. The template for creation of the cartilaginous construct can be fashioned from a silicone model created by impression of the contralateral ear, or more simply, by creating a map of the normal ear out of clear radiograph film.[15,16] In addition to the cartilage used for creation of the auricular construct, a block of cartilage can be stored in the subcutaneous tissue of the chest wall to aid with achieving projection in the second stage.

As an alternative to autologous cartilage, alloplastic sources are available such as the Medpor (Stryker, Kalamazoo, MI) silastic auricular implant. This option offers many benefits, including shorter surgery time, shorter recovery, lower cost, and in cases, easier patient acceptance. In addition, it circumvents the concerns regarding morbidity associated with harvest of costal cartilage (pneumothorax, chest wall deformity, pain associated with harvest, scarring, and so forth). However, as a foreign body, it is associated with slightly higher rates of graft exposure, or outright failure.

Soft tissue reconstruction Much of the complexity associated with auricular reconstruction depends on the condition of the surrounding periauricular soft tissues.[5] This variable is largely dependent on the conditions under which the defect was acquired. For instance, the condition of the surrounding soft tissues is generally favorable in the case of oncologic resection or trauma, compared with burn injuries. Similarly, auricular reconstruction in the patient with multiple previous reconstructive attempts may present additional soft tissue restrictions not only as a result of scarring but also because this situation requires consideration for the soft tissue options that have been exhausted on previous operations.

When the periauricular soft tissues are in good condition, the cartilage graft can usually be placed under a posteriorly based flap of mastoid skin. During the second stage, several months later, when the auricular construct is released from the side of the head, a temporoparietal fascia flap provides an excellent source of abundant, well-vascularized local tissue. This procedure is often followed by split-thickness skin graft for epithelial coverage.[17] In cases in which there is inadequate periauricular skin, temporoparietal fascia can sometimes be used for the initial coverage of the autologous cartilage graft. This tissue is readily adapted to the underlying hard tissue construct because of its minimal thickness. This technique has also been proposed to accomplish a single-staged reconstruction.[18]

In patients for whom skin grafting or temporoparietal fascia flaps are unacceptable, the use of tissue expanders for soft tissue coverage has been described. In this technique, 1 or 2 kidney-shaped tissue expanders are placed in a plane just below the subcutaneous fat through a radial incision in the scalp paralleling the hairline. At a second stage 3 to 6 months later, the expanded skin is used to cover and auricular construct without the need for fascial flaps or skin grafting.[19]

In cases in which the periauricular skin is severely compromised as with extensive burning, other options can be considered. This is a scenario in which prosthetic reconstruction (discussed elsewhere in this article) must be considered. An alternative is microvascular free-tissue transfer, provided that suitable recipient vessels are available.

Implant-retained Prosthetic Reconstruction

Patient selection

The evaluation of the patient with a missing ear is important; losing an ear can have a profound impact on their emotional state, because it affects facial aesthetics and function.[6,20] The extent of the surgery may or may not obliterate the ear canal, diminishing the ability to hear. It can also affect the patient's vision if the patient uses glasses; this seems most problematic in patients with bifocals.[6] Often, the patients have to be creative with the use of Velcro or some kind of band around the head to hold their glasses in place.

Patients with congenital defects may be more difficult to reconstruct prosthetically because of the lack of an ideal site to work with. These patients present with microtia, irregular, malformed and asymmetrical ears, which can be associated with craniofacial syndromes. These patients may have undergone multiple surgeries to try to reconstruct the ear or prepare the site to receive a prosthesis and may be frustrated with the process. Thus, good communication is required with the young and growing patient and their parents.

In the case of planed surgical ablation, the patient can be seen preoperatively. The information gathered can help facilitate the reconstructive phase.[3,5,21] The following information is usually obtained:

Diagnostic bilateral auricular impressions
Facial photograph (frontal, lateral, and posterior views)
Maxillofacial CT scan

Surgical technique

The use of osseointegrated implants in the temporal bone was first reported in 1981.[22,23] There have been multiple reports of titanium implants being a successful option for retention of maxillofacial implants.[2,24–27] The advantages of facial implants include:

- Improved retention when compared with adhesive
- Less time needed to place the prosthesis
- Ease of use
- Improved life span of the prosthesis
- Less skin irritation when compared with adhesives
- Less dependence on other to help place the prosthesis
- Proper positioning of the device
- Can be placed in irradiated bone

The disadvantages include:

- Care and maintenance of the implants
- Possibility of infection and inflammation around the implants
- Need for a surgical procedure to place the implants

The surgical procedure can be performed in an outpatient setting, but many surgeons choose to perform this procedure in the operating room, because of the proximity to the brain of the surgical site and the occasional need for navigation during surgery.[28] A preoperative CT scan is needed to evaluate the thickness of available bone. A surgical guide is used to allow for proper implant placement (**Fig. 5**). A curvilinear incision is made approximately 2 to 2.5 cm superior and posterior to the external auditory canal (EAC), extending inferiorly. A skin flap is elevated just below the dermis. The underlying fat, fascia, muscle, and periosteum are excised from the region of the EAC to approximately 3 to 3.5 cm superior, posterior, and inferior to the EAC. Debulking the soft tissue at the planned implant site is necessary to reduce inflammation and improve the long-term survival of the implants. The general guidelines for implant placement for an auricular prosthesis are 18 to 20 mm from the center of the EAC and 15 mm apart. The implants are usually placed at the 2, 3, and 4 o'clock positions. The region superior to the EAC is usually too thin for implant placement, and in the region directly inferior to the EAC, there is no available bone. The surgical guide is placed and the pilot holes are prepared using a drill with a 3-mm to 4-mm stop, depending on available bone (Vistafix Cochlear Bone Anchored Solutions AB, Macquarie Park, New South Wales). The

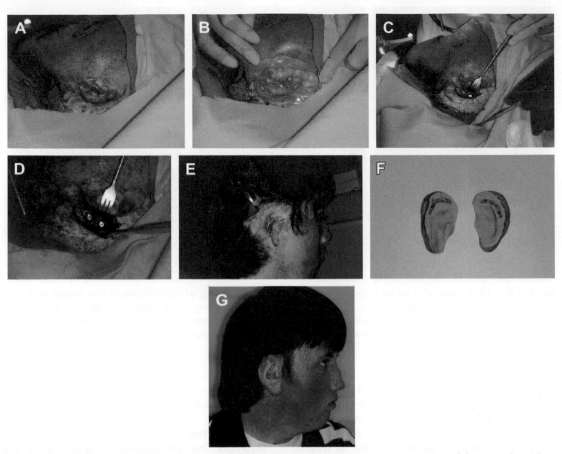

Fig. 5. (*A*) Patient with missing right ear and failed previous autogenous reconstruction. (*B*) Surgical guide in place. (*C*) Surgical flap raised and 2 endosseous implants in place. (*D*) Close-up of the surgical field. Note the implant position in the 2 and 4 o'clock position. (*E*) Lateral view of the patient with implant superstructure in place. (*F*) Bilateral ear prosthesis, showing the undersurface with attachment in place. (*G*) Lateral view of the patient with the implant-retained ear prosthesis in place. Note the excellent contour and color match.

osteotomy must be visually inspected for available depth. If there is inadequate bone thickness, then an alternative site must be chosen based on the CT scan. The final drill is used and a self-tapping implant is placed. A flat healing cap is placed for a 2-stage procedure. The incision is closed with a long-lasting resorbable deep suture, and fast-absorbing-gut suture can be used on the skin. If a 1-stage technique is used, a taller healing cap is placed. The flap is closed in a similar fashion and small punctures are made over the implants for the implants to protrude. A bolster dressing is placed with Xeroform (Covidien, Kendall, Mansfield, MA) gauze and RestOn Foam. (3M, St Paul, MN) This dressing helps the flap to heal without hematoma formation. This dressing is generally removed after 7 days. A minimum of 2 implants are placed. When there is abundant bone, a third implant is placed (**Fig. 6**). This implant can be incorporated into the prosthesis or used as

a sleeper in case any of the other implants has to be taken out of service. In the 2-stage technique, the implants are allowed to heal for 3 months before uncovering and placement of the second-phase healing cap. In the single-stage technique, the implants are not loaded for at least 3 months.

Postoperative care

The patient is instructed to keep the site dry while the bolster dressing is in place. The patient is placed on antibiotics and analgesics postoperatively. On postoperative day 7, the bolster dressing is removed, and any residual sutures can be removed. The wound can be cleansed with soap and water. Once the implants are exposed, they are cleaned twice a day with peroxide and water and medical grade alcohol. Chlorhexadine skin scrub can also be used twice daily. The implants are not engaged by the prosthesis for at least 3 months.

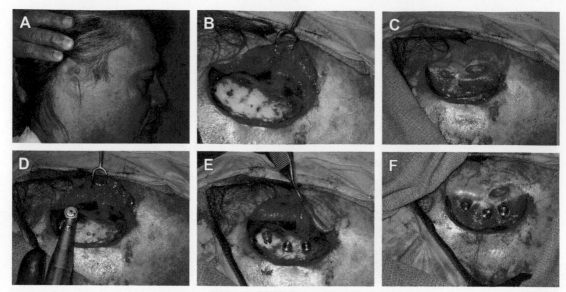

Fig. 6. (*A*) Lateral view of a patient missing the right ear. (*B*) Close-up of right postauricular region with flap elevated and thinned and pilot holes in place. (*C*) Surgical field showing the thinned surgical flap. (*D*) Osteotomies being created for the endosseous implants. (*E*) Endosseous implants in place at the 1, 3, and 5 o'clock positions. (*F*) Endosseous implants in place with the thinned surgical flap positioned for a single-stage procedure.

Complications

Studies show a low complication rate for temporal bone implants and a high success rate. Some studies have shown a success rate between 98% and 100% in irradiated and nonirradiated bone.[29–31] Loss of implants can occur as a result of breakdown of interface between the soft tissue and implants. This finding is common in burn victims (**Fig. 7**). Loss of implants can also occur in previous irradiated bone, especially those situations in which the local dose exceeds 40 cGy.

Prosthetic technique

Materials The most popular materials are medical grade silicones. These silicones have many lifelike properties; they are easily manipulated, can be

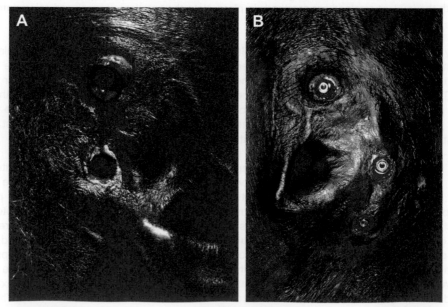

Fig. 7. (*A, B*) Burned victim. Repeated complications were observed in this patient around the implant tissue junction.

intrinsically colored, and can be extrinsically stained and sealed. Their life span varies according to their use and care. Although improvements have been made in the tear strength of the material, this remains the most significant weakness. It also can become discolored as a result of exposure to the elements, such as sunlight. A patient should expect to have the prosthesis replaced every 2 years. There are 2 main groups of silicones: heat-temperature vulcanizing silicone and room temperature vulcanizing (RTV) silicone, the latter being the most popular for facial prosthesis.[6,20]

Evaluation of the defect The defect is evaluated by observation of the face and finding useful landmarks to help position the missing pinna. When the tragus and the EAC are present, these landmarks help determine the position of the wax trial auricular or future prosthesis. These 2 landmarks are located in the center of the ear and help divide the ear in 2 parts and determine the position of the future prosthesis relative to the other ear. When the tragus or ear canal is not present, the Frankfort horizontal plane (a line that runs from the infraorbital rim to just above the EAC), as measured from the opposite side, can be useful in positioning the prosthesis.[32]

The symmetry of the eyebrows is another important landmark. The eyebrows aid in positioning the superior border of the wax trial auricular and future prosthesis. For the inferior border of the auricular, an imaginary line is drawn from the base of the nose to the inferior border of the opposite ear and is used for comparison.[6]

Prosthetics The prosthetic technique is divided in 2 phases: a provisional phase and a definitive phase.

The provisional or healing phase entails fabrication of a prosthesis for the patient to use while healing from the initial surgery. This initial prosthesis is used from 4 to 6 months.[6] The advantage is that the patient has a smooth transition during the postsurgical healing period. This prosthesis also may give the patient a better understanding of what the retention will be like with the adhesive-retained prosthesis. This strategy may help the patient to decide if they desire osseointegrated implants (Vistafix), which enhances retention, ease of placement, and orientation of the auricular prosthesis (**Fig. 8**).[33] The main disadvantage posed in this phase is the inability to modify the provisional prosthesis, because it can be costly and time consuming to have multiple wax trials and casting as tissues settle.

Once the tissues have healed, the defect area should be reevaluated for useful undercuts, the presence of the tragus, or EAC, and texture of the skin; especially if it has been irradiated. Radiation, depending on the dose, increases the risk of failure of craniofacial implants, thus limiting their use. The patient should be informed that the final prosthesis requires a total of 5 to 7 appointments.[34,35]

Impressions Mark landmarks with a Thompson's color transfer applicator (Great Plains Dental Products, Kingman, KS) or indelible pen. Block off the EAC with a cotton pellet infused with petroleum jelly. Lubricate the hair around the ear and drape the patient's shoulders. Seat the patient looking straightforward. Select the impression material that best suits the needs; the preferred materials are slow-set alginate for facial impression (J-638 [Factor II, Lakeside, AZ]); type 0 putty consistency and polyvinyl siloxanes type 2 medium body Aquasil Monophase (Densply, Caulk, Milford, DE) may be best suited to copy detail and incorporate craniofacial implants, when present.

Apply the impression material in uniform layers, starting from top to bottom. Try to dam the material when possible. If craniofacial implants are incorporated in the plan, use impression copings at this time (**Fig. 9A–D**). Before the material reaches the total setting time, apply the putty layer and incorporate mechanical retention, as shown in **Fig. 9E**, then cover the impression material with a mixture of laboratory plaster. To expedite the setting of the plaster, replace plain water with slurry water or add salt to it. The addition of the plaster gives support to the impression (see **Fig. 9F**). Once the materials have set completely, gently remove the impression without separating the layers. The patient can assist in the removal of the impression material by performing facial movement. Pour the impression with improved extrahard die stone type IV, preferable white (Whip Mix, Louisville, KY) (see **Fig. 9G**).

Wax-up of the prosthesis Once the cast has been obtained and trimmed, begin the sculpting of the ear by using the marks obtained from landmarks and the opposite ear. Apply a thin layer of separating media on the cast and let it dry. Make wax for sculpting by using a mixture of pink base plate wax and clear rope wax in a ratio of 1:1 (True Wax Pink Type II and Utility Wax White [Densply]). Heat to fuse the 2 together, and wait until it has hardened enough to start layering. This strategy allows excellent sculpting and margin adaptation. Sculpt the ear to full shape, then try it on the patient. Have the patient make suggestions and modify accordingly. This stage may take several attempts. Have the patient approve the final wax-up (**Fig. 10**).

Implant component verification When craniofacial implants are used, evaluate the vertical space

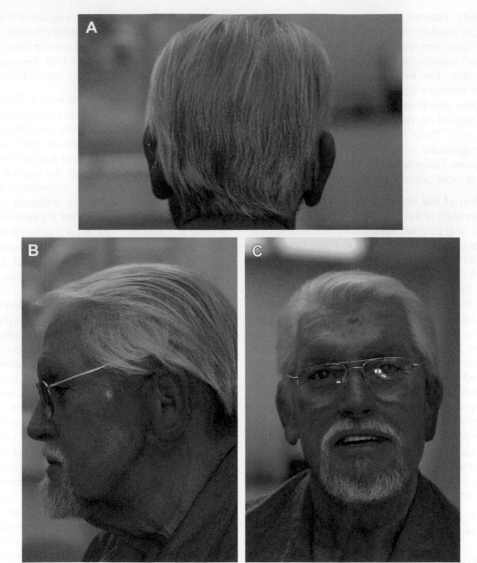

Fig. 8. (*A–C*) Multiple views of the patient showing the provisional prosthesis phase that is adhesive retained.

for the craniofacial components. The rationale for the verification at this time is that the wax-up of the auricle has been accomplished. Duplicate the wax-up and pour in stone. Make a vacuum form matrix, cut and fit it on to a working cast, and verify adequate space for bars, magnets, locator attachments and acrylic resin keepers (**Fig. 11**).[36]

Implant superstructure Once the verification of space has been achieved, the choice of retentive superstructure is made. Choices include individual abutments or a bar.

For direct use, select standard abutments, console magnets abutments, or Magnabutments (Vistafix). When using a bar, the choices include a round prefabricated (Vistafix) or Hadder wax pattern for casting. The other choice for bar

fabrication is to use a computer-aided design (CAD)/computer-aided manufacturing (CAM) system such as Cgenix (**Fig. 12**).

The bar is tried on. If it fits, then incorporate the retentive elements chosen with metal housings. Wax up and process an acrylic resin keeper (Lucitone Clear and Lucitone 199 [Densply]) in clear acrylic resin or a mixture of clear and pink acrylic resin for a more natural outcome. Incorporate, trim, and try it on the patient. Then incorporate this keeper to the waxed ear. Both components must be tried on the patient. Verify that the wax-up is still what both the patient and the doctor envisioned.

Mold fabrication For auricular prosthesis, the mold should be made in 3 pieces. This strategy enables visualization of all parts and retrieval of

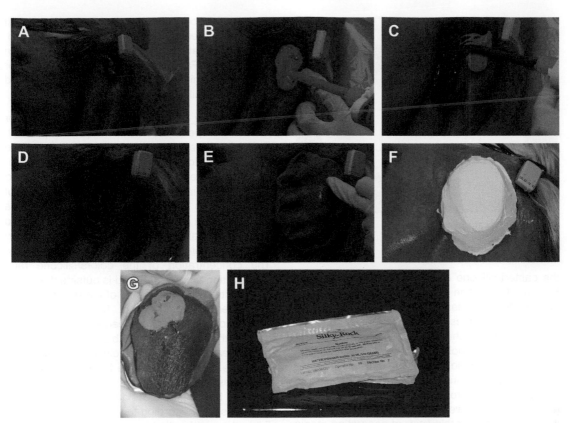

Fig. 9. (*A–H*) Sequence of the impression technique and materials when patient has craniofacial implants. (*A*) Tapered impression copings. (*B*) Application of Aquasil Ultra LV. (*C, D*) Application of Aquasil Monophase. (*E*) Application of putty and mechanical retention. (*F*) Application of laboratory plaster. (*G*) Stone for pour-up of working cast. (*H*) Silky Rock (Whip Mix, Louisville, KY) extrahard die stone.

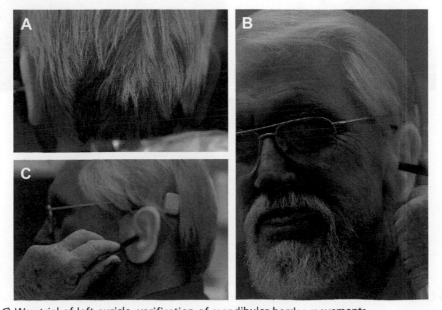

Fig. 10. (*A–C*) Wax trial of left auricle, verification of mandibular border movements.

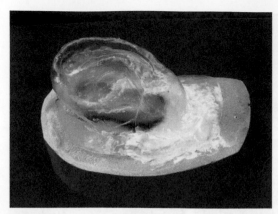

Fig. 11. Verification of space with a vacuum form matrix over wax-up for keeper.

the casted silicone once it has been vulcanized. For the fabrication of this mold, use a metal denture flask (Hanau, Pearson Dental Products, Sylmar, CA) or plastic round container that can be cut off the stone once it sets. This strategy creates durable molds for more than 1 casting. All parts of the mold need to be indexed and well fitted with their counterpart (**Fig. 13**).

The wax needs to be boiled out, and the mold has to be cleaned well with soap and water. Before it dries off, another thin layer of separating media

(Factor II) should be applied, and air dried. If a keeper is used, this too has to be cleaned, dried, and a thin coat of primer needs to be applied on it (A-330-G, Factor II), which needs to set for 1.5 hours. This procedure enhances the bond between the silicone and the acrylic resin.

Intrinsic color matching Intrinsic silicone color matching is performed with the patient present. Select the type of silicone, then create the palate of colors, which is unique for each patient. For this procedure, use RTV platinum silicone and functional intrinsic paint (Factor II). The ratio of the silicone to paint is 10:1. The average silicone amount for an auricular prosthesis is about 40 to 60 g of base and catalyst. The basic colors used for human skin are white, red, blue, and yellow. The concentration of the colors/silicone ratio varies among individuals and is outside the scope of this article. The base tone of the skin is attained first, then the chroma of the base color is increased or changed as needed for the different parts of the ear. In general, a base shade is needed plus at least 5 variants. The closer the shades are to all the auricular parts the better, because this minimizes extrinsic staining.

Apply the palate of colors into the mold with paintbrushes, according to your coloring diagram. Fill in the mold entirely and assemble all parts of

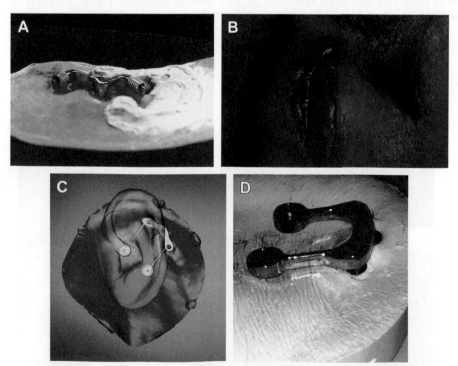

Fig. 12. (*A*) Casted Hadder bar. (*B*) Soldered prefabricated bar. (*C, D*) CAD CAM bar, verification stent, and final product.

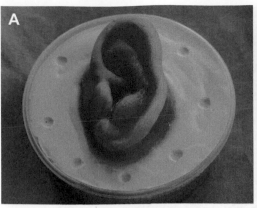 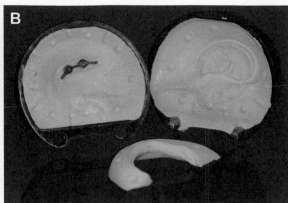

Fig. 13. (*A*) Waxed auricle with lower part of the mold with removable plastic container. (*B*) Three-piece mold, with duplicate bar made out of technique metal.

the mold created. Once closed, place the mold under pressure so the excess material can flow out. Maintain under pressure while vulcanizing with a champ.

Vulcanization Depending on the type of silicone used (RTV platinum silicones VST-50 or A-588-1; A-588-2 [Factor II]), if expedited vulcanization is desired, a dry heat oven may be used. At all times the mold needs to be under pressure regardless of the route of vulcanization. RTV without the stimulus of heat vulcanization takes 8 to 10 hours: with the help of a dry heat oven at a constant temperature of 119°F, it takes 2 to 3 hours. When the time is up, let the mold cool at room temperature and remove the auricular prosthesis gently out of the mold. Evaluate its integrity (**Fig. 14**).

Extrinsic staining and sealing Trim excess and remove any unwanted seams from the prosthesis. Wash with soap and water, dry and clean the

prosthesis with acetone, and let it air dry. If implants have been used, this is a good opportunity to evaluate the prosthesis for passive fit and retention. Evaluate the color and where it needs to be enhanced; use FE Extrinsic stain kit paints (Factor II). In order for these stains to work, use them in conjunction with the FE 100 solvent.

The sealing process requires a few steps and takes at least 80 to 90 minutes. Each layer of sealant needs to set for 20 to 30 minutes. To help in the setting of each layer, the dry heat oven can be used at 119°F. The sealants fall into the category of acetoxy silicones (Factor II). The sealing process is as follows: apply a thin layer of TS-564 with a disposable brush and let it set for 20 to 30 minutes (**Fig. 15**). Then apply another thin layer of the A-564. Apply it with a disposable brush, and blot with a humid gauze, then let it set for 20 to 30 minutes. Then mix 10 g of MD-564 with 2 g of A-564 and apply gently and evenly on the prosthesis. Let this set for 20 to 30 minutes. Apply the layer that gives the final finish of MD-564; this provides a matting finish and has an appearance of white chalk. Let it set for another 20 to 30 minutes, then wash the prosthesis with soap and water. Dry and deliver to patient.

Maintenance and care Instructions of care for skin vary depending on whether the prosthesis is retained by adhesive or craniofacial implants. With an adhesive-retained prosthesis, the skin needs to be cleaned, wiped off with an alcohol wipe, and air dried. The prosthesis needs to be clean with soap and water and air dried. The water-based adhesive (B-200-30 Daro Hydrobond [Factor II]) has to be applied around the border or area assigned for retention. As adhesive is applied it is white, and as it dries, it turns clear, when it is ready to be oriented on the patient's face. Sometimes, the patient needs help from a spouse or

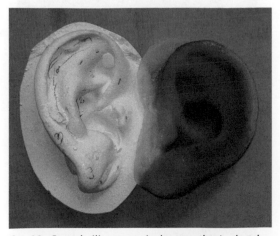

Fig. 14. Casted silicone auricular prosthesis that has been intrinsically colored, using RTV A588-1.

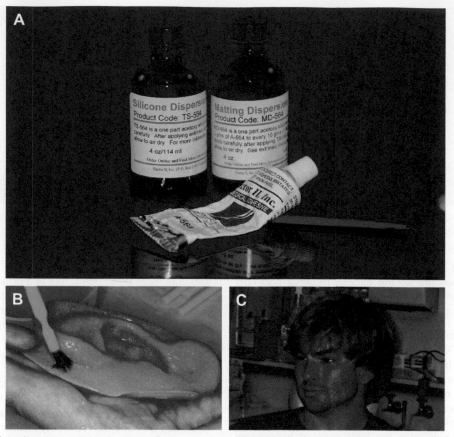

Fig. 15. (*A*) Sealing kits. (*B*) Application of sealers. (*C*) Finished product.

caregiver to orient the prosthesis properly until they become proficient at placement. The adhesive lasts between 6 and 8 hours under most weather conditions. On removal, the prosthesis and skin need to be cleaned with water and soap.[37]

An implant-retained prosthesis requires more care around the interface between the implant abutments and the skin. This prosthesis can be cleaned with a cotton swab and peroxide diluted with water, on a daily base to avoid crusting from the oil and keratin produced by the skin (**Fig. 16**). The prosthesis is then pressed into place and retained by the implant components. The auricular prosthesis needs to be cleaned daily with soap and water and air dried. Most patients prefer implant-retained prosthesis because of the retention and ease of orientation.

Replacement and repair Most of the maintenance is geared toward the implant-retained prosthesis. The retentive nylon elements wear out and their housings become loose and sometimes lost. These elements can be easily replaced. Failure of the implants can occur, especially if the tissues

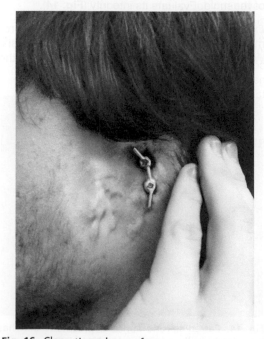

Fig. 16. Clean tissue bar surface.

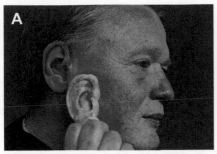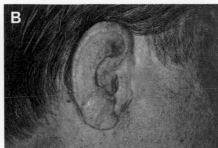

Fig. 17. (*A*) New prosthesis and discolored auricular silicone prosthesis after 2 years of continued use. (*B*) Restrained and resealed prosthesis. ([*A*] *Courtesy of* Dr Don Leopoldo Jayanetti.)

have been irradiated or the implants are not properly cleaned. The bar components wear out or fracture and require replacement.

Other issues are related to the integrity of the margins and changes in color of the prosthesis.[38] These issues apply to both types of prosthesis. At times, the color issues can be addressed by restaining the prosthesis and resealing. When this solution is not possible, another casting from the original mold can be made, if there are no tissue volumetric changes (**Fig. 17**).

ACKNOWLEDGMENTS

We would like to thank all of those who have contributed to the care of our patients. Without your collaboration, this small segment would not have been possible; this includes those who have strived to provide us with the best and cutting-edge materials, the artist and mentors who guide us with their techniques and tips, the interaction with the surgical partners and colleagues, the fellows who challenge our imagination on daily bases, and last but most importantly our patients, who trust in our abilities to return back their dignity.

REFERENCES

1. Templer J, Renner GJ. Injuries of the external ear. Otolaryngol Clin North Am 1990;23(5):1003–18.
2. Guo G, Schwedtner O, Klein M. A retrospective study of implant-retained auricular prostheses. Int J Oral Maxillofac Implants 2008;23(3):539–43.
3. Steffen A, Katzbach R, Klaiber S. A comparison of ear reattachment methods: a review of 25 years since Pennington. Plast Reconstr Surg 2006; 118(6):1358–64.
4. Wilkes GH, Wolfaardt JF. Osseointegrated alloplastic versus autogenous ear reconstruction: criteria for treatment selection. Plast Reconstr Surg 1994; 93(5):967–79.
5. Luo X, Yang J, Yang Q, et al. Classification and reconstruction of posttraumatic ear deformity. J Craniofac Surg 2012;23(3):654–7.
6. McKinstry R, Allen R. Fundamentals in facial prosthetics. Arlington (VA): ABI Professional Publications; 1995.
7. Antia NH, Buch VI. Chondrocutaneous advancement flap for the marginal defect of the ear. Plast Reconstr Surg 1967;39(5):472–7.
8. Bialostocki A, Tan ST. Modified Antia-Buch repair for full-thickness upper pole auricular defects. Plast Reconstr Surg 1999;103(5):1476–9.
9. Masud D, Tzafetta K. The 'double headed slug flap': a simple technique to reconstruct large helical rim defects. J Plast Reconstr Aesthet Surg 2012; 65(10):1410–3.
10. Fata JJ. Composite chondrocutaneous advancement flap: a technique for the reconstruction of marginal defects of the ear. Plast Reconstr Surg 1997;99(4):1172–5.
11. Schonauer F, Vuppalapati G, Marlino S, et al. Versatility of the posterior auricular flap in partial ear reconstruction. Plast Reconstr Surg 2010;126(4): 1213–21.
12. Tanzer RC. Total reconstruction of the auricle. The evolution of a plan of treatment. Plast Reconstr Surg 1971;47(6):523–33.
13. Brent B. Ear reconstruction with an expansile framework of autogenous rib cartilage. Plast Reconstr Surg 1974;53(6):619–28.
14. Nagata S. A new method of total reconstruction of the auricle for microtia. Plast Reconstr Surg 1993; 92(2):187–201.
15. Tanner PB, Mobley SR. External auricular and facial prosthetics: a collaborative effort of the reconstructive surgeon and anaplastologist. Facial Plast Surg Clin North Am 2006;14(2):137–45, vi–vii.
16. Gault D. Post traumatic ear reconstruction. J Plast Reconstr Aesthet Surg 2008;61(Suppl 1):S5–12.
17. Pearl RA, Sabbagh W. Reconstruction following traumatic partial amputation of the ear. Plast Reconstr Surg 2011;127(2):621–9.

18. Ali SN, Khan MA, Farid M, et al. Reconstruction of segmental acquired auricular defects. J Craniofac Surg 2010;21(2):561–4.

19. Zhang GL, Zhang JM, Liang WQ, et al. Implant double tissue expanders superposingly in mastoid region for total ear reconstruction without skin grafts. Int J Pediatr Otorhinolaryngol 2012;76(10):1515–9.

20. Beumer J, Manirick MT, Esposito SJ. Maxillofacial rehabilitation. Hanover Park (IL): Quintessence; p. 255–313.

21. Euvrard S, Kanitakis J, Claudy A. Skin cancers after organ transplantation. N Engl J Med 2003;348(17): 1681–91.

22. Tjellstrom A, Lindstrom J, Nylen O, et al. The bone-anchored auricular episthesis. Laryngoscope 1981; 91(5):811–5.

23. Tjellstrom A, Lindstrom J, Hallen O, et al. Osseointe-grated titanium implants in the temporal bone. A clinical study on bone-anchored hearing aids. Am J Otol 1981;2(4):304–10.

24. Parel SM, Holt GR, Branemark PI, et al. Osseointe-gration and facial prosthetics. Int J Oral Maxillofac Implants 1986;1(1):27–9.

25. Tjellstrom A, Rosenhall U, Lindstrom J, et al. Five-year experience with skin-penetrating bone-anchored implants in the temporal bone. Acta Otolaryngol 1983;95(5–6):568–75.

26. McCartney JW. Osseointegrated implant-supported and magnetically retained ear prosthesis: a clinical report. J Prosthet Dent 1991;66(1):6–9.

27. Demir N, Malkoc MA, Ozturk AN, et al. Implant-re-tained auricular prosthesis. J Craniofac Surg 2010; 21(6):1795–7.

28. Verma SN, Schow SR, Stone BH, et al. Applications of surgical navigational systems for craniofacial bone-anchored implant placement. Int J Oral Maxil-lofac Implants 2010;25(3):582–8.

29. Tolman DE, Taylor PF. Bone-anchored craniofacial prosthesis study. Int J Oral Maxillofac Implants 1996;11(2):159–68.

30. Wolfaardt JF, Wilkes GH, Parel SM, et al. Craniofacial osseointegration: the Canadian experience. Int J Oral Maxillofac Implants 1993;8(2):197–204.

31. Parel SM, Tjellstrom A. The United States and Swedish experience with osseointegration and facial prostheses. Int J Oral Maxillofac Implants 1991;6(1): 75–9.

32. Anderson JD, Szalai JP. The Toronto outcome measure for craniofacial prosthetics. A condition-specific quality-of-life instrument. Int J Oral Maxillofac Implants 2003;18:531–8.

33. Kouyoumdjian J, Chalian VA, Moore BK. A comparison of the physical properties of a room temperature vulcanizing silicone modified and unmodified. J Prosthet Dent 1985;53(3):388–91.

34. Granstrom G. Osseointegration in irradiated cancer patients: an analysis with respect to implant failures. J Oral Maxillofac Surg 2005;63(5):579–85.

35. Jacobsson M, Tjellstrom A, Fine L, et al. A retrospective study of osseointegrated skin-penetrating titanium fixtures used for retaining facial prostheses. Int J Oral Maxillofac Implants 1992;7(4): 523–8.

36. Disantis WS. Technique for using an acrylic resin insert to simulate a cartilaginous structure in a silicone prosthetic ear. J Prosthet Dent 1984;52(6):889–91.

37. Kiat-amnuay S, Gettleman L, Khan Z, et al. Effect of adhesive retention on maxillofacial prostheses. Part I: skin dressings and solvent removers. J Prosthet Dent 2000;84(3):335–40.

38. Haug SP, Andres CJ, Munoz CA, et al. Effects of environmental factors on maxillofacial elastomers: part III–Physical properties. J Prosthet Dent 1992; 68(4):644–51.

Microsurgical Reconstruction of the Trigeminal Nerve

Roger A. Meyer, DDS, MS, MD[a,b,c,e],
Shahrokh C. Bagheri, DMD, MD[b,c,d,e],*

KEYWORDS

- Nerve injury • Maxillofacial trauma • Ablative tumor surgery • Trigeminal nerve
- Sensory dysfunction • Nerve repair • Microneurosurgery • Nerve graft

KEY POINTS

- The peripheral branches of the second (maxillary) and third (mandibular) divisions of the trigeminal nerve supply sensation to the midface, upper lip, maxilla and palate, lower face, lower lip, mandible, and tongue.
- These nerves are at risk of avulsive injury with loss of continuity from maxillofacial trauma or ablative surgical procedures. Sensory recovery from such injuries seldom occurs spontaneously.
- Peripheral trigeminal nerve injuries can result in permanent sensory dysfunction (decreased or lost sensation, painful sensation, or a combination of both).
- Sensory dysfunction of many of the peripheral branches of the second and third divisions of the trigeminal nerve interferes with performance of orofacial activities of daily living, and may adversely affect the quality of life of afflicted patients.
- In selected patients, microsurgical repair of injured peripheral trigeminal nerve injuries can be helpful in regaining functional sensory recovery and in improving their quality of life.

INTRODUCTION

Patients who sustain avulsive injuries from motor vehicle trauma, missile injuries, interpersonal violence, or military combat, or those who undergo ablative tumor operations in the oral and maxillofacial region often suffer loss of continuity of 1 or more peripheral branches of the trigeminal (fifth cranial) nerve (TN5). The infraorbital nerve (IFN; branch of the maxillary division of TN5) and the inferior alveolar (IAN), mental (MN), and lingual (LN) nerves (branches of the mandibular division of TN5) are especially vulnerable, and are frequently accidentally injured during maxillofacial trauma or intentionally sacrificed during the excision of tumors. Injury to these important sensory branches of TN5 not only causes many patients bothersome or unacceptable loss of sensation (hypoesthesia, anesthesia) to the upper and lower lips, maxilla, mandible, tongue, and chin, but may also initiate onset of prolonged or permanent painful sensation (dysesthesia) or hypersensitivity (hyperesthesia) in these areas.

Altered, lost, or painful sensations (**Box 1**) interfere with normal sensory feedback to the central nervous system and seriously interfere with the afflicted patient's ability to perform normal everyday

Funding Sources: None for either author.
Conflict of Interest: None for either author.
[a] Maxillofacial Consultations Ltd, 1021 Holt's Ferry, Greensboro, GA 30642, USA; [b] Georgia Oral and Facial Surgery, 1880 West Oak Parkway, Suite 215, Marietta, GA, USA; [c] Department of Oral and Maxillofacial Surgery, School of Dental Medicine, Georgia Health Sciences University, 1430 John Wesley Gilbert Drive, Augusta, GA 30912, USA; [d] Division of Oral and Maxillofacial Surgery, Department of Surgery, School of Medicine, Emory University, 1365-B Clifton Road, Atlanta, GA 30322, USA; [e] Division of Oral and Maxillofacial Surgery, Department of Surgery, Northside Hospital, 1000 Johnson Ferry Road, Atlanta, GA 30342, USA
* Corresponding author. Georgia Oral and Facial Surgery, 1880 West Oak Parkway, Suite 215, Marietta, GA.
E-mail address: sbagher@hotmail.com

Oral Maxillofacial Surg Clin N Am 25 (2013) 287–302
http://dx.doi.org/10.1016/j.coms.2013.01.002
1042-3699/13/$ – see front matter © 2013 Elsevier Inc. All rights reserved.

<table>
<tr><td colspan="2">
Box 1
Sensory symptoms of peripheral trigeminal nerve injuries
</td></tr>
</table>

Box 1

Sensory symptoms of peripheral trigeminal nerve injuries

Numbness

Tingling

Itching

Crawling

Pain

Burning

Hypersensitivity

Shock-like sensations

Table 1

Medical Research Council Scale for grading sensory function of peripheral nerves as applied to the trigeminal nerve

Grade	Description
S0	No sensation
S1	Deep cutaneous pain in an autonomous zone
S2	Some superficial pain and touch sensation
S2+	Pain and touch sensation with hyperesthesia
S3	Pain and touch sensation without hyperesthesia; static 2pd >15 mm
S3+	Same as S3 with good stimulus localization and static 2pd 7–15 mm
S4	Normal sensation

Grades S3, S3+, and S4 are considered functional sensory recovery. See text for discussion.

Abbreviation: 2pd, 2-point discrimination.

Adapted from Birch R, Bonney G, Wynn Parry CB. Surgical disorders of the peripheral nerves. Philadelphia: Churchill Livingstone; 1998. p. 405–14.

oral and facial functions (**Box 2**). For many patients, such sensory dysfunction seriously detracts from their quality of life, despite having an otherwise successful operation to repair maxillofacial injuries or remove a tumor and reconstruct lost segments of the jaw, lip, face, or tongue.[1] Just as the reconstruction of the facial (seventh cranial, CN7) nerve is an integral part of the rehabilitation to restore functional facial animation of the patient following its resection along with a malignant tumor of the parotid gland, so is the reconstruction, when possible, of injured branches of TN5 to achieve functional sensory recovery[2] of the tongue or lips.

Functional sensory recovery (FSR) is based on the Medical Research Council Scale (MRCS) for grading sensory nerve function,[3] adapted to the oral and maxillofacial region.[4,5] FSR is defined as an MRCS score of 3.0 or greater (**Table 1**). Sensory function of the TN5 is scored using the results of standard neurosensory testing (**Fig. 1**)

Box 2

Common orofacial functions that are interfered with by lost or altered sensation from peripheral trigeminal nerve injuries

Chewing food

Swallowing

Shaving

Applying lipstick, make-up

Kissing

Drinking fluids

Speaking

Washing

Tooth brushing

Playing wind musical instruments

as proposed by Zuniga and Essick[6,7] and validated by clinical experience.[8,9] Further discussion of the evaluation of trigeminal nerve injuries is beyond the scope of this article, and the reader is referred to the aforementioned references.

INDICATIONS AND TIMING FOR TRIGEMINAL NERVE RECONSTRUCTION

The patient who is undergoing repair of maxillofacial trauma or ablative oncologic surgery will often have the injured or intentionally resected nerve directly exposed and visible (open injury). Because tumor cells often spread externally along nerve sheaths, and malignant tumors spread by intraneural invasion, nerves in the vicinity of locally aggressive tumors such as ameloblastoma or myxoma,[10] as well as those involved by malignant tumors,[11,12] are routinely sacrificed by most surgeons during ablative tumor operations. This point in time is ideal for repair of the nerve (immediate primary repair), if microsurgical expertise is available (either the primary surgeon responsible for the patient's care or a microsurgeon who is called in consultation). On the other hand, if conditions are unfavorable at this time, nerve reconstruction may be deferred (delayed primary repair, within 1 week, or early secondary repair, after appearance of visible granulation tissue in the wound), with a prognosis for sensory recovery as good as

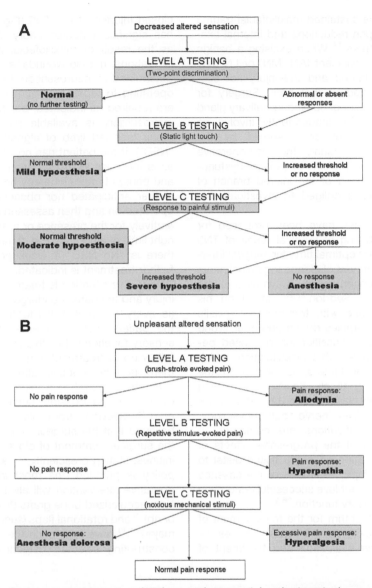

Fig. 1. Algorithms for neurosensory testing (NST) to evaluate peripheral trigeminal nerve injuries and their recovery: (*A*) Evaluation of the patient with decreased altered sensation. (*B*) Evaluation of the patient with unpleasant/painful altered sensation. Allodynia, hyperpathia, and hyperalgesia are examples of hyperesthesia referred to in the Medical Research Council Scale (MRCS). Results from NST are used to score nerve function according to the MRCS. See text for discussion.

for that following immediate primary repair.[13,14] Common indications to delay reconstruction of an open traumatic nerve injury include: (1) compromised physical status, which makes the patient a poor risk for additional, non–life-saving surgery; (2) a contaminated wound in which there is high risk of infection (especially true in combat injuries); and (3) the lack of ready availability of a surgeon with microsurgical training/skills.[15] In the patient who has a large soft-tissue and/or osseous maxillofacial surgical defect following

malignant tumor excision, immediate reconstruction with vascularized free flaps is highly successful and significantly improves the patient's quality of life. In patients who will have restoration of their defect including nerve repair with nonvascularized grafts, the reconstruction is much less likely to be successful whether that reconstruction is immediate or delayed, especially if adjunctive chemotherapy or radiation are required.[16]

A nerve injury may be unsuspected or unobserved (closed nerve injury), particularly when patients who have sustained maxillofacial trauma do not require open reductions and internal fixation of their fractures.[17] When excising a benign tumor or cyst, an adjacent IAN, MN, or LN may be unavoidably injured and the injury not suspected or visualized at that time. Surgery for benign submandibular or sublingual salivary gland disease may likewise inadvertently involve an adjacent LN and not be observed by the surgeon.[18,19] When during the postoperative period the patient complains of sensory dysfunction in the distribution of the injured branch of TN5, the surgeon is obliged to investigate the situation.

Although guidelines have been proposed for indications and timing of surgical repair of TN5 injuries,[20] the exact optimal time for surgical intervention in the treatment of closed trigeminal nerve injuries remains uncertain, as shown by a recent literature review.[21] Seddon,[22,23] based on his extensive experience with treatment of missile injuries to the extremities during and after World War II, proposed a classification of closed peripheral nerve injuries. This classification, which emphasizes clinical factors, is helpful to the clinician in making timely decisions regarding treatment. Another classification devised by Sunderland[24] emphasizes nerve pathophysiology, and these 2 classifications are compared in **Table 2**. Because of the progressive effects of Wallerian degeneration on nerve tissue distal to the site of nerve injury,[25] time is of the essence when attempting to achieve successful restoration of satisfactory sensory function.[26,27]

The authors' algorithm for the management of patients with maxillofacial trauma[17] serves as one guide for the evaluation and treatment of closed injuries of the TN5 (**Fig. 2**). If the patient has significant neurosensory dysfunction (NSD) as the result of maxillofacial injuries (fractures, lacerations, missile wounds, and so forth), this is determined by neurosensory testing (NST) before operating to repair the injuries. The injuries then are repaired as indicated, depending on whether microsurgery is available for immediate nerve repair (see left limb of algorithm, **Fig. 2**, under "NSD"). If the patient has no NSD preoperatively, as is the case in many patients with large cysts and benign tumors whereby nerve involvement is neither anticipated nor observed, the patient is operated on and then assessed with NST postoperatively for the presence or absence of NSD (see right limb of algorithm, **Fig. 2**, under "No NSD"). If there is "No NSD" 1 week postoperatively, no further treatment is indicated. However, if there is "NSD," this situation is treated as a closed nerve injury and the patient undergoes frequent periodic (ie, every 2–4 weeks) NST for the next 3 months. If the patient makes an acceptable recovery of sensory function within this time frame, no further follow-up or treatment is necessary. If, however, there is unacceptable altered sensation after 3 months, referral to a microsurgeon for further evaluation and possible nerve repair is considered.[28] Seddon, from his clinical experience, believed that the surgeon must be aggressive in the surgical treatment of closed peripheral nerve injuries, stating presciently, "if a purely expectant policy is pursued, the most favorable time for operative intervention will always be missed."[23] Nonvascularized bone grafts (from the ilium, tibia, or rib)[16] and rotational flaps (such as the pectoralis major)[29,30] have long been the workhorses in reconstructing selected defects of the mandible

Table 2
Comparison of Seddon's[22,23] and Sunderland's[24] classifications of peripheral nerve injuries as applied to the trigeminal nerve

Seddon	Neurapraxia	Axonotmesis	Neurotmesis
Sunderland	I	II, III, IV	V[a]
Nerve sheath	Intact	Intact	Interrupted
Axons	Intact	Some interrupted	All interrupted
Wallerian degeneration	None	Yes, some distal axons	Yes, all distal axons
Conduction failure	Transitory	Prolonged	Permanent
Potential for spontaneous recovery	Complete	Partial	Little or none
Time to spontaneous recovery	Within 4 wk	Begins at 5–12 wk; may take months	None, if not begun by 12 wk

Seddon's classification is most helpful to clinicians in making timely decisions regarding surgical intervention.
[a] Sunderland also has a class VI (complex) injury, which is a combination of classes I–V within the same injured nerve.

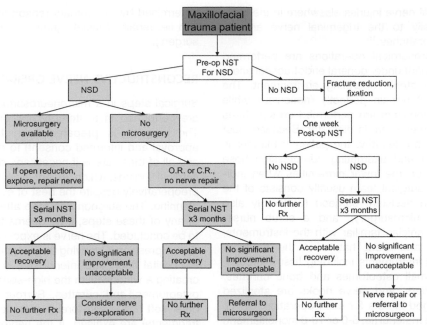

Fig. 2. Algorithm for the management of patients with maxillofacial trauma with injury of peripheral branches of the trigeminal nerve, which is adaptable to all closed nerve injuries. The white boxes indicate management of a closed nerve injury regardless of the cause. See text for discussion. C.R., closed reduction of fracture; NSD, neurosensory dysfunction, including hypoesthesia, anesthesia, and/or hyperesthesia; NST, neurosensory testing; O.R., open reduction of fracture; Rx, treatment. (*Adapted from* Bagheri SC, Meyer RA, Khan HA. Microsurgical repair of peripheral trigeminal nerve injuries from maxillofacial trauma. J Oral Maxillofac Surg 2009;67:1791–9; with permission.)

and other maxillofacial areas. In such cases, a separate donor site was necessary to obtain an autogenous nerve graft to reconstruct a nerve gap in a TN5 peripheral branch. This additional surgery was often eschewed until the work of Hausamen in the 1970s showed that restoration of sensation in the soft tissues associated with a reconstructed mandible after ablative tumor surgery was not only desirable but also highly successful.[31–33] Subsequently, Wessberg and colleagues[34] presented a case of reconstruction of a mandibular discontinuity defect caused by osteomyelitis in a comminuted fracture and repair of the IAN in a single operation, with good results. Noma and colleagues[35] reported a series of cases of resection of ameloblastoma with successful reconstruction of the mandible and the IAN during the same operation. This approach established, for the time being, the standard of treatment for reconstruction of the mandible and the IAN after traumatic or ablative surgical loss of continuity.

In recent years, however, the vascularized free flap has become the preferred method of reconstructing larger defects (>6 cm) of the mandible and all large soft-tissue defects unable to be restored by local rotational flaps.[16] Because free flaps often contain sensory nerves suitable as

grafts to reconstruct important branches of the TN5 resected along with a tumor, they provide an excellent opportunity to restore important sensation to the tongue, lip, or face during the same operation. For instance, a microvascularized osseomyocutaneous scapulolatissimus dorsi free flap containing the long thoracic nerve has been used to successfully reconstruct mandibular defects and restore the sensation of the IAN after resection of oral carcinomas.[36] A radial free forearm flap[37] containing either the medial antebrachial nerve[38] or the lateral forearm cutaneous nerve[39] provides a well-matched donor nerve to reconstruct the IAN or the LN after ablative cancer surgery. Many cancer reconstructive teams now include a microsurgeon, which enhances the opportunity for restoration of optimum osseous continuity, soft-tissue coverage, and nerve function.[40,41]

SURGICAL PRINCIPLES

Surgical treatment of peripheral nerve injuries has benefited from increased knowledge of neuropathophysiology and technical advances in equipment and surgical nuances over the past 30 years.[13,14,28,42,43] The principles of treatment of peripheral nerve injuries elsewhere in the body apply equally to the trigeminal nerve and its peripheral branches.[15]

Microneurosurgical operations are performed with the patient under general endotracheal anesthesia in a sterile operating environment. The patient must remain perfectly motionless while delicate maneuvers are performed on structures often less than 2 mm in diameter. Because most procedures are lengthy, the patient's bladder is catheterized and alternating compression hose are placed on the lower extremities when indicated. The surgical team usually consists of the surgeon, an assistant surgeon (preferably also trained in microsurgery), and a scrub nurse/ surgical technician familiar with the instruments, objectives, and work habits of the surgeon. Specialized instruments including tissue forceps, scissors, small osteotomes and bone curettes, needle holders, and nerve hooks are sterilized and packaged in sets for each operation. Small, nonreactive material (ie, 8-0 or 10-0 monofilament) is used for suturing nerves. In repair of the peripheral branches of the TN5, a polyfascicular nerve, sutures are generally placed only within the epineurium.[15,44] The operating microscope with foot-pedal controls and multiple ports for surgeon, assistant, and/or camera and surgical loupes (2.5–5.0×) are essential for adequate magnification and visualization of delicate nerve structure. The surgeon and assistant are often seated, and supportive rests for the wrists and forearms help to minimize tremorous hand movements during surgical manipulations. Good hemostasis is required to aid in visualization and to minimize later formation of scar tissue in the operative site surrounding the repaired nerve. Hemostasis is achieved by control of the patient's blood pressure by the anesthesiology team, elevation of the operative site (ie, the head), placement of bone wax to staunch oozing from medullary bone, injection of epinephrine-containing local anesthetic solution, and the judicious use of bipolar cautery for electrocoagulation of small vessels within or adjacent to the nerve.

Whereas the IFN is generally exposed via an incision within or inferior to the lower eyelid, and the LN and MN are exposed transorally, the IAN may be approached either transorally or through a submandibular skin incision. The decision regarding which incision to use is largely determined by the degree of access and visualization afforded by a particular approach and, in some instances, by the surgeon's personal preference and experience.[15] In the case of reconstructive procedures, which are the subject of this issue of the *Clinics*, the approach will usually be determined by the primary reason for the operation (ie, repair of facial injuries or ablative tumor surgery).

RECONSTRUCTIVE NERVE OPERATIONS

Surgical steps in a microneurosurgical operation are performed in a stereotypical order (**Fig. 3**). The surgeon is prepared (with the patient's approval and informed consent) to complete any and all of these steps if necessary, depending on surgical findings, which are not always predictable preoperatively despite the best of evaluation, and planning. The surgeon can stop after completion of any of these steps, if he deems the operation to be concluded. The nerve is exposed by external decompression. Overlying bone (eg, the mandible, the orbital floor, and inferior rim) is removed by creating a window with the high-speed drill, small osteotomes, and curettes. Surrounding scar or other soft tissue and foreign material (eg, missile fragments) are excised. If the nerve injury is not fresh, there may be lateral neuromas, which are removed. If the nerve appears externally to be anatomically intact, the interior of the nerve can be examined by opening the epineurium axially and examining the internal structure for scar tissue or discontinuity of individual fascicles. Scar tissue is removed and discontinuous fascicles are sutured (seldom) or simply placed passively into good alignment without suturing (internal neurolysis). If there is a discontinuity defect of the entire diameter of the nerve, the proximal and distal nerve stumps are prepared for suturing. Stump neuromas and scar tissue are excised and normal-appearing nerve tissue is exposed. The

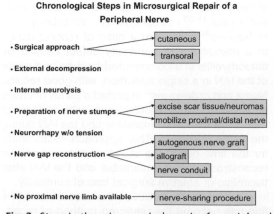

Chronological Steps in Microsurgical Repair of a Peripheral Nerve

- Surgical approach → cutaneous / transoral
- External decompression
- Internal neurolysis
- Preparation of nerve stumps → excise scar tissue/neuromas / mobilize proximal/distal nerve
- Neurorrhaphy w/o tension
- Nerve gap reconstruction → autogenous nerve graft / allograft / nerve conduit
- No proximal nerve limb available → nerve-sharing procedure

Fig. 3. Steps in the microsurgical repair of a peripheral nerve are completed in chronologic order, and the surgeon can conclude the operation at any step, if he deems the procedure to be completed. See text for discussion.

proximal and distal nerve limbs are mobilized by freeing them from adjacent connective tissue. In the case of nerves within bony canals (eg, the IAN within the inferior alveolar canal, the IFN within the inferior orbital canal), the amount of mobilization that can be achieved may be minimal.[28] Nerves residing in soft tissue (the LN, the mental nerve, the IFN after it exits the infraorbital foramen) may be able to be mobilized significantly. For example, the somewhat tortuous course of the LN in the floor of the mouth often allows, after its mobilization, for its proximal and distal nerve limbs to be brought together easily for a tension-free neurorrhaphy.[26] However, such is not usually the case in patients with large traumatic avulsive or ablative surgical LN nerve defects.

The sine qua non of successful direct repair of a nerve discontinuity defect (neurorrhaphy) is the lack of tension across the suture line.[45,46] Tension of greater than 25 g creates adverse conditions for regeneration of the nerve. Either the tension tends to pull the nerve stumps apart or additional sutures are required to overcome the tension to hold them together, which increases scar-tissue proliferation and obstruction to the path of regenerating axons attempting to progress from the proximal nerve stump across the area of approximation and into the distal stump.[47] Nerve stumps held together under tension may undergo attenuation of vascular elements creating an ischemic segment, which after necrosis becomes scar tissue, itself an impediment to nerve continuity and conductivity. In the case of avulsive injuries or ablative oncologic operations, lost nerve tissue seldom is able to be repaired by neurorrhaphy. The resulting nerve gap requires reconstruction.

The gold standard for reconstructing a peripheral nerve gap, when it is not possible to perform a neurorrhaphy and regardless of its etiology, has long been the autogenous nerve graft.[4] A nerve graft interposed between the proximal and distal nerve stumps eliminates tension across the repair, and distal nerve regeneration approximates that occurring across a tension-free neurorrhaphy.[48] In the oral and maxillofacial regions, the great auricular nerve (GAN) in the upper lateral neck for nerve gaps of less than 3 cm, and the sural nerve (SN) in the lower extremity for longer nerve gaps, have long been the most frequently harvested donors for peripheral nerve reconstruction (**Fig. 4**).[49] The superficial peroneal nerve in the lower extremity is a valuable donor nerve when a lengthy graft or multiple grafts are required.[50] When the lost soft tissue or bone included in a tumor resection or an avulsive injury are to be reconstructed with a vascularized free flap, nerves contained in such flaps, including the long thoracic nerve (in a scapulolatissimus dorsi flap for reconstruction of the mandible)[36] or the medial antebrachial[38] or lateral cutaneous nerve of the forearm (in a forearm flap for reconstruction of the tongue, palate or lip),[39] provide easily accessible material for simultaneous TN5 reconstruction during the same operation. If the diameter of the donor nerve is less than that of the recipient, 2 or more cable grafts can be placed side by side to match the recipient nerve diameter and maximize neurotization of the distal nerve limb (**Fig. 5**).

Critical to the success of interpositional nerve grafting is the availability of healthy proximal and distal nerve limbs. When the proximal nerve has been rendered inaccessible owing to infection, missile injury, tumor resection, or for other reasons, a nerve-sharing procedure can be used to reconstruct a sensory conduit from an intact distal nerve.[51,52] For example, a distal IAN or LN can be reconstructed by exposing the GAN in the ipsilateral neck and then bridging it to the distal nerve with an autogenous SN graft sutured to the GAN proximal stump, tunneled through the upper cervical and submandibular soft tissue, and sutured to the distal nerve stump (**Fig. 6**). Another clinical situation that has lent itself to successful nerve-sharing operations includes connecting a distal IAN nerve limb to the LN in its location adjacent to the medial surface of the molar region of the mandible after sacrifice of a segment of the IAN during excision of a large cyst or tumor.[53] Kaban and Upton[54] reported successful restoration of lower lip sensation following a nerve-sharing procedure between a normal right mental nerve and a left mental nerve distal stump whose ipsilateral IAN was atrophied proximally into the pterygomandibular space because of previous surgery and nerve injury, and thus unavailable for reconstruction. An autogenous sural nerve graft (ASNG) was used to connect the most posterior of the 3 branches of the right mental nerve to the main stump of the left mental nerve (**Fig. 7**). Nerve sharing between an IFN and the ipsilateral MN using an interpositional ASNG was used to restore sensation to the lower lip after the IAN had been avulsed in a traumatic injury,[55] and a cross-over ASNG can be placed between the injured right and intact left IFNs to restore sensation to the right upper lip (**Fig. 8**).[56]

Reconstruction of the nerve gap with a processed allograft shows promise in laboratory research.[57] A product consisting of a human decellularized allograft, which has been made to be nonimmunogenic and inert in the recipient's body but which provides a biological substrate for nerve regeneration (Avance; AxoGen Inc,

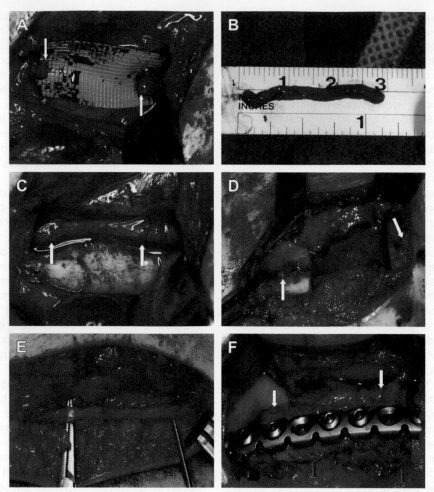

Fig. 4. Autogenous nerve grafting in reconstruction of nerve gaps of the inferior alveolar nerve (IAN): (*A*) IAN proximal and distal limbs (*arrows*) prepared for nerve grafting of a nerve gap. Note the presence of fascicles in nerve stumps; (*B*) Great auricular nerve (GAN) graft harvested for repair of a 2-cm gap. (*C*) IAN gap reconstructed with GAN graft; suture lines are marked by arrows. (*D*) Right mandibular defect after resection of tumor and sacrifice of IAN. IAN proximal and distal stumps are indicated by arrows. (*E*) Sural nerve (SN) graft obtained to replace 6-cm gap. (*F*) Mandible and IAN reconstructed with iliac crest bone graft (*black arrows*) and SN graft (*white arrows*), respectively.

Alachua, FL), is now available for clinical practice. Recently a successful case of IAN reconstruction with a decellularized nerve allograft was reported,[58] and early results with repair of small TN5 gaps (<3 cm) are favorable in the authors' practice. This product is currently used to repair longer nerve gaps in the extremities. Although at present this experience has not been reported for the reconstruction of large TN5 gaps and the ultimate maximal length of a nerve gap that can be restored with the processed allograft has yet to be determined, it will undoubtedly play a larger role in nerve reconstruction in the maxillofacial region in the future.

Guided nerve regeneration with an autogenous vein graft conduit has been used to reconstruct short gaps in small digital nerves in the hand.[59–62] This technique is successful only in short nerve gaps (<3 cm) when used in peripheral trigeminal nerve repairs.[63–65] An alloplastic nerve conduit (polyglycolic acid or polytetrafluoroethylene) has been used with limited success in TN5 injuries, but only in minimal nerve gaps.[66,67] Such distances are commonly exceeded when reconstructing traumatic avulsive or oncologic surgical defects with nerve gaps of the TN5, therefore guided nerve regeneration has limited applicability. For a thorough discussion of the management of the smaller nerve gap in the TN5 from all causes (which is beyond the scope of this article), the reader is referred to recent reviews in the literature.[28,55]

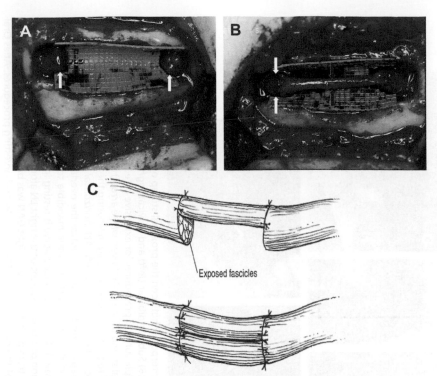

Fig. 5. Use of cable grafts when there is a discrepancy between the diameter of a donor nerve graft and its recipient nerve. (*A*) Right IAN gap requiring reconstruction; proximal and distal nerve ends (*arrows*) prepared to receive an autogenous nerve graft. (*B*) GAN graft (*black arrows*) has only one-half the diameter of proximal stump of IAN (*white arrows*), which will decrease the potential for neurotization of the distal IAN. (*C*) Parallel cable grafts can be placed to maximize the number of axons that cross the graft from the proximal nerve stump to the distal nerve stump. (*From* Meyer RA. Nerve harvesting procedures. Atlas Oral Maxillofac Surg Clin North Am 2001;9:77–91; with permission.)

POSTOPERATIVE CARE AND REHABILITATION

The operation to reconstruct the TN5 is only the first permissive step in the patient's recovery, giving such patients the opportunity to regain acceptable sensory input to the central nervous system and redevelop acceptable functional capacity when performing everyday orofacial activities. Aside from the usual medications for antibacterial prophylaxis and pain relief, attention to wound care (donor and recipient sites), assistance with ambulation (if an ilium or lower extremity was used for a graft or free-flap donor harvest), and provision of adequate nutrition, measures to allow the patient to achieve the maximum potential recovery of sensation and orofacial function are an integral and essential part of the rehabilitation of the patient who has undergone reconstruction of traumatic or ablative surgical defects.

After a successful peripheral nerve reconstruction, despite normal or near normal responses to NST, the patient may still continue to complain of subjective feelings of "numbness," and experience frustration over difficulty performing orofacial functions that are dependent on adequate sensory input from the lips or tongue.[68] Such symptoms are undoubtedly caused by new connections in the healed nerve, slower than normal conduction time in regenerating axons, and arrival of impulses in new or different areas of the central nervous system (CNS) than existed before TN5 injury and repair.[5] This situation is even more challenging for the patient who has undergone a nerve-sharing procedure,[49] as the proximal limb of the regenerating nerve relays sensory impulses back to a different area of the brain from the GAN (via the second, third, and fourth cervical nerves), rather than to the trigeminal ganglion from the proximal limb of the IAN, for example.

The CNS, even as it ages, has been found to retain its capacity for adaptation and learning, a concept termed neural plasticity.[69,70] Wynn Parry[71,72] first realized the potential of neural plasticity in devising a rehabilitation program ("sensory reeducation") for patients with sensory nerve injuries of the hand. This program, through a series

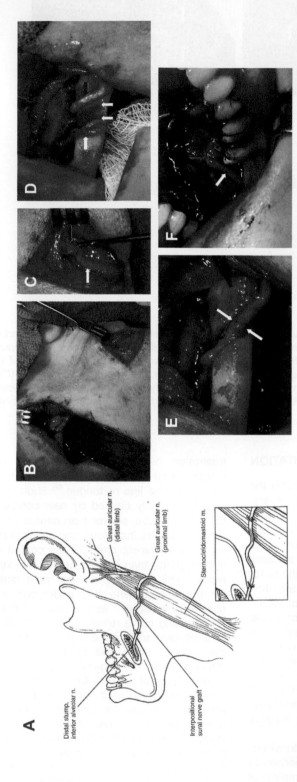

Fig. 6. The nerve-sharing procedure. (*A*) Schematic representation. An autogenous SN graft is interposed between the proximal stump of the GAN and the distal stump of the IAN when the proximal limb of the IAN is inaccessible or unsuitable for reconstruction. (*B*) Submandibular (*left*) and cervical (*right*) incisions for exposure of the IAN and the GAN in a patient whose left IAN proximal limb was not available secondary to multiple surgical procedures for extensive osteomyelitis of the left mandibular ramus and posterior body. (*C*) The SN graft (*upper, black arrow*) has been sutured to the proximal stump of the GAN (*lower, white arrow*) and brought from the left neck to the left mandible through a soft tissue tunnel beneath the platysma muscle. The length of SN required is determined by measuring the distance between the proximal GAN stump and the distal IAN stump and adding an additional 25% to the graft length. (*D*) The distal stump of the left IAN (*horizontal white arrow*) and the stump of the SN (*horizontal black arrow*) are draped over the inferior border of the left mandible in preparation for suturing. Notice the overlapping lengths of the 2 nerves, which facilitates suturing without tension. A groove (*vertical white arrows*) has been created in the lateral surface of the mandible to receive the sutured nerve. (*E*) The SN (*right of arrows*) has been sutured (*arrows*) to the distal stump of the left IAN (*left of arrows*). The reconstructed nerve is resting in a groove in the lateral surface of the mandible to protect it from external compression or trauma. (*F*) A patient who had resection of a large segment of the right LN along with tumor of right submandibular salivary gland. The right LN was reconstructed with a nerve-sharing procedure. SN graft from proximal stump of right GAN was brought (via a soft-tissue tunnel) into the right floor of the mouth (*white arrow*), and sutured (*black arrow*) to the distal stump of the right LN. (*From* Meyer RA. Nerve harvesting procedures. Atlas Oral Maxillofac Surg Clin North Am 2001;9:77–91; with permission.)

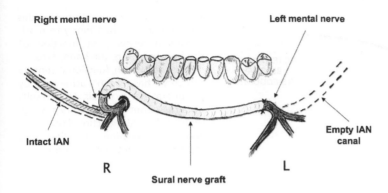

Fig. 7. A cross–mental nerve-sharing procedure. The left IAN is unavailable for repair, owing to prior injury and atrophy. The viable left mental nerve is bridged to the normal right IAN via an autogenous sural nerve graft to the most posterior branch of the intact right mental nerve, to restore sensation in the patient's left lower lip. (*Adapted from* Kaban LB, Upton J. Cross mental nerve graft for restoration of lip sensation after inferior alveolar nerve damage: report of case. J Oral Maxillofac Surg 1986;44: 649–51; with permission.)

of daily sensory exercises continued for a year or more following surgical repair, aims to retrain the CNS to normalize its interpretation of sensory impulses from the recovering peripheral nerve, and to realize as much as possible the potential for functional recovery in the affected body part.[3] The program has been shown to be highly successful (**Fig. 9**).[73] Sensory reeducation has been modified for the TN5, where it has proved to be of benefit to sensory function and the performance of orofacial activities once responses to pain and light touch have returned to the reconstructed nerve.[5,74] Sensory reeducation has thus become an integral part of the care and rehabilitation of the patient who has undergone surgical reconstruction of the TN5. For an in-depth discussion

of the theory and techniques for sensory reeducation in the orofacial region, the reader is referred to the references already cited in this section.

In addition to sensory rehabilitation, patients with ablative or traumatic defects may require the coordinated expertise of a physiatrist, physical therapist, speech pathologist or myofunctional therapist, clinical psychologist, psychiatrist, dentist and dental hygienist, and/or algologist, making the care of such patients a true team effort.

RESULTS

Analyzing, interpreting, and comparing the results of microsurgical repair of TN5 injuries from multiple studies have frequently been difficult

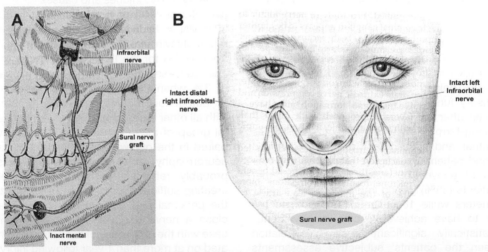

Fig. 8. Nerve sharing involving the infraorbital nerve (IFN). (*A*) An autogenous sural nerve graft (ASNG) is used to connect the left IFN nerve with the ipsilateral mental nerve to restore lower-lip sensation after an injury to the ipsilateral proximal inferior alveolar nerve has rendered it unavailable for repair. (*B*) An ASNG is used as a bridging conduit from the intact nasal branch of the left IFN to the distal limb of the right IFN to restore sensory input from the right upper lip. The ASNG is placed through a soft-tissue tunnel in the upper lip. ([*A*] *From* Wolford LM, Rodrigues DB. Autogenous grafts/allografts/conduits for bridging peripheral trigeminal nerve gaps. Atlas Oral Maxillofac Surg Clin North Am 2011;19:91–107; with permission. [*B*] *From* Epker BN, Gregg JM. Surgical management of maxillary nerve injuries. Oral Maxillofac Surg Clin N Am 1992;4:439–45; with permission.)

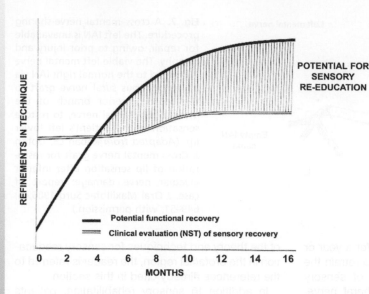

POTENTIAL FOR
SENSORY
RE-EDUCATION

Fig. 9. Sensory reeducation provides the patient the opportunity to reach maximum recovery of function of the body part (eg, the hand, face, or mouth) for which functional sensory recovery has been achieved by peripheral nerve repair. NST, results obtained from neurosensory testing. (*From* Dellon AL. Functional sensation and its reeducation. Clin Plast Surg 1984;11:95–9; with permission.)

Potential functional recovery

Clinical evaluation (NST) of sensory recovery

tasks in the past, because of a lack of standardized methods of evaluating neurosensory function and a uniform grading system for surgical outcomes. With the development, application, and acceptance of a clinically proven method of NST[6–9] and modification and use of the MRCS,[4,5] an established system for grading surgical outcomes originally developed for the extremities,[3] this effort will become less problematic going forward.

In the last 10 years studies conducted by experienced clinicians have established that microsurgical repair of trigeminal nerve injuries can result in improved sensory function for a large majority of selected patients. Pogrel[75] reviewed his results, based on NST, from microsurgical repair of 51 TN5 injuries (IAN = 17, LN = 34), and reported that 28 (54.9%) gained "some" or "good" improvement in sensory function. Nerve repair at longer than 10 weeks after injury was less likely to be successful. A long-term follow-up of repair of 20 LN injuries by Rutner and colleagues[76] using standardized NST and patients' subjective evaluations of their degree of recovery of sensory function found that 15 patients (85%) gained improvement in all NST parameters while 18 patients (90%) judged the repair to have achieved "some improvement," a statistically significant positive correlation between the patients' subjective assessments and NST. Microsurgical repair of 28 IAN injuries evaluated by NST produced "slight" (n = 12, 42.9%) or "significant" (n = 14, 50%) improvement, whereas only 2 repairs resulted in "no improvement" (7.1%).[77]

Subsequent studies have used NST for preoperative and postoperative assessment of sensory function and have graded the outcome of surgical intervention of TN5 according to the MRCS described earlier. In a review of 60 surgically repaired TN5 injuries (IAN = 4, LN = 56), 45 (75%) were found to have achieved FSR (ie, an MRCS score of ≥3.0 or greater) 1 year postoperatively.[2] The time from nerve injury to surgery did not statistically correlate with outcome, although all patients were operated on at less than 1 year after injury. Bagheri and colleagues[17] have reported their extensive experience with microsurgical repair of a variety of TN5 injuries and causes.[26,27,78] Among the total of 429 nerve repairs (IAN = 186; LN = 222; MN = 12; IFN = 7; LBN = 2), the success rate (achieving FSR, MRSC grade of ≥3.0) varied from 81.7% for the IAN[27] to 90.5% for the LN.[26] The success rate for IAN repair increased to 87.3% when the nerve was reconstructed with an autogenous nerve graft (ANG) in comparison with all other types of repair. In the most successful group of nerve repairs, the LN nerve was repaired in the overwhelming majority of cases by neurorrhaphy rather than an ANG.[26] This result probably reflects the much greater ease of creating sufficient mobilization of the LN to bring the proximal and distal nerve limbs together to close a nerve gap without tension than is the case with the IAN. Many of the patients were operated on at more than 1 year following injury, allowing for an analysis of the effect of time on the outcome of nerve repair. At more than 9 months following LN repair[26] or 12 months after IAN repair,[27] there was a statistically significant decrease in successful outcome. Patient age was also a significant factor in outcome, with significant drop-off in success rate for IAN repair after

51 years of age,[27] and a similar decline in favorable outcome for LN repair after age 45 years.[26]

FUTURE PERSPECTIVES

Susarla and colleagues[79] found a strong correlation between improvement in NST after microsurgical repair of the IAN or LN and patient satisfaction with the surgical outcome. Those patients who experienced greater improvement in NST also reported a lower frequency of dysfunction of related orofacial activities. In a long-term follow-up of a series of patients seen for evaluation and treatment of TN5 injuries, some patients who received surgical treatment continued to be dissatisfied with their condition, whereas others who either declined or were offered no treatment were able to accommodate to previously distressing sensory symptoms.[80] Going forward in the quest for improvement in the management of TN5 injuries, it is hoped that clinicians and researchers will use standard methods of evaluation of neurosensory function and of grading of surgical outcomes, and that patients' subjective evaluation of their own condition will be given appropriate attention (patient-oriented research) when making decisions regarding treatment.[81]

Within the past century, armed conflicts and the care of the wounded by military surgical personnel have produced treatment methods that have subsequently greatly influenced civilian medical and surgical practice. A recent report summarizing US military personnel casualties in the combat campaigns in Iraq and Afghanistan showed that improved modern body armor had significantly reduced mortality attributable to chest and abdominal wounds in comparison with previous battlefield experience.[82] However, 26% of US service members sustained injuries to the craniomaxillofacial region, an impressive increase over their incidence previously in World War II, Korea, and Vietnam.[83] As a result of improved immediate resuscitation on or near the battlefield, more casualties of all types, including those with seriously injured extremities, are surviving and requiring reconstructive procedures to rebuild lost sections of the face, mouth, and jaws, and to replace lost limbs. These challenges have been met with an extensive research effort by the US Armed Forces Institute of Regenerative Medicine to develop more successful methods of reconstructing lost segments of the jaws and face, replacing lost extremities with functional prosthetics, and creating alloplastic conduits for the regeneration of lost nerve tissue to the extremities.[84] This situation has also stimulated a response in the civilian sector, where an ongoing bioengineering project is hoping to develop a satisfactory conduit for improved regeneration or reconstruction of TN5 injuries.[85] To fully rehabilitate a patient with extensive osseous and soft-tissue loss from traumatic injury or ablative surgery, restoration of a satisfactory level of sensory function of areas critical to orofacial activities (eating, drinking, swallowing, speaking, and so forth) and an acceptable quality of life are important components of enlightened treatment for civilians and military personnel alike. It is hoped that, as the result of the dedication of clinicians and researchers, this ideal will be realized in the not too distant future.

SUMMARY

Patients who sustain large traumatic avulsive injuries or defects from ablative tumor surgery in the oral and maxillofacial region often have lost sensory function caused by injury or avulsion of 1 or more peripheral branches of the TN5. Such injuries result in altered and/or painful sensation in the tissues previously supplied by these important sensory nerves. Normal orofacial functions such as eating, drinking, oral hygiene, swallowing, and speaking are dependent on adequate sensory input. Loss of this input creates significant orofacial dysfunction and seriously jeopardizes the quality of life of afflicted patients.

Whenever possible, repair or reconstruction of injured branches of the TN5 should be planned and performed in conjunction with reconstruction of other lost osseous or soft tissues in the oral and maxillofacial region. After surgery, an important aspect of global rehabilitation of such patients is a well-planned program of daily sensory reeducation exercises to assist in achieving maximum potential sensory recovery and associated orofacial function and, thus, an improved quality of life.

REFERENCES

1. Fernandes R, Pirgousis P. Contemporary methods in tongue reconstruction. In: Bagheri SC, Bell RB, Khan HA, editors. Current therapy in oral and maxillofacial surgery. St Louis (MO): Elsevier/Saunders; 2012. p. 508–15.

2. Susarla SM, Kaban LB, Donoff RB, et al. Functional sensory recovery after trigeminal nerve repair. J Oral Maxillofac Surg 2007;65:60–5.

3. Birch R, Bonney G, Wynn Parry CB. Surgical disorders of the peripheral nerves. Edinburgh (United Kingdom): Churchill Livingstone; 1998. p. 405–14.

4. Dodson TB, Kaban LB. Recommendations for management of trigeminal nerve defects based on a critical appraisal of the literature. J Oral Maxillofac Surg 1997;55:1380–6.

5. Meyer RA, Rath EM. Sensory rehabilitation after trigeminal nerve injury or nerve repair. Oral Maxillofac Surg Clin N Am 2001;13:365–76.

6. Zuniga JR, Essick GK. A contemporary approach to the clinical evaluation of trigeminal nerve injuries. Oral Maxillofac Surg Clin N Am 1992;4:353–68.

7. Essick GK. Comprehensive clinical evaluation of perioral sensory function. Oral Maxillofac Surg Clin N Am 1992;4:504–26.

8. Zuniga JR, Meyer RA, Gregg JM, et al. The accuracy of clinical neurosensory testing for nerve injury diagnosis. J Oral Maxillofac Surg 1998;56:2–8.

9. Meyer RA, Bagheri SC. Clinical evaluation of nerve injuries. In: Miloro M, editor. Trigeminal nerve injuries. Heidelberg (Germany):Springer; in press.

10. Williams TP. Aggressive odontogenic cysts and tumors. Oral Maxillofac Surg Clin N Am 1997;3: 329–38.

11. Lydiatt DD, Lydiatt WM. Advances in the surgical management of carcinoma of the oral cavity. Oral Maxillofac Surg Clin N Am 1997;9:375–83.

12. Brown J. Mechanism of cancer invasion of the mandible. Curr Opin Otolaryngol Head Neck Surg 2003;11:96.

13. Jabaley ME. Current concepts of nerve repair. Clin Plast Surg 1981;8:33–44.

14. Mackinnon SE. Surgical management of the peripheral nerve gap. Clin Plast Surg 1989;16:587–603.

15. Meyer RA. Applications of microneurosurgery to the repair of trigeminal nerve injuries. Oral Maxillofac Surg Clin N Am 1992;4:405–16.

16. Potter JK. Mandibular reconstruction. In: Bagheri SC, Bell RB, Khan HA, editors. Current therapy in oral and maxillofacial surgery. St Louis (MO): Elsevier/Saunders; 2012. p. 483–96.

17. Bagheri SC, Meyer RA, Khan HA, et al. Microsurgical repair of peripheral trigeminal nerve injuries from maxillofacial trauma. J Oral Maxillofac Surg 2009;67:1791–9.

18. Catone GA, Merrill RG, Henny FA. Sublingual gland mucus-escape phenomenon—treatment by excision of sublingual gland. J Oral Surg 1969;27:774.

19. Chidzonga MM, Mahomva L. Ranula: experience with 83 cases in Zimbabwe. J Oral Maxillofac Surg 2007;65:79–82.

20. Meyer RA, Ruggiero SL. Guidelines for diagnosis and treatment of peripheral trigeminal nerve injuries. Oral Maxillofac Surg Clin N Am 2001;13: 365–76.

21. Ziccardi V, Steinberg M. Timing of trigeminal nerve microsurgery: a review of the literature. J Oral Maxillofac Surg 2007;65:1341–5.

22. Seddon HJ. Three types of nerve injury. Brain 1943; 66:237–88.

23. Seddon HJ. Nerve lesions complicating certain closed bone injuries. J Am Med Assoc 1947;135: 691–3.

24. Sunderland S. A classification of peripheral nerve injuries producing loss of function. Brain 1951;74: 491–516.

25. Waller AV. Experiments on the glossopharyngeal and hypoglossal nerves of the frog and observations produced thereby in the structure of their primitive fibres. Phil Trans Roy Soc London 1850; 140:423.

26. Bagheri SC, Meyer RA, Khan HA, et al. Retrospective review of microsurgical repair of 222 lingual nerve injuries. J Oral Maxillofac Surg 2010;68: 715–23.

27. Bagheri SC, Meyer RA, Cho SH, et al. Microsurgical repair of the inferior alveolar nerve: success rate and factors that adversely affect outcome. J Oral Maxillofac Surg 2012;70:1978–90.

28. Bagheri SC, Meyer RA. Management of trigeminal nerve injuries. In: Bagheri SC, Bell RB, Khan HA, editors. Current therapy in oral and maxillofacial surgery. St Louis (MO): Elsevier/Saunders; 2012. p. 224–37.

29. Ariyan S. The pectoralis major myocutaneous flap. A versatile flap for reconstruction in the head and neck. Plast Reconstr Surg 1979;63:73–81.

30. Baur DA, Horan MP, Rodriguez JC. The pectoralis major myocutaneous flap. In: Bagheri SC, Bell RB, Khan HA, editors. Current therapy in oral and maxillofacial surgery. St Louis (MO): Elsevier/Saunders; 2012. p. 566–72.

31. Hausamen JE, Samii M, Schmidseder R. Repair of the mandibular nerve by means of autologous nerve grafting after resection of the lower jaw. J Maxillofac Surg 1973;1:174–8.

32. Hausamen JE, Samii M, Schmidseder R. Restoring sensation to the cut inferior alveolar nerve by direct anastomosis or by free autologous nerve grafting. Plast Reconstr Surg 1974;54:83–7.

33. Hausamen JE, Samii M, Schmidseder R. Indication and technique for the reconstruction of nerve defects in the head and neck. J Maxillofac Surg 1974;2:159–67.

34. Wessberg GA, Wolford LM, Epker BN. Simultaneous inferior alveolar nerve graft and osseous reconstruction of the mandible. J Oral Maxillofac Surg 1982;40: 384–90.

35. Noma H, Kakizawa T, Yamane G, et al. Repair of the mandibular nerve by autogenous nerve grafting after partial resection of the mandible. J Oral Maxillofac Surg 1986;44:31–6.

36. Schultes G, Gaggl A, Karcher H. Vascularized transplantation of the long thoracic nerve for sensory reinnervation of the lower lip. Br J Oral Maxillofac Surg 2000;38:138–41.

37. Woo BM, Kim DD. Radial forearm free flap. In: Bagheri SC, Bell RB, Khan HA, editors. Current therapy in oral and maxillofacial surgery. St Louis (MO): Elsevier/Saunders; 2012. p. 572–9.

38. McCormick SU, Buchbinder D, McCormick SA, et al. Microanatomic analysis of the medial antebrachial nerve as potential donor nerve in maxillofacial grafting. J Oral Maxillofac Surg 1994;52:1022–5.

39. Shibahara T, Noma H, Takasaki Y, et al. Repair of the inferior alveolar nerve with a forearm cutaneous nerve graft after ablative surgery of the mandible. J Oral Maxillofac Surg 2000;58:714–7.

40. Hoffman GR, Islam S, Eisenberg RL. Microvascular reconstruction of the mouth, jaws and face: experience of an Australian oral and maxillofacial surgery unit. J Oral Maxillofac Surg 2012;70:e371–7.

41. Salama AR, McClure SA, Ord RA, et al. Free-flap failures and complications in an American oral and maxillofacial surgery unit. Int J Oral Maxillofac Surg 2009;38:1048–53.

42. Dellon AL. Management of peripheral nerve injuries: basic principles of microneurosurgical repair. Oral Maxillofac Surg Clin N Am 1992;4:393–403.

43. Zuniga JR, Zenn MR. Principles of microsurgery. Oral Maxillofacial Clin N Am 2001;13:331–42.

44. Ziccardi VB. Microsurgical techniques for repair of the inferior alveolar and lingual nerves. Atlas Oral Maxillofac Surg Clin North Am 2011;19:79–90.

45. Terzis J, Faibisoff B, Williams H. The nerve gap: suture under tension vs. graft. Plast Reconstr Surg 1975;56:166–70.

46. Miyamoto Y. Experimental study of results of nerve suture under tension versus nerve grafting. Plast Reconstr Surg 1979;64:54–8.

47. Millesi H. Interfascicular grafts for repair of peripheral nerves of the upper extremity. Orthop Clin North Am 1977;8:405–10.

48. Mackinnon SE, Dellon AL. Surgery of the peripheral nerve. New York: Thieme; 1988. p. 91.

49. Meyer RA. Nerve harvesting procedures. Atlas Oral Maxillofac Surg Clin North Am 2001;9:77–91.

50. Buntic RF, Buncke HJ, Kind GM, et al. The harvest and clinical application of the superficial peroneal sensory nerve for grafting motor and sensory nerve defects. Plast Reconstr Surg 2001;109:145–51.

51. Hall EJ, Buncke HJ. Microsurgical techniques to reconstruct irreparable nerve loss. Orthop Clin North Am 1981;12:381.

52. LaBanc JP, Epker BN. Trigeminal nerve microreconstructive surgery using the great auricular nerve transfer technique. Oral Maxillofacial Surg Clin N Am 1992;4:459–63.

53. Haschemi A. Partial anastomosis between the lingual and mandibular nerves for restoration of sensibility of the mental nerve area after injury to the mandibular nerve. J Maxillofac Surg 1981;9: 225–7.

54. Kaban LB, Upton J. Cross mental nerve graft for restoration of lip sensation after inferior alveolar nerve damage: report of case. J Oral Maxillofac Surg 1986;44:649–51.

55. Wolford LM, Rodrigues DB. Autogenous grafts/allografts/conduits for bridging peripheral trigeminal nerve gaps. Atlas Oral Maxillofac Surg Clin North Am 2011;19:91–107.

56. Epker BN, Gregg JM. Surgical management of maxillary nerve injuries. Oral Maxillofac Surg Clin N Am 1992;4:439–45.

57. Whitlock EL, Tuffaha SH, Luciano JP, et al. Processed allografts and type 1 collagen conduits for repair of peripheral nerve gaps. Muscle Nerve 2009;39:787–99.

58. Shanti RM, Viccardi VB. Use of decellularized nerve allograft for inferior alveolar nerve reconstruction. J Oral Maxillofac Surg 2011;69:550–3.

59. Walton RL, Brown RE, Matory WE Jr, et al. Autogenous vein graft repair of digital nerve defects in the finger: a retrospective clinical study. Plast Reconstr Surg 1989;84:944–9.

60. Chiu DT, Strauch B. A prospective clinical evaluation of autogenous vein grafts used as a nerve conduit for distal sensory nerve defects of 3 cm or less. Plast Reconstr Surg 1990;86:928–34.

61. Tang JB, Gu YQ, Song YS. Repair of digital nerve defect with autogenous vein graft during flexor tendon surgery in zone 2. J Hand Surg Br 1993; 18:449–53.

62. Tang JB, Shi D, Zhou H. Vein conduits for repair of nerves with a prolonged gap or in unfavorable conditions: an analysis of three failed cases. Microsurgery 1995;16:133–7.

63. Miloro M. Inferior alveolar nerve regeneration through an autogenous vein graft. J Oral Maxillofac Surg 1996;54(Suppl 3):65–6.

64. Pogrel MA, Maghen A. The use of autogenous vein grafts for inferior alveolar and lingual nerve reconstruction. J Oral Maxillofac Surg 2001;59:985–8.

65. Miloro M. The use of autogenous vein grafts for inferior alveolar and lingual nerve reconstruction: discussion. J Oral Maxillofac Surg 2001;59:988–93.

66. Crawley WA, Dellon AL. Inferior alveolar nerve reconstruction with a polyglycolic acid bioabsorbable nerve conduit. Plast Reconstr Surg 1992;90:300–2.

67. Pogrel MA, McDonald AR, Kaban LB. Gore-Tex tubing as a conduit for inferior alveolar and lingual nerve repair: a preliminary report. J Oral Maxillofac Surg 1998;56:319–21.

68. Zuniga JR. Perceived expectation, outcome, and satisfaction of microsurgical nerve repair. J Oral Maxillofac Surg 1991;49(Suppl 1):77–8.

69. Cotman CW, Anderson KJ. Neural plasticity and regeneration. In: Siegal W, editor. Basic neurochemistry. New York: Raven; 1989. p. 507–22.

70. Bach-Y-Rita P. Brain plasticity as a basis for recovery of function in humans. Neuropsychologia 1990;28: 457.

71. Wynn Parry CB. Rehabilitation of the hand. London: Butterworth; 1966.

72. Wynn Parry CB, Salter RM. Sensory re-education after median nerve lesions. Br J Hand Surg 1976; 8:250–7.

73. Dellon AL. Functional sensation and its reeducation. Clin Plast Surg 1984;11:95–9.

74. Phillips C, Blakely G, Essick GK. Sensory retraining: a cognitive behavioral therapy for altered sensation. Atlas Oral Maxillofac Surg Clin North Am 2011;19: 109–18.

75. Pogrel MA. The results of microneurosurgery of the inferior alveolar and lingual nerve. J Oral Maxillofac 2002;60:485–9.

76. Rutner TW, Ziccardi VB, Janal MN. Long-term outcome assessment for lingual nerve microsurgery. J Oral Maxillofac Surg 2005;63:1145–9.

77. Strauss ER, Ziccardi VB, Janal MN. Outcome assessment of inferior alveolar nerve microsurgery: a retrospective review. J Oral Maxillofac 2006;64:1767–79.

78. Bagheri SC, Meyer RA, Khan HA, et al. Microsurgical repair of the peripheral trigeminal nerve after mandibular sagittal split osteotomy. J Oral Maxillofac Surg 2010;68:2770–82.

79. Susarla SM, Lam NP, Donoff RB, et al. A comparison of patient satisfaction and objective assessment of neurosensory function after trigeminal nerve repair. J Oral Maxillofac Surg 2005;63:1138–44.

80. Pogrel MA, Jergensen R, Burgon E, et al. Long-term outcome of trigeminal nerve injuries related to dental treatment. J Oral Maxillofac Surg 2011;69:2284–8.

81. Meyer RA, Bagheri SC. Long-term outcome of trigeminal nerve injuries related to dental treatment [letter]. J Oral Maxillofac Surg 2011;69:2946.

82. Lew TA, Walker JA, Wenke JC, et al. Characterization of craniomaxillofacial battle injuries sustained by United States service members in the current conflict of Iraq and Afghanistan. J Oral Maxillofac Surg 2010;68:3–7.

83. Hale RG. Craniomaxillofacial battle injuries: the limitations of conventional treatment, a call for regenerative medicine technologies and face regeneration: concept to reality. Georgia Soc Oral Maxillofac Surg. Greensboro, August 21, 2011.

84. Vandre R. Annual report: our science for their healing. Armed Forces Inst Regen Med 2009.

85. Steed MB, Mukhatyar V, Valmikinathan C, et al. Advances in bioengineered conduits for peripheral nerve regeneration. Atlas Oral Maxillofac Surg Clin North Am 2011;19:119–30.

Static and Dynamic Repairs of Facial Nerve Injuries

Hilliary White, MD[a,b], Eben Rosenthal, MD[c,*]

KEYWORDS

- Static repair • Dynamic repair • Facial nerve paralysis

KEY POINTS

- Understanding and use of the House-Brackmann scale to communicate the degree of facial nerve weakness is important in documentation and communication to monitor for changes in function.
- Patients presenting with facial nerve weakness of gradual onset (weeks or months) should be considered to have a tumor until proved otherwise.
- Management of functional issues, especially eye closure, is critical and should be addressed aggressively; cosmetic concerns should be addressed secondarily.
- Primary facial nerve grafting at the time of injury or resection wherever possible provides the best long-term outcome.

INTRODUCTION

Facial expression is critical for daily communication. As a result, facial nerve dysfunction can be a catastrophic condition by imposition of numerous negative effects on the cosmetic, functional, social, psychological, and economic aspects of a person's life. The facial nerve is the most commonly paralyzed nerve in the human body. Facial paralysis can inhibit and mar facial expression, communication, symmetric smile, eye protection, and oral competence.[1]

A thorough evaluation includes a complete history and physical examination and directs the surgeon to the appropriate treatment modality. The surgeon must decide on the most appropriate method of reconstruction based on the findings of a detailed medical assessment of the patient, a thorough evaluation of the disease process, and sound judgment. History should include a determination of the location, extent, and degree of paralysis; cause of the nerve injury; duration of paralysis; and time delay between injury and presentation. Patient history is critical to differentiate paralysis likely to recover spontaneously, such as Bell palsy or a temporary iatrogenic injury, from paralysis that is related to permanent injury or undetected malignancy. The cause of the paralysis determines the best course of management. However, treatment must be individualized based on life expectancy, age, patient preferences, and cosmetic or functional deficits.

FACIAL NERVE ANATOMY

The nerve is divided into 3 main segments: intracranial, intratemporal, and extratemporal. The intracranial segment originates in the pons and is a 23-mm to 24-mm segment from the cerebellopontine angle to the internal auditory canal. The nerve then courses through the temporal bone, where it is divided into multiple named segments: the meatal portion (8–10 mm), the labyrinthine portion (3–5 mm), the tympanic/horizontal segment (8–11 mm), and the mastoid/vertical segment (10–14 mm). The extratemporal segment exits the skull base at the stylomastoid foramen and travels within the parotid gland, then

[a] Head & Neck Surgery Center of Florida, Florida Hospital Celebration Health, Suite 305, 410 Celebration Place, FL 34747, USA; [b] Otolaryngology Head and Neck Surgery, University of Central Florida College of Medicine, 6850 Lake Nona Boulevard, Orlando, FL 32827; [c] University of Alabama at Birmingham, 563 Boshell Building, 1808 7th Avenue South, Birmingham, AL 35294, USA
* Corresponding author.
E-mail address: erosenthal@uabmc.edu

Oral Maxillofacial Surg Clin N Am 25 (2013) 303–312
http://dx.doi.org/10.1016/j.coms.2013.02.002
1042-3699/13/$ – see front matter © 2013 Elsevier Inc. All rights reserved.

subsequently divides at the pes anserinus into the upper and lower divisions, which then divide further into the 5 branches of the facial nerve: frontal, zygomatic, buccal, marginal mandibular, and cervical.[2]

ASSESSMENT OF INJURY

After traumatic injury, it is critical to determine if the nerve has been transected. This assessment can often be made by a good physical examination (**Figs. 1** and **2**). Even heavily sedated and uncooperative patients grimace in response to stimuli and this is often sufficient to assess nerve continuity. The suspected location of the nerve transection also determines the need for intervention. Distally located injuries in the end-organ musculature are not so amenable to primary repair compared with more proximal injuries.[3,4] The lateral canthus is used as an anatomic landmark and any transection medial to this landmark is generally not amenable to repair. In the early stage of injury, nerve function is either absent or present, but it is critical to perform assessments over time to determine any warranted secondary interventions. A standard reporting system that is simple, but clinically meaningful, is critical to reporting and following facial nerve function. The most widely accepted nerve classification system is the House-Brackmann scale. This scale assesses the degree of voluntary movement present to document the grade of facial paralysis. The House-Brackmann scoring system was established by the American Academy of Otolaryngology-Head and Neck Surgery as the

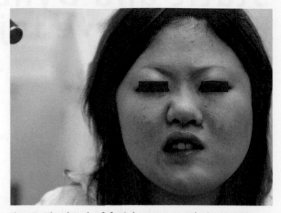

Fig. 2. The level of facial nerve paralysis was House-Brackmann grade V. (*From* Tanigawa T, Tanaka H, Sato T, et al. Craniometaphyseal dysplasia unnoticed until 19 years of age: First diagnosed from facial nerve paralysis. Auris Nasus Larynx 2011;38(3):408.)

standard means of reporting facial nerve function and recovery after facial nerve injury (**Table 1**).

ELECTRODIAGNOSTIC TESTING

Electrodiagnostic testing is a method of evaluating the degree of injury to the facial nerve and the integrity of the facial musculature. This test can add valuable information about the nature of the injury, especially in those circumstances in which the extent of injury is unclear (iatrogenic) or the patient is a poor historian. This information can be used to determine if the nerve injury will benefit from surgical intervention or may be best managed conservatively. A variety of electrical tests are

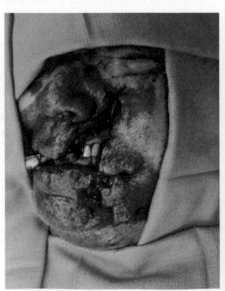
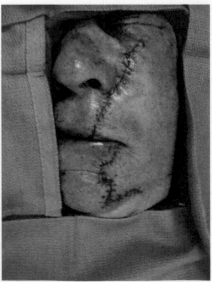

Fig. 1. Traumatic injury to left face with injury to the facial nerve located medial to the left lateral canthus.

Table 1
House-Brackmann scoring system

Grade	Description	Characteristics
I	Normal	Normal facial function
II	Mild dysfunction	Gross: slight weakness on close inspection, normal symmetry and tone at rest, may have slight synkinesis Motion: forehead: moderate to good function; eye: complete closure with minimal effort; mouth: slight asymmetry
III	Moderate dysfunction	Gross: obvious difference between sides, noticeable synkinesis contracture, or hemifacial spasm, normal symmetry and tone at rest Motion: forehead: slight to moderate movement; eye: complete closure with effort; mouth: slightly weak with maximal effort
IV	Moderately severe dysfunction	Gross: obvious weakness or disfiguring asymmetry; normal symmetry and tone at rest Motion: forehead: none; eye: incomplete closure; mouth: asymmetric with maximum effort
V	Severe dysfunction	Gross: only barely perceptible motion; asymmetry at rest Motion: forehead: none; eye: incomplete closure; mouth: slight movement
VI	Total paralysis	No movement

From House JW, Brackmann DE. Facial nerve grading system. Otolaryngol Head Neck Surg 1985;93:146–7.

available, but the most commonly used tests are the maximum stimulation test, the nerve excitability test, electroneuronography (ENOG), and electromyography (EMG). These tests are most commonly used when there is uncertainty about the status of the nerve or additional documentation of the nerve status is required. Those tests most often used include the ENOG and EMG.[5]

ENOG evaluates the integrity of the nerve and muscle together as a unit. A supramaximal electrical stimulation of the facial nerve at the level of the stylomastoid foramen is used to produce a compound muscle action potential. If intact axons are present in the muscles of facial expression, where the surface electrodes are placed (typically the nasolabial muscles), then an action potential is generated and recorded. The results are expressed as a percentage of the amplitude of the action potentials on the abnormal side compared with the normal side. The timing for performing this test should allow for complete Wallerian degeneration, which normally is complete around 3 days after the insult. Monitoring the change in action potential over time may be most critical because it provides information on the progressive loss or gain of function.[5]

EMG of the facial musculature is a useful diagnostic study after 3 weeks of facial paralysis. It can show the presence or absence of viable facial muscle tissue, as well as the gross functional integrity between nerve and muscle. This test is performed by inserting needle electrodes into the orbicularis oculi and orbicularis oris muscles while monitoring voluntary contractions of these muscles. Fibrillation potentials correlate with a poor prognosis, whereas polyphasic reinnervation potentials correlate with potential recovery of facial nerve function.[1]

Once sufficient diagnostic and clinical information has been obtained to determine that surgical intervention is needed, a discussion with the patient is warranted to determine the nature of the intervention.

GOALS OF REANIMATION

When discussing surgical options for facial reanimation, existing functional and cosmetic deficits should be discussed in relation to their effects on overall quality of life. Potential surgical and anesthetic risks related to the procedure(s) must also be taken into consideration. Establishing patient expectations and goals for functional and cosmetic recovery of reconstructive surgery may be most critical in surgical planning. One of the priorities in planning is not only to identify functional deficits, such as incomplete eye closure, drooling, speech difficulties, and nasal airway obstruction, but also to determine which of these most significantly affects their quality of life. Once the functional deficits are managed, the cosmetic aspects of this devastating problem need to be clearly recognized and addressed. The numerous techniques that are discussed throughout this article may be divided into general categories based on the nature of repair, dynamic versus static, and the subunit of the face involved. Typically, a combination of both static and dynamic procedures is used to achieve a satisfactory result.

FACIAL NERVE REPAIR

Primary repair of the facial nerve is the most effective procedure to restore facial function. Timely repair of the nerve is indicated in all patients who have suffered acute traumatic transection or unplanned injury to the nerve during surgery. Early identification and repair are key in achieving desirable postoperative function. Studies have shown that the regenerative process begins soon after the injury occurs, and therefore, most advocate repair within the first 30 days.[6]

Primary Repair and Cable Grafting

After suspected traumatic transection of the nerve, it is critical to explore the wound to identify the distal and proximal nerve ends to attempt a primary nerve repair or cable graft. When possible, a primary neurorrhaphy is considered the optimal repair technique. A primary neurorrhaphy may be performed if the repair is tension free and the defect is less than or equal to 17 mm. Multiple different techniques have been attempted to improve the success of primary neurrophaphy. These techniques include epineural versus perineural neurorraphy, trophic factors, tissue adhesives, laser neurorrhaphy, and tubulization. No 1 factor has been found to be superior to the other. The most common methods of neurorraphy include perineural (fascicular) and epineural repair with 2 or 3 interrupted 9-0 nylon sutures. Most surgeons have abandoned the perineural repair because of its increased technical difficulty, without proof of its superiority over epineural repair.[7] However, evidence has shown that cutting the nerve ends at a 45° angle exposes more neural tubules and improves regrowth of the nerve.[8,9]

Although the prognosis for facial nerve regeneration after direct repair is better than that for other motor nerves, there are several primary factors that directly affect outcome: proximity of the injury to the cell body, type of neural injury, timing of repair, and type of repair. There are also a host of secondary factors that affect long-term results, including patient age, previous chemotherapy or radiation, nutrition, and underlying comorbidities. Of these prognosticators, the surgeon influences only the timing and type of repair.[10] The single

most important prognostic factor, apart from neurorrhaphy technique, is tension-free coaptation of the stumps.[11] A tension-free primary repair of the nerve can achieve good results, even in the very elderly and previously radiated patient.

When end-to-end approximation is not feasible, an interposition graft may be used. Nerve grafts are indicated when the proximal and distal cut stumps of the facial nerve are clearly identifiable, but the intervening gap is too wide to achieve a tension-free repair. A common rule is that any defect greater than 2 cm should be repaired with a nerve graft. The sural, greater auricular, medial antebrachial cutaneous, or lateral antebrachial cutaneous nerves are all acceptable donors. The greater auricular nerve is readily available, because it is often within the operative site and has approximately the same diameter as the facial nerve. However, if a length greater than 8 to 10 cm is required, the medial antebrachial or sural nerve should be considered. Nerve selection may depend on ancillary procedures being performed. For example, if an anterior lateral thigh graft is being used for reconstruction, the nerve to the vastus lateralis muscle may be harvested for cable graft repair. When a cable graft is used, recovery typically becomes first noticeable around 6 months, with a full recovery expected around 12 to 18 months after repair. Most patients should expect to reach a House-Brackmann III level of function. Recent literature has shown that 97% of patients receiving nerve grafts have some return of function at a median of 6.2 months postoperatively and most (63.6%) have good function (House-Brackmann score ≤4).[12] A recent study[13] investigated the factors that were effectual in the recovery of facial nerve function after repair with grafting, and preoperative deficit duration was found to be the only significant factor that affected the prognosis.

Cross-Facial Nerve Grafting

When the proximal facial nerve stump is unavailable for primary repair, the reconstructive surgeon may use a cross-facial nerve graft. In this technique, axons from the contralateral facial nerve are diverted to the injured distal facial nerve stump via a free nerve graft. Usually, 1 or 2 branches that cause elevation of the oral commissure and upper lip are chosen. Noticeable facial movement is not typically evident until at least 9 to 12 months after the procedure. Cross-face grafting was introduced in the 1970s, but has fallen out of favor for numerous reasons. One of the most notable drawbacks is donor site morbidity and synkinesis (involuntary movement) on recovery of the paralyzed side. This technique is mainly used as part of a free-muscle transposition procedure. In this technique, a tunneled cable nerve graft uses contralateral buccal branches of the intact facial nerve to innervate a microvascular free flap. This technique can be performed in a 1-stage or 2-stage fashion.

Crossover Grafts

Nerve transfer techniques are most useful in the intermediate period after nerve injury (3 weeks–2 years). The following conditions are required for a successful nerve crossover graft: intact proximal donor nerve, intact distal facial nerve, and intact muscles of facial expression. The hypoglossal-facial jump graft is most frequently used and has been shown to achieve substantial facial reinnervation (House-Brackmann grade III or better) in 83.3% of patients.[14] This procedure places an interpositional nerve graft between a partially transected hypoglossal nerve trunk and the distal facial nerve trunk. Partial transection of the hypoglossal nerve, as opposed to complete transection, decreases the amount of donor nerve deficit, but achieves similar facial movement seen with the XII to VII crossover. It has been reported that as little as 8% of patients undergoing jump grafting experienced permanent tongue deficits, compared with 100% of nerve transfer patients.[15] As with any form of surgical repair, patients must undergo biofeedback and motor sensory rehabilitation to learn voluntary control of movement, to decrease synkinesis, and to limit facial grimacing that can occur with mastication.

DYNAMIC RECONSTRUCTION TECHNIQUES

Although not appropriate in the acute setting, a variety of reconstructive techniques are available after initial repair. Dynamic reconstruction procedures tend to be more successful and fruitful than static techniques and should be offered to each patient considering reconstruction, unless health risk contraindications exist. The most common approaches for dynamic reconstruction, aside from direct nerve repair and nerve grafting, include regional and free-muscle transfer. This patient population includes those with facial nerve dysfunction greater than 18 months, congenital facial paralyses, and severe neurofibrosis and myofibrosis of the distal neuromuscular unit.[16]

The area of the face most amenable to muscle transfer is the perioral region, where the primary goals are to restore symmetry of the smile and improve oral function.

Regional Muscle Transfer

Dynamic slings may be used to restore facial and oral motor function. Numerous different muscles and techniques have been described, with various success rates. The mainstay of this technique is the temporalis muscle transfer, because of its length, contractility, and favorable vector of pull.

Temporalis

In long-standing facial paralysis, temporalis muscle transfer gives a dependable and quick result. This procedure is possible only in patients with intact trigeminal motor function. There are key advantages to the temporalis flap. No distant surgical sight is required, the scar is camouflaged in the hairline, the technique limits the surgical field to the involved hemiface, and the flap is easily harvested and transferred. It can be transferred in a manner that does not create an unsightly donor defect.[17] Its primary limitation is that it is used almost exclusively for mouth animation.

First described in 1934 by Gillies,[18] the procedure traditionally included the transfer of all or a portion of the origin of the muscle. However, there are some drawbacks to this standard surgical technique. By removing the muscle from its fan-shaped origin on the squamous portion of the temporal bone, an unsightly defect is created in the temporal region. In addition, if the muscle is reflected over the arch of the zygoma, a soft tissue protrusion overlying the zygomatic arch results in obvious facial asymmetry. Each of these protrusions can be lessened by using only the central third of the muscle belly, placing a temporal implant to fill in the depression, or even removing the zygomatic arch to lesson the protrusion.[17]

Transfer of the temporalis tendon provides improved function and elimination of the tell-tale signs of temporalis muscle transfer produced by the classic technique. The technique for orthodromic temporalis tendon transfer involves release and mobilization of the muscle at its insertion into the coronoid. The tendon is then transferred to the oral commissure, which avoids the unsightly depression in the temple and tissue protrusion lateral to the zygomatic arch.

Cosmetic deficiencies associated with temporalis muscle transfer can also be lessened by using the transoral approach described by McLaughlin.[19] This approach involves transecting the temporalis muscle from its insertion at the coronoid process of the mandible and attaching it to the perioral region using a fascia lata graft. This concept was then later modified by Labbé and Huault[20] by using a temporal approach to transfer the insertion of the muscle to the oral commissure without an extension graft. This technique required releasing the origin of the muscle and allowing the entire muscle to slide through the buccal region.

Overcorrection is necessary with this technique for an optimal result, much like with static sling procedures. This overcorrection typically settles and has a more natural/symmetric appearance by 3 to 6 weeks. The results of the transposition should be evident by 4 to 6 weeks. Patients should be warned of possible complications such as infection, hematoma, and seroma, as well as gradual relaxation of the sling secondary to the long-term effects of age and gravity.[21]

Other Regional Flap Options

The masseter muscle is another option for dynamic facial reanimation. It is suboptimal, because rerouting of its insertion to the region of the oral commissure results in a vector of contraction that is too horizontal for optimal function. Furthermore, the defect at the angle of the mandible left by rotation of the muscle is highly visible. Transfer of the masseter muscle is performed by detaching the anterior portion of the masseter muscle from its mandibular insertion, bisecting it, and then securing it to the modiolus. The facial irregularity produced at the oral commissure is bulky and a considerable drawback of this technique. Aggressive postoperative physical therapy is required to produce a less than natural smile.[22]

The marginal mandibular branch of the facial nerve is the most frequently injured division of cranial nerve VII. It is particularly vulnerable because of its location overlying the mandible but also is at risk from iatrogenic trauma during parotidectomy, submandibular gland excision, face lift, and neck dissections. Functional difficulties secondary to injury of this nerve include biting of the lower lip and oral incompetence. The modern reanimation technique for lower lip paralysis was developed by Conley. This technique involved transposing the tendon of the anterior belly of the digastric muscle to the orbicularis muscle of the lower lip.[23] The goal of this procedure is to mimic the depressor function without exaggerating it. Patients are able to achieve great static repositioning of the lower lip and occasionally some dynamic function.[24]

Free-Muscle Transfer

Free-muscle transplantation offers the advantage of restoration of some emotional animation, in addition to good tone at rest and some voluntary facial movement. Numerous muscles have been investigated for free transfer to the paralyzed face, including the gracilis, serratus, pectoralis minor, latissimus dorsi, platysma, rectus abdominis, rectus femoris, and extensor digitorum brevis. The first report of free-muscle transfer for facial paralysis was described by Harii in 1976[25] and involved the use of the gracilis muscle. The gracilis continues to be the muscle of choice for numerous reasons, including its ease of dissection, adequate neurovascular pedicle, and muscle fiber length. Its blood supply is derived from the medial femoral circumflex artery and it is innervated by the anterior branch of the obturator nerve, which can be dissected to a length of 10 to 12 cm.

Free-muscle transplantation can be performed in a single-stage or 2-stage manner. For single-stage procedures, the obturator nerve branch of the gracilis muscle can yield a length of 12 cm, which allows primary anastomosis of this nerve to the contralateral facial nerve. Others have reported primary anastamosis to the masseter nerve as well. Incorporating the masseter nerve with free-tissue transfer in this single-stage strategy has become a reasonable alternative (and may become the criterion standard) to the dual-stage approach with cross-facial nerve grafting. The enormous advantage of using the masseter nerve is that, unlike the cross-facial nerve graft, the masseter nerve can elicit muscle movement (in relation to smile and commissure excursion) in a near-normal range with consistent movement.[26]

Two-stage procedures use a cross-facial nerve graft in the first procedure from contralateral buccal branches and a free-muscle transposition in the second stage. Free-muscle transfer is usually performed 9 to 12 months after the nerve graft. Movement can be expected in 6 to 9 months after muscle transfer, with improvement over the following 2 to 3 years. The disadvantages of the 2-stage approach are unpredictability of the function of the transplanted muscle, long delay awaiting the second stage, and scar formation on the nonparalyzed side of the face.[7]

Numerous studies have evaluated the results of microvascular free-tissue transfer for management of facial palsy. Kumar and Hassan[27] compared single-stage free-tissue transfer with dual-stage free-tissue transfer for facial reconstruction in their study of 25 patients. These investigators found that the single-stage transfer has fewer complications and a reduced recovery time with decreased rehabilitation, but the dual-stage approach achieved better overall symmetry. Good to excellent results in 51% of 47 patients treated by microvascular free-muscle transfer were reported by O'Brien and colleagues[28]; these surgeons most commonly used cross-facial nerve grafts and gracilis muscle transfers in their technique.

STATIC RECONSTRUCTION TECHNIQUES

Static techniques can be used to suspend the soft tissue structures of the face, but do not provide facial reanimation. They are often used as adjunctive maneuvers with dynamic techniques to enhance facial symmetry. In patients who are not suitable candidates for dynamic reanimation procedures secondary to medical comorbidities, static procedures can be useful in restoration of facial symmetry for functional reasons. Static suspension procedures are designed to most importantly protect the cornea by restoring eyelid competence, and to a lesser extent to enhance mastication and speech, and restore facial symmetry at rest. It is helpful to describe the various static procedures available based on the facial subunit to be addressed.

Brow

Ptosis of the brow can have both cosmetic and functional consequences. Hooding of the upper eyelid can lead to lateral visual field compromise. The midforehead lift is a commonly used technique and is effective in men and the elderly. Alternatively, the direct brow lift can be used for unilateral brow ptosis, with good results. This technique involves direct skin excision with suspension of the orbicularis oculi muscle to the underlying periosteum. Endoscopic brow lifts in select patients are offered by many as a less invasive procedure to achieve brow symmetry (**Fig. 3**).[29]

Orbital Complex

One of the most critical elements in facial reanimation surgery is management of the paralyzed upper lid. The ocular sequelae of facial paralysis include lagophthalmos, with corneal exposure, lower lid ectropion, and decreased tear production. Inadequate corneal protection can cause exposure keratitis, corneal ulceration, and blindness. Failure to use conservative measures, such as ointment and artificial tears, often results in exposure keratitis, which typically presents as a subjective complaint of foreign body sensation and significant scleral edema and vascular injection on examination. Tarsorrhaphy is an effective method of eye protection when there is evidence of keratitis, but is not suitable for long-term management secondary to visual field disturbances. It should be offered only to those patients at a severe risk for exposure keratitis.[30]

Gold weight lid loading is a simple procedure that relies on gravitational pull to passively close the lid and may be performed under local anesthesia. It has been shown to have a greater than 90% success rate, with low complication rates.[31] A retrospective analysis of 45 patients over a 5-year period revealed extrusion of the gold weight in 1 (2.2%) patient and delayed infections in 3 (6.6%).[32] Early implantation should be considered in all patients with facial nerve paralysis, even if recovery is anticipated. The weight can be easily removed if upper lid function returns. Although preoperative testing can help to identify the ideal

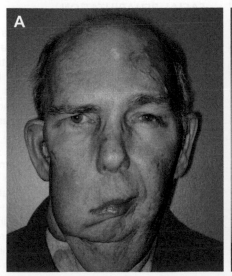
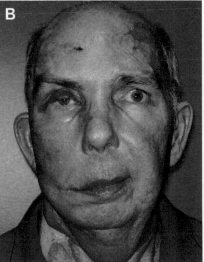

Fig. 3. Facial nerve static reconstruction. (*A*) Patient status after resection of malignant right parotid tumor with complete right facial paralysis. Note the significant facial ptosis. (*B*) Patient status after right browlift, placement of gold weight right upper lid, right commissure of the lip suspension. Note the improved brow and lip position. (*Courtesy of* Patrick J. Louis, DDS, MD, Birmingham, AL.)

implant weight, a 1.2-g gold weight is appropriate in most patients and is often used empirically. The palpebral wire spring is rarely used, because it has a significantly higher extrusion and infection rate than gold weight implantation.[33]

Patients may experience ectropion or epiphora secondary to lower lid laxity. This condition is best addressed at the time of upper lid weight loading. Techniques frequently used include medial or lateral canthoplasty, lid tightening procedures, and lid suspension. Lateral lid laxity may be addressed by a full-thickness wedge resection, lateral canthoplasty, or tarsal strip procedure. Over time, lid sagging may recur as a result of poor orbicularis tone, and these procedures may be repeated as needed. If further elevation of the lower lid is needed, then spacer grafts (palate mucosa, conchal cartilage, acellular human dermis) may be used to provide vertical height to the eyelid.[34]

Nose

Paralysis of the nasalis muscles leads to nasal collapse, resulting in unilateral nasal airway obstruction and internal valve collapse. This condition may be corrected by a nasal lateralization procedure, in which a sling is secured to the deep tissue of the lateral alar base and then suspended laterally to the ascending maxillary buttress.[35] Another approach to address internal valve collapse is with placement of a spreader graft.

Midface and Oral Commissure

A static sling is used most commonly for creation of the nasolabial fold and restoration of cheek and mouth symmetry. It may improve oral competence, but provides no dynamic benefit when smiling. A variety of materials have been used. Autologous tissue, such as fascia lata or plantaris tendon, is easily harvested and affords adequate length and strength. Fascia lata is preferred because multiple strips can be acquired. Initial overcorrection is necessary to compensate for expected stretching over time. More recently, alloplastic materials, such as acellular dermis, Gore-Tex, and polypropylene mesh, have been used. They eliminate donor site morbidity, but have been associated with higher complication rates as a result of infection and extrusion.[36]

The static sling procedure for midface lifting typically involves 2 incisions: 1 in the nasolabial fold and 1 either preauricularly or at the temporal hairline. The material of choice is then tunneled between the 2 incisions and sutured in place at the desired level of suspension, with care being taken to overcorrect with autologous sling materials. The suture technique has been described as another method to achieve static suspension. Sutures are placed through a multi-vector approach, resulting in functional and aesthetic improvements. This technique is less invasive than other static techniques and can be accomplished percutaneously.[37]

Drooping of the oral commissure can be aesthetically and functionally problematic. This drooping may be addressed by static sling suspension to either the zygomatic arch or the orbital rim in a similar manner to the cheek and midface. Exposure of the oral commissure can be achieved via incisions at the vermilion border of the upper and lower lip or at the nasolabial fold. An extended subciliary incision or a vertical incision anterior to the sideburn provides exposure to the orbital rim and zygomatic arch. The sling material of choice is sutured to the modiolus or may be split into 2 and fixed to the orbicularis muscle fibers of the upper and lower lips. By analyzing the position of the mouth on the unaffected side, the suspension vector is determined and the free end of the sling is suspended and fixed to the zygomatic arch or infraorbital rim by a permanent suture, screw, or miniplate.[1]

Residual lip asymmetry may be addressed by a full-thickness V or W wedge excision. Cheiloplasty may also be beneficial in some patients. This technique is performed by resecting redundant paralyzed lip tissue and exchanging it for normal orbicularis and lip from the contralateral unaffected side.

FACIAL REHABILITATION

Previously, facial rehabilitation has not been widely available or considered to be of benefit. The emerging presence of rehabilitation science and neuromuscular reeducation has been a key factor in the overall success rates of all of these procedures. Evidence for the efficacy of facial neuromuscular reeducation, a process of facilitating the return of intended facial movement patterns and eliminating unwanted patterns of facial movement and expression, may provide patients with facial paralysis with the opportunity for improved overall recovery of facial movement and function.

Facial retraining is essential to optimize results in most patients undergoing facial reanimation. Although the benefit of facial retraining has not been proved, several studies have suggested a positive effect on outcomes. Lindsay and colleagues[38] reported statistically significant improvements in Facial Grading Scale scores after facial rehabilitation, and these were long-lasting with continued treatment. This finding indicated that patients can successfully manage symptoms with rehabilitation and underscored the importance of specialized therapy in the management of facial paralysis.

In general, the coordinated care of a physical therapist with expertise in facial retraining is recommended. Neuromuscular facial retraining therapy can address loss of strength, loss of isolated motor control, muscle tension hypertonicity, or synkinesis. Techniques frequently used combine patient education in basic facial anatomy, physiology, and kinesiology; relaxation training; sensory stimulation; EMG biofeedback; and spontaneously elicited facial movements.

SUMMARY

The patient with facial paralysis presents a daunting challenge to the reconstructive surgeon. A thorough evaluation is key in directing the surgeon to the appropriate treatment methods. Aggressive and immediate exploration with primary repair of the facial nerve continues to be the standard of care for traumatic transection of the facial nerve. Secondary repair using dynamic techniques is preferred over static procedures, because the outcomes have proved to be superior. However, patients should be counseled that facial movement and symmetry are difficult to mimic and none of the procedures described is able to restore all of the complex vectors and overall balance of facial movement and expression.

REFERENCES

1. Hoffman WY. Reanimation of the paralyzed face. Otolaryngol Clin North Am 1992;25(3):649–67.
2. Feng Y, Zhang YQ, Liu M, et al. Sectional anatomy aid for improvement of decompression surgery approach to vertical segment of facial nerve. J Craniofac Surg 2012;23(3):906–8.
3. Hwang K, Suh MS, Lee SI, et al. Zygomaticotemporal nerve passage in the orbit and temporal area. J Craniofac Surg 2004;15(2):209–14.
4. Hwang K, Cho HJ, Chung IH. Pattern of the temporal branch of the facial nerve in the upper orbicularis oculi muscle. J Craniofac Surg 2004;15(3):373–6.
5. Yamada H, Hato N, Murakami S, et al. Facial synkinesis after experimental compression of the facial nerve comparing intratemporal and extratemporal lesions. Laryngoscope 2010;120(5):1022–7.
6. Bascom DA, Schaitkin BM, May M, et al. Facial nerve repair: a retrospective review. Facial Plast Surg 2000;16(4):309–13.
7. Clark MA, William W, editors. Facial plastic and reconstructive surgery. 3rd edition. New York: Thieme Medical Publishers; 2009.
8. Gidley PW, Gantz BJ, Rubinstein JT. Facial nerve grafts: from cerebellopontine angle and beyond. Am J Otol 1999;20(6):781–8.
9. Yamamoto E, Fisch U. Experiments on facial nerve suturing. ORL J Otorhinolaryngol Relat Spec 1974;36(4):193–204.
10. Piza-Katzer H, Balogh B, Muzika-Herczeg E, et al. Secondary end-to-end repair of extensive facial nerve defects: surgical technique and postoperative functional results. Head Neck 2004;26(9):770–7.
11. Millesi H. Nerve grafting. Clin Plast Surg 1984;11(1):105–13.
12. Iseli TA, Harris G, Dean NR, et al. Outcomes of static and dynamic facial nerve repair in head and neck cancer. Laryngoscope 2010;120(3):478–83.
13. Ozmen OA, Falcioni M, Lauda L, et al. Outcomes of facial nerve grafting in 155 cases: predictive value of history and preoperative function. Otol Neurotol 2011;32(8):1341–6.
14. Hammerschlag PE. Facial reanimation with jump interpositional graft hypoglossal facial anastomosis and hypoglossal facial anastomosis: evolution in management of facial paralysis. Laryngoscope 1999;109(2 Pt 2 Suppl 90):1–23.
15. Hadlock TA, Greenfield LJ, Wernick-Robinson M, et al. Multimodality approach to management of the paralyzed face. Laryngoscope 2006;116(8):1385–9.
16. Glickman LT, Simpson R. Cross-facial nerve grafting for facial reanimation: effect on normal hemiface motion. J Reconstr Microsurg 1996;12:99. J Reconstr Microsurg 1996;12(3):201–2.
17. Byrne PJ, Kim M, Boahene K, et al. Temporalis tendon transfer as part of a comprehensive approach to facial reanimation. Arch Facial Plast Surg 2007;9(4):234–41.
18. Gillies H. Experiences with fascia lata grafts in the operative treatment of facial paralysis: (section of otology and section of laryngology). Proc R Soc Med 1934;27(10):1372–82.
19. McLaughlin CR. Surgical support in permanent facial paralysis. Plast Reconstr Surg (1946) 1953;11(4):302–14.
20. Labbe D, Huault M. Lengthening temporalis myoplasty and lip reanimation. Plast Reconstr Surg 2000;105(4):1289–97 [discussion: 1298].
21. Snow J, Wackym PA, editors. Ballenger's otorhinolaryngology head and neck surgery. 17th edition. Shelton (CT): People's Medical Publishing House; 2008.
22. Garanhani MR, Rosa Cardoso J, Capelli Ade M, et al. Physical therapy in peripheral facial paralysis: retrospective study. Braz J Otorhinolaryngol 2007;73(1):106–9.
23. Conley J, Baker DC, Selfe RW. Paralysis of the mandibular branch of the facial nerve. Plast Reconstr Surg 1982;70(5):569–77.

24. Sckolnick J, Schaitkin B. Digastric transposition for unilateral lower lip weakness after injury to the marginal mandibular nerve. Operative Techniques in Otolaryngology 2008;19(4):237–9.

25. Harii K, Ohmori K, Torii S. Free gracilis muscle transplantation, with microneurovascular anastomoses for the treatment of facial paralysis. A preliminary report. Plast Reconstr Surg 1976;57(2):133–43.

26. Bianchi B, Copelli C, Ferrari S, et al. Use of the masseter motor nerve in facial animation with free muscle transfer. Br J Oral Maxillofac Surg 2012;50: 650–3.

27. Kumar PA, Hassan KM. Cross-face nerve graft with free-muscle transfer for reanimation of the paralyzed face: a comparative study of the single-stage and two-stage procedures. Plast Reconstr Surg 2002; 109(2):451–62 [discussion: 463–4].

28. O'Brien BM, Pederson WC, Khazanchi RK, et al. Results of management of facial palsy with microvascular free-muscle transfer. Plast Reconstr Surg 1990;86(1):12–22 [discussion: 23–4].

29. Ducic Y, Adelson R. Use of the endoscopic forehead-lift to improve brow position in persistent facial paralysis. Arch Facial Plast Surg 2005;7(1):51–4.

30. Scoppetta C. Non-surgical tarsorraphy in peripheral facial nerve paralysis. Ital J Neurol Sci 1981;2(1):97.

31. May M, Levine RE, Patel BC. Eye reanimation techniques. In: The facial nerve: May's second edition.

2nd edition. New York: Georg Thieme Verlag; 2000. p. 677–774.

32. Linder TE, Pike VE, Linstrom CJ. Early eyelid rehabilitation in facial nerve paralysis. Laryngoscope 1996; 106(9 Pt 1):1115–8.

33. May M. Gold weight and wire spring implants as alternatives to tarsorrhaphy. Arch Otolaryngol Head Neck Surg 1987;113(6):656–60.

34. Taban M, Douglas R, Li T, et al. Efficacy of "thick" acellular human dermis (AlloDerm) for lower eyelid reconstruction: comparison with hard palate and thin AlloDerm grafts. Arch Facial Plast Surg 2005; 7(1):38–44.

35. Soler ZM, Rosenthal E, Wax MK. Immediate nasal valve reconstruction after facial nerve resection. Arch Facial Plast Surg 2008;10(5):312–5.

36. Constantinides M, Galli SK, Miller PJ. Complications of static facial suspensions with expanded polytetrafluoroethylene (ePTFE). Laryngoscope 2001; 111(12):2114–21.

37. Winslow CP, Wang TD, Wax MK. Static reanimation of the paralyzed face with an acellular dermal allograft sling. Arch Facial Plast Surg 2001;3(1):55–7.

38. Lindsay RW, Robinson M, Hadlock TA. Comprehensive facial rehabilitation improves function in people with facial paralysis: a 5-year experience at the Massachusetts Eye and Ear Infirmary. Phys Ther 2010;90(3):391–7.

Surgical Navigation in Reconstruction

Wolfram M.H. Kaduk, MD, DDS[a],*,
Fred Podmelle, MD, DDS[a], Patrick J. Louis, DDS, MD[b]

KEYWORDS

- Real-time image-guided surgical navigation • Equipment • Function and performance
- Maxillofacial and reconstructive surgery • Quest for imaging • Case reports • Scientific capability

KEY POINTS

- Equipment required to perform surgical navigation (SN) includes: (1) infrared camera, (2) advanced images of the patient on computer using the navigation software, and (3) an interactive display monitor.
- Steps in SN include: (1) advanced imaging, (2) data analysis, (3) planning phase, (4) surgical phase, and (5) assessment of results.
- Because of the complexity of SN a series of check lists have been developed: (1) preoperative, (2) preoperative planning, (3) operating room, (4) intraoperative imaging, and (5) postoperative.
- SN can be used to manage simple and complex cases.
- As the surgeon becomes more familiar with SN, more surgical cases can be aided by the use of this technology.

SURGICAL NAVIGATION: HISTORY AND DEFINITION

Different terms are currently used to describe surgery guided by real-time imaging: computer-assisted surgery, image-guided surgery, navigational surgery, and surgical navigation (SN). The first term includes the application of surgery robots and is not addressed in this article, which instead focuses on real-time image-guided SN. SN has its origin in neurosurgical demands and was first used in stereotactic procedures together with a stereotactic human brain atlas.[1] A precondition for further progress of this technique was the development of 3-dimensional (3D) imaging in medicine. With computed tomography (CT) and later, magnetic resonance imaging (MRI) other imaging modalities, the way was paved for the development of SN in neurosurgery, beginning in the 1990s. With the experience of frameless stereotaxy[2] or neuronavigation and the development of robot systems in medicine, the idea arose to combine both techniques, initially called computer-assisted surgery, by early 2000. Computer-navigated robots such as the Da Vinci system did not increase daily use in maxillofacial

a Department of Maxillofacial Surgery/Plastic Surgery, Greifswald University, Sauerbruchstr./ Bettenhaus MKG, Greifswald D-17487, Germany; b Department of Oral and Maxillofacial Surgery, University of Alabama at Birmingham, 1919 7th Avenue South, SDB 419, Birmingham, AL 35294-0007, USA
* Corresponding author.
E-mail address: kaduk@uni-greifswald.de

Oral Maxillofacial Surg Clin N Am 25 (2013) 313–333
http://dx.doi.org/10.1016/j.coms.2013.01.003
1042-3699/13/$ – see front matter © 2013 Elsevier Inc. All rights reserved.

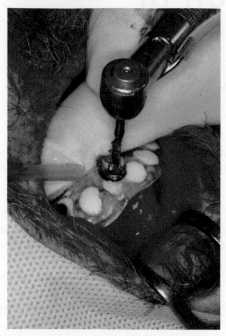

Fig. 1. Template to guide dental implants into their predicted position in the lower jaw.

development of specialized software in maxillofacial and reconstructive surgery. For a basic review of this topic an article entitled "Navigational Surgery of the Facial Skeleton" by Schramm and colleagues[3] is recommended, which also contains a comprehensive collection of references.

Two kinds of navigation techniques are practiced in maxillofacial surgery: template-guided navigation (TGN) and real-time image-guided surgical navigation (SN). TGN uses computer-aided design/manufacture (CAD/CAM) or rapid prototyping technology to produce templates that guide dental implants into the right position (**Fig. 1**). Disadvantages of TGN are less flexibility, in terms of producing a new modified template during surgery if the surgical situation becomes altered suddenly. SN has a wide variety of indications in reconstructive and maxillofacial surgery. It is applicable for dental implantations as an adapted system, with reduced software functions for dental implant guiding only (http://www.robodent.de). The reader is referred to a downloadable video; RoboDent NaviPanel Video (Avi, DivX, MP3, 58 MB) by RoboDent GmbH (Gleissenweg 1, D-85737 Ismaning, Germany) to learn more.

EQUIPMENT AND FUNCTION OF REAL-TIME IMAGE-GUIDED SURGICAL NAVIGATION

surgery for routine procedures, because of the ease and predictability of endoscopic and transoral procedures.

SN has become much more common in oral and maxillofacial surgery in Germany, owing to the

SN consists of 3 components: (1) an infrared camera, (2) advanced images of the patient on computer using the navigation software, and (3) an interactive display monitor. The infrared camera (eg, Brain LAB; brainlab.com) acts as an

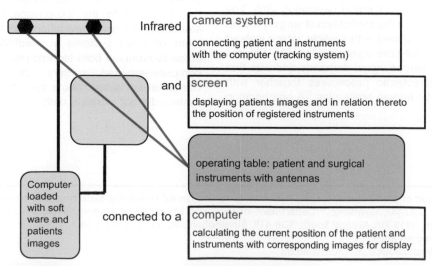

Fig. 2. Schematic pattern of real-time image-guided surgical navigation (SN).

Table 1
Performance ability of surgical navigation (SN)

SN Performance	Application and Surgical Procedure
Search, find, and remove	Foreign bodies, alterations, tumors
Mark and save	Nerve and vessel surgery
Guide, take out, and remove	Tumors, alterations, foreign bodies
Ensure adequate removal	Tumors, alterations, foreign bodies, transplants
Drill and cut exactly, direction, and depth	Implants, osteotomies, tumors, alterations
Choose the best surgical access	All surgeries
Evaluate hidden regions	Cysts, foreign bodies, deep layers, tumors, skull base surgery, joint surgery
Transposition and repositioning	Malformations, transplants, implants
Reshape surfaces	Modeling and aesthetic surgery
Document and correlate during surgery	Radiotherapies and histopathology, all surgery
Collect experience for future surgery, filter or percolate information	All surgery
Make the right decision and avoid mistakes	All surgery
Compare preoperative and postoperative situations, compare and control surgical quality	All surgery
Measure, filter, mirror, document, collect, replace, create, etc	Scientific capability

optical passive connection (tracking system) between the patient, surgical instruments, and computer. The link between instruments and computer varies between companies: optically active (eg, Stryker; stryker.com) electromagnetically (eg, GE Healthcare; gehealthcare.com), or via ultrasound.[4] The software calculates the current positions of the patients and instruments,

chooses the correlating images of the patient together with the preoperative planning, and displays all on the screen. The display can have touch-screen function for input and control (**Fig. 2**).

Most important for SN is the development of an accurate model of the patient, which can be conducted by several medical imaging technologies

Table 2
Selection of companies offering SN systems

Company Name	SN System Names
Brain LAB (brainlab.com)	Curve, Caliber, Vector Vision
Stryker (stryker.com)	eNlite Navigation System, Nav Suite
Medtronic (medtronic.com)	Stealth Station, Fusion ENT
GE Healthcare (gehealthcare.com)	Insta Track 3500
Karl Storz (karlstorz.de)	ENT Surgical Cockpit
Collin (www.collinmedical.fr)	DigiPointer
RoboDent GmbH (www.robodent.de)	RoboDent NaviPanel
DenX (denx.com)	Image-Guided Implantology (IGI)

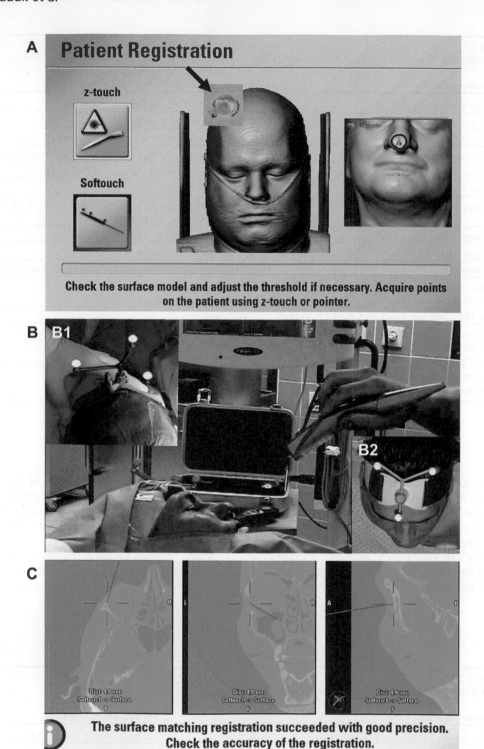

Fig. 3. (*A*) Surface check for registration (*black arrow—universal marker*). (*B*) Laser surface scan. (*B1*) Screw-fixed antenna. (*B2*) Rubber-band–fixed antenna. (*C*) Registration check by SN pointer.

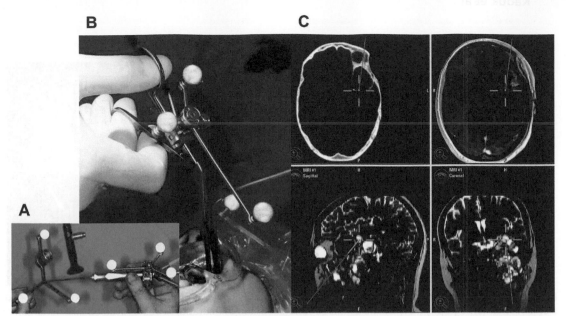

Fig. 4. (*A*) The easiest way of instrument registration. The authors' new temporomandibular joint (TMJ) arthroscope shows a mold in the midpoint of the patient's antenna for pivoting the tip of the instrument that should be registered. (*B*) SN to reduce a slow-growing teratoma in the brain and retromaxillary with access across the maxillary sinus by Blakesley nasal forceps. (*C*) Merged computed tomography (CT) and magnetic resonance imaging (MRI) scans to navigate forceps during surgery.

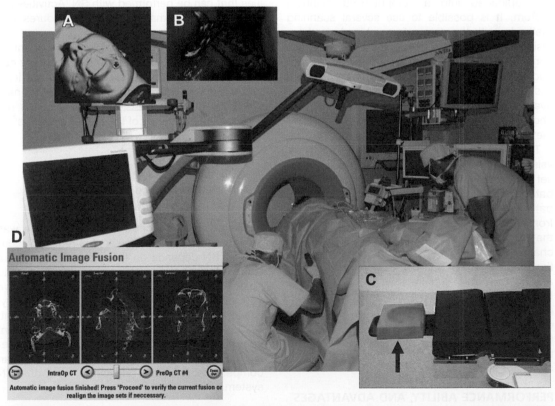

Fig. 5. Intraoperative imaging by cone-beam CT (CB-CT). (*A*) To reproduce the position of the moveable mandible during SN, the patient must wear a jaw separator during imaging. (*B*) The authors' self-constructed mandible-positioning plate for intraoperative imaging. (*C*) Self-constructed table top with (*arrow*) carbon headrest. (*D*) Intraoperative imaging fusion with preoperative images.

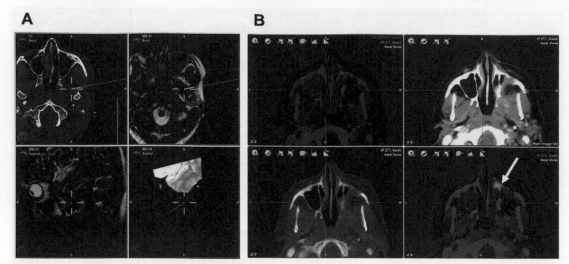

Fig. 6. (*A*) CT-MRI image fusion; injection needle in sagittal MRI plane is located close to the optic nerve. (*B*) Positron emission tomography (PET)-CT and CT image fusion in a case of midfacial sarcoma revealed additional tumor spreading in the bone of the right upper jaw medially (*white arrow*).

including CT, MRI, ultrasonography, and other modalities. The area of interest has to be scanned and uploaded into a computerized planning system. It is possible to use several scanning methods, with the data sets combined via data-fusion techniques. The final objective is the creation of a 3D data set that reproduces the exact geometric situation of the normal and pathologic tissues and structures of the patient. Among the available scanning methods, CT is often the first choice.[5] MRI data sets are known for having volumetric deformations that may lead to inaccuracies.

The next step after image creation is image analysis. When using special planning software, a data set can be rendered into a virtual 3D model of the patient; this involves the manipulation of the patient 3D model to extract relevant information from the data. Based on differing contrast levels, the varying tissues within the model can be changed to show more hard structures or soft tissues. By doing so, the surgeon can better assess the case and improve the diagnostics. Before surgery occurs, the intervention can be planned and simulated virtually. The best way to document the SN process in the operating room (OR) would be through video streaming. Unfortunately, in most current SN systems only screenshots are available.

PERFORMANCE ABILITY, AND ADVANTAGES AND DISADVANTAGES OF SN

In principle SN can be used in the same manner as any other surgical instrument such as a forceps,

knife, or scissors. The clinician should not hesitate to use SN if it is needed. **Table 1** contains all activities that can be performed with SN. Activities are assigned to the main surgical procedures and applications.

The accuracy of SN is exceedingly important for the operating surgeon. The highest accuracy can be achieved with image slices of 1 mm or less, and is reported with approximate sizes of 1.5 mm. The intraoperative precision of SN systems depends on the accuracy of the following factors[3]:

- CT data set
- SN system
- Pointer localization
- Patient registration system
- Patient registration procedure

The accuracy reported in recent articles was around 1 mm.[6,7] Nevertheless, the required accuracy of SN depends on the type of surgery, but should always be as precise as possible. This credo holds especially true for skull-base surgery, nerve and vessel surgery, and dental implant surgery, whereby deviations of 1 or 2 mm are very important.

The experience of the surgeon and constant control are important and crucial factors for superior results with SN. An experienced surgeon can compensate for small inaccuracies of the SN system.

Advantages of SN[8,9]

- Decrease invasiveness of surgery
- Decrease morbidity

Table 3
Daily SN cases

Case No.	Figure No.	Task for SN	Case Description
1	—	Find, remove	Unnoticed lost screw in left maxillary sinus during osteosynthesis of fractured zygoma, later removed with SN
2		Find position	Dental implant insertion into sella turcica for reconstruction of a tumor caused midface defect
3	—	Find, remove	Osteoma removed transnasally
4		Find, remove	Calculus removed of submandibular gland
5		Find, remove	Shortening of styloid process in case of eagle syndrome
6	7	Find	Treatment of anterior cranial fossa fracture with cerebrospinal fluid leak transnasally by application of fibrin glue
7	—	Find, remove	SN-assisted ultrasound-based removal of parotid gland calculus and small lymph nodes
8		Control, save	SN to check distance from lymph node metastasis to lung and to major subclavicular vessels during neck dissection level 5
9		Find, remove	SN-assisted removal of bone erosion caused by pleomorphic adenoma in maxillary sinus, to find the inner side of zygoma
10		Correlate, document	SN to excise floor of the mouth for tumor staging to correlate and document biopsy with report of radiologist
11	8	Control, document	SN to control and document suitable resection margins (area of pterygoideus medialis muscle) in a case of midface carcinoma
12		Control, document, determine	SN to determine resection margins in a carcinoma of the mandible. Parts of the chin and the right mentalis nerve revealed by SN must be removed together with appropriate parts of the mandible and surrounding soft tissues
13		Save, find	SN for biopsy near the internal carotid artery and the cervical spine by intraoral access
14		Find, remove	SN to find retained and dislocated teeth in cleft palate patient
15		Show	SN to show the best excess and the area for osteotomy in a case of carcinoma of the midface
16		Find position	SN for insertion of difficult dental implants (eg, in augmented cleft palate patients)
17	4C	Find, remove, save	SN used for access to retromaxillary regions through maxillary sinus without resection of maxilla in a case of growing teratoma

- Faster recovery, shorter hospital stay
- Better disease or cancer control
- High flexibility and adaptability
- Modifications during surgery
- Templates not always necessary
- Unplanned is possible if appropriate imaging available
- Versatile and universal applicable
- Excellent teaching tool

When SN is not needed it should not be used. This guideline is based on the experience of the surgeon.

Disadvantages of SN

- Cost of the equipment
- Need for education and training
- Sometimes more time consuming
- Soft-tissue reconstruction is limited

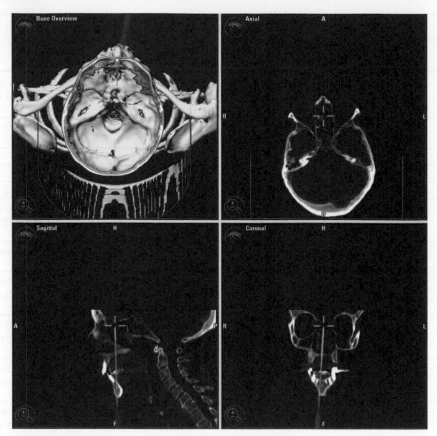

Fig. 7. SN-assisted transnasal treatment of anterior cranial fossa fracture with cerebrospinal fluid leak.

PURCHASE OR SHARE A SURGICAL NAVIGATION SYSTEM

When starting with SN, the decision between purchasing and sharing an existing system with other specialties of the hospital has to be made. Neurosurgery has the most specialty experience with SN. The most economical way to start with SN is to share a system.

If a new system has to be purchased, it is important to list all needed requirements. In addition to hardware described in previous sections, additional items include: antennas for the patient and instruments; devices to fix the antennas; a pointer and/or a laser for registration; and an ultrasound device. Package deals may include software and instrumentation. It is common to pay extra for different single features such as preoperative planning image fusion or intraoperative image fusion, advanced planning tools such as automatic segmentation, networking, and other useful software. Technical support by a trained technician is paramount. **Table 2** shows a selection of companies and the names of the SN systems offered.

QUEST FOR IMAGING AND CLINICAL IMPLEMENTATION OF SN (WORKFLOW CHECKLISTS)

When an SN system is available in the hospital, preconditions necessary for routine surgery must first be established. Selection of procedures that will benefit from SN is the decision of the surgeon. It is thus indispensable for the surgeon to know what the available SN systems are able to accomplish. To determine for which cases SN would be indicated, an adequate image database must be obtained. The radiologist needs specific information to deliver the best possible scans for navigation, thus avoiding exposure of the patient to repeat imaging and delays in surgery.

When starting with SN it is absolutely essential to stay abreast of the development of modern imaging in medicine. The surgeon, in conjunction with the radiologist, has to correlate imaging possibilities with the demands of SN to be able to select the best imaging modality. When planning SN for the mandible, it is necessary to fix the mandible during imaging in the same position

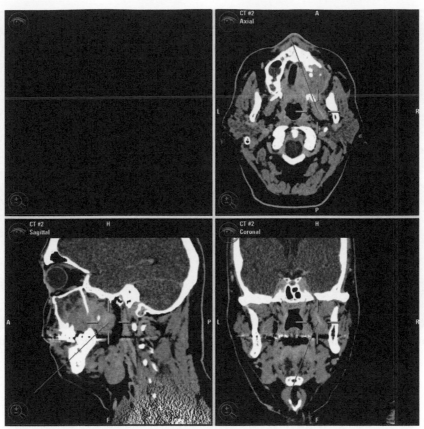

Fig. 8. SN-assisted control and documentation of suitable resection margins (area of pterygoideus medialis muscle) in a case of midface carcinoma.

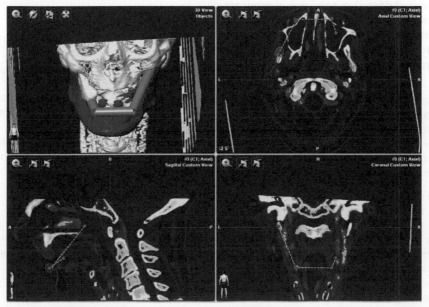

Fig. 9. Reset of mandible after resection, planning, and navigation of microsurgical reconstruction by a fibula transplant with advanced SN planning tools.

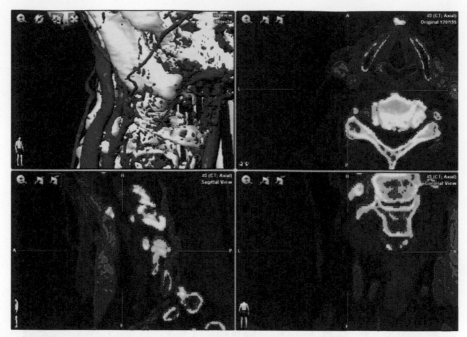

Fig. 10. SN of vessels in a routine CT angiography for microsurgical secondary reconstruction of the mandible.

that it will be in during surgery, to ensure accuracy.

Thus far this article has emphasized the importance of imaging for SN. Along with imaging, checklists help to avoid omissions in performing successful surgery. Not all steps for SN cases are listed here. Adapted details and appropriate explanations are given in the section dealing with case reports. The following 5 checklists should help in performing SN. The checklists are subdivided according to the following topics:

1. Preoperative SN checklist
2. Preoperative planning SN checklist
3. Operating room (OR) SN checklist
4. Intraoperative imaging (cone-beam CT [CB-CT]) SN checklist
5. Postoperative SN checklist

Once the decision has been made that SN is of benefit for the surgery, it is most important to check the preoperative scans for registration possibilities (**Fig. 3**A) and to determine the registration method. Surface matching (see **Fig. 3**B) is often sufficient and should be tried first. If this does not work, registration markers will have to be used (see **Fig. 3**A, black arrow), which must be applied before additional imaging (universal self-sticking markers are currently available for

CT, MRI, and CB-CT). Self-drilling 1.5-mm osteosynthesis screws as a marker or dental splint registration are also available.

Modern navigation software allows for defining registration points during surgery, but this is time consuming, less accurate, and not recommended.

Preoperative SN Checklist

- Determine patient registration method
- Decide on diagnostic imaging
- Place marker and/or fix the mandible if needed
- Employ the radiologist in SN imaging
- Evaluate Digital Imaging and Communication in Medicine (DICOM) data
- DICOM data available at planning computer
- If yes, follow Preoperative planning list
- If not, follow OR planning list

Preoperative Planning SN Checklist

- Load DICOM data set(s) into SN planning software
- Check data set for surface quality
- Match data set(s) and align
- Allow planning software to perform segmentations and check accuracy
- Create objects, points and trajectories for surgery

Table 4
Advanced SN cases

Case No.	Figure No.	Task for SN	Case Description
1	**11**	Outline, find, remove, save	Outlined T4 carcinoma of the floor of the mouth and tongue with proposed tumor margins and major vessels for appropriate resection; documentation for histologic examination and radiotherapy
2	**9** and **10**	Segmentation, object creation, trajectories, measure	Planning and navigation of microsurgical reconstruction by fibula transplant with advanced SN planning tools, SN planning tools to reset of the resected mandible from preoperative imaging
3	**12**	Outline, planning, save	SN to plan the osteotomy for access and to save the optic nerve (black arrow) during resection of a neurofibroma
4	**13**	Object creation, trajectories	Secondary reconstruction of traumatic orbit and midface deformity with 3-dimensional imaging (3D MD, Atlanta, GA, USA), CAD/CAM modeling, and advanced SN, but before autosegmentation and mirroring in SN planning software was available on the market
5	**14**	Object creation, mirroring	Double vision in a case of orbital floor fracture after overcorrection with titanic mesh; advanced SN planning with autosegmentation revealed the badly fitted titanic mesh, and only removal solved the problem. (Caution! do not overindicate titanic meshes, because in most of the fractures of the orbital floor PDS foils are superior) If the titanic mesh is already ingrown, required removal can destroy the orbital floor substantially
6	**15**A, B	Object creation, mirroring, measuring	12-y-old boy with 6-mo-old trauma of both orbits and the nasoethmoidal region, standard values of the orbit acquired by autosegmentation from 5 CT scans of previous imagings from hospital pool (PACS), superposition of the self-created standard orbit revealed a mainly left-sided surplus of orbital volume and deformity; decision for remodeling of the left orbit only by reosteotomy of the lateral floor and lateral wall (**Fig. 16**A) with advanced SN control (the pointer shows the achieved result after finishing surgery nearby the green standard orbit). Another possibility in case of volume deficiency of the orbit and enophthalmos: calculation of orbit volume and planning reconstruction of loss with hydrocolloid osmotic expander, fits best between lateral and inferior orbital muscle (see **Fig. 16**B)

(continued on next page)

Table 4 (continued)			
Case No.	Figure No.	Task for SN	Case Description
7	**17**	Object creation, mirroring, marking, determination, orientation	Surgical therapy for endocrine orbitopathy[14,15] supported by advanced SN for determination of osteotomy lines and amount of orbital wall alterations, mirroring to achieve a good symmetry, marking of infraorbital and optic nerve before surgery for orientation
8	**18**	Find, determination of drill direction	The advanced SN autopilot could help to find the region of interest or the predicted implant position exactly and in a short time
9	**19**		First step is the production of an implant; this needs very close cooperation with the technicians of the CAD/CAM company. Main problem in 1-step surgical reconstruction is to make sure that the prefabricated CAD/CAM implant fits during surgery into the defect. SN could make it possible and allow control if intraoperative imaging is available. Nevertheless the authors prefer ceramic rather than titanium implants if possible, because they are easier to adapt during surgery if finally necessary
10	—		Placement of TMJ endoprosthetics
11	—	Shape, modeling	Modeling osteotomy in case of fibrous dysplasia[16]

Abbreviations: CAD/CAM, computer-aided design/manufacture; CT, computed tomography; PACS, picture archive and communication system; PDS, polydioxanone; TMJ, temporomandibular joint.

- If useful; create, load, or use STL (stereolithography) files
- Search for individual solutions in each case (use, eg, self-created reference values from similar patients)
- Save and transfer SN preoperative planning to OR computer system
- Follow OR SN checklist

OR SN Checklist

- Send SN data set by network or USB stick to OR SN system
- Position SN system so that the surgical field is in view of the tracking system (infrared camera)

- Position the patient
- Attach the patient antenna (see **Fig. 3**B1, 3B2)
- Register the patient (see **Fig. 3**B) and check accuracy (see **Fig. 3**C)
- If needed, register additional instruments (**Fig. 4**A), check accuracy
- Navigate and use intraoperative imaging if beneficial (**Fig. 5**), send data to SN system, and match with preoperative data (see **Fig. 5**D)
- Take screenshots/movies for documentation
- Save data and finish SN

Patient registration is a very important step. The navigation pointer is a preregistered instrument and is always available without intraoperative

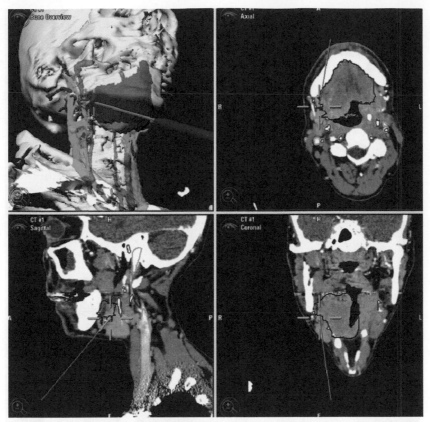

Fig. 11. Advanced SN with proposed tumor margins and vessels for appropriate resection and documentation for pathologist and radiotherapy. Outlined large carcinoma in the floor of the mouth with major arteries during SN of margins.

registration. Additional instruments must be registered during surgery by a special procedure. The patient and one instrument can be navigated at the same time in optical passive SN systems. More instruments can be registered, depending on the number of different antennas available, but only one is active. Optical passive referenced SN recognizes the instrument (pointer, drill, forceps, suction, injection needle, knife, endoscope, laser, diathermia, and so forth) by the shape of the antenna.

If 3D imaging in the operating room is available, preoperative and intraoperative imaging can be acquired. Such images allow one to start with SN at any time, for example, if during surgery problems arise that can be solved easier with navigation or if during SN there is a need for new imaging showing the current state of surgery. CT or CB-CT is the best choice for intraoperative imaging in maxillofacial reconstructive surgery.[10] The SN system must

be loaded with the patient's DICOM data, and the patient antenna must be adapted. If the imaging machine is preregistered in the SN system, the patient does not have to be registered. Systems currently registered in SN systems include ultrasonography, c-arm, CT, and MRI.

Intraoperative Imaging SN Checklist

- Check the quality of CB-CT 3D surface for applicability to surface registration. (New Tom 3G: imaging and surface reconstruction suitable for SN; New Tom 5G: system is unreliable)
- Change OR table top into carbon head rest (see **Fig. 5C**)
- Position patient for CB-CT scan (see **Fig. 5**)
- Acquire CB-CT DICOM data set and transfer to SN
- If needed, change table top for further surgery

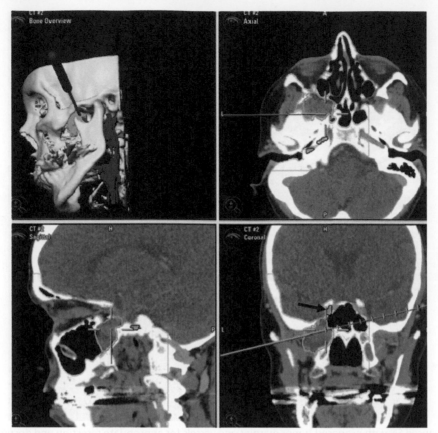

Fig. 12. SN-assisted resection of a neurofibroma; the optic nerve (*black arrow*) must be saved.

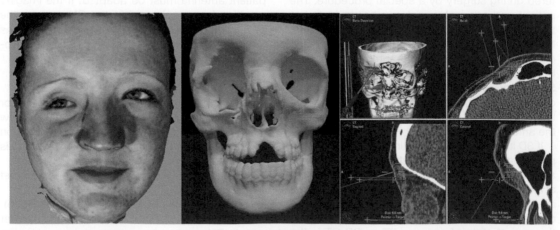

Fig. 13. Secondary reconstruction of traumatic orbit and midface deformity with 3-dimensional imaging (3D MD, Atlanta, GA, USA), computer-aided design/manufacturing (CAD/CAM) modeling, and advanced SN. This case was performed before autosegmentation and mirroring in SN was available on the market.

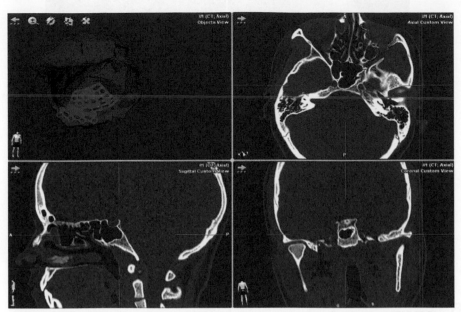

Fig. 14. Double vision after overcorrection with titanic mesh in a case of orbital floor fracture. Advanced SN planning with autosegmentation revealed the poor-fitting titanic mesh. Removal only of the titanium mesh solved the problem.

After finishing SN there are some postoperative demands before leaving the OR.

Postoperative SN Checklist

- Remove patient antenna (if it was fixed with osteosynthesis screw, 1 stitch may be needed)
- Check SN documentation
- Use documentation for patient's chart (**Fig. 6**A, B)
- Use experience for next SN[11] and further education
- Share documentations with colleagues, eg, pathologist, radiotherapist
- Save data, eg, for later CAD/CAM reconstructions

DAILY SURGICAL NAVIGATION: DEFINITION AND CASE REPORTS

Daily surgical navigation means immediate start of SN by data transfer from imaging to navigational system without preoperative computer planning. There are a wide variety of SN cases without need of computer planning efforts especially if imaging is of good quality. Otherwise spontaneous decision for SN is often limited by the quality of routine imaging. This aspect must be discussed with the radiologist to consistently obtain navigable imaging.

The first task in daily SN is "find and remove." All tasks and cases listed and described in **Table 3**. Depending on the case SN could be essential or at least really helpful.

ADVANCED SURGICAL NAVIGATION: DEFINITION AND CASE REPORTS

Advanced SN not only needs data transfer but also preoperative planning, and cannot be performed spontaneously. There is a large variety of tools, functions, and processes that can be combined to solve different tasks in surgery.[12] Thorough engagement and creativity is required by the surgeon to plan each advanced case individually. Furthermore, new imaging methods must be considered. For example, use of a novel positron emission tomography/CT tracer further aids in tumor surgery if imaging is combined with SN. Current advantages of SN in tumor surgery and reconstruction are as follows.

- Find the areas of interest for biopsies, staging, and especially restaging in the deep layers of tongue and floor of mouth
- Real time with high accuracy to control resection margins
- Documentation of resection margins for further diagnosis and therapy (pathology, radiotherapy)

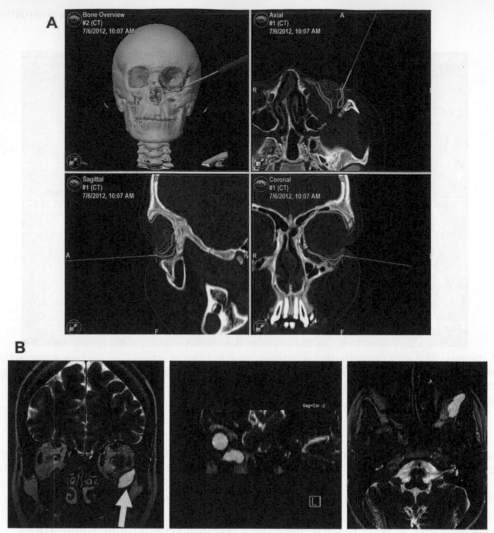

Fig. 15. (*A*) A 12-year-old boy with a 6-month-old trauma of both orbits and the nasoethmoidal region: primary reconstruction by resorbable sonic weld system only. Reexamination with SN tools showed moderate volume excess of left orbit and associated left enophthalmus. Secondary reconstruction is indicated only on the left side. The green pointer shows the achieved result at the end of surgery nearby the green target object. (*B*) Another possibility in the case of volume deficiency of the orbit and enophthalmus: Calculation of orbit volume and planning reconstruction of loss with (*arrow*) hydrocolloid osmotic expander fits best between lateral and inferior muscle.

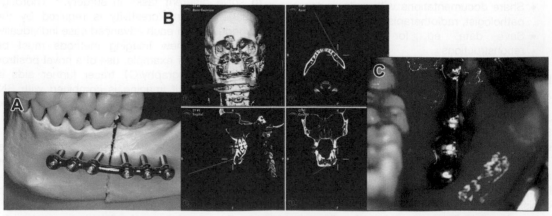

Fig. 16. (*A*) Development of a transmucosal osteosynthesis system inspired by SN. (*B*) SN could help to control closed bone reposition and to avoid mandible nerve and teeth lesions during osteosynthesis. (*C*) Intraoral view on a transmucosal osteosynthesis plate.

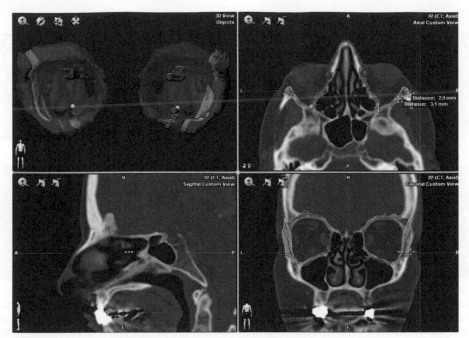

Fig. 17. Surgical therapy for endocrine orbitopathy. Advanced SN for determination of osteotomy lines and amount of orbital wall alterations, mirroring to achieve a good symmetry, and marking of infraorbital and optic nerve before surgery for orientation.

- Measurements, planning, and template construction for bone and soft-tissue reconstruction
- Assistance in search for suitable vessels, especially for microsurgical secondary reconstructions after primary tumor resection, neck dissection, and radiotherapy
- Assistance in CAD/CAM reconstruction of tumor-associated defects

Immediate reconstruction as described by Zheng and colleagues[13] requires virtual surgical simulation or SN in primary reconstruction of the mandible. By contrast, delayed reconstruction avoids radiation of the transplant and allows for a "12-month recurrence-free patient." Direct measurement of the resected specimen is always possible in obtaining the right amount of fibula transplant to replace lost parts of the mandible in

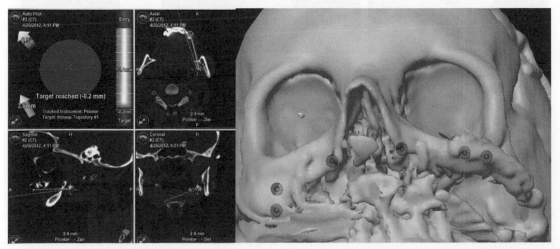

Fig. 18. The advanced SN autopilot could help to find the region of interest or the predicted implant position precisely and within a short time.

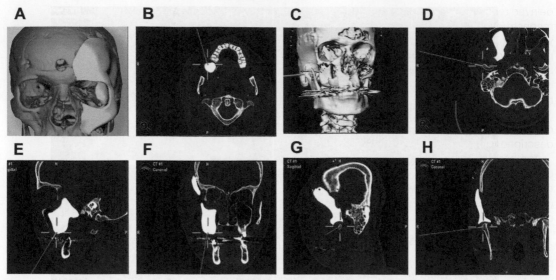

Fig. 19. (*A*) The first step in surgical reconstruction is the production of an implant, which needs very close cooperation with the technicians of the CAD/CAM company. The main problem in 1-step surgical reconstruction is to make sure that the prefabricated CAD/CAM implant fits into the defect during surgery. (*B–H*) SN makes this possible and allows control if intraoperative imaging is available. The authors prefer ceramic rather than titanium implants because they are easier to adapt during surgery.

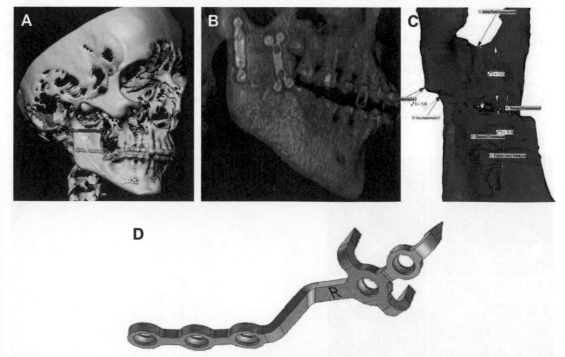

Fig. 20. (*A, B*) Parallel to occlusal plane proposed supraforaminal osteotomy line, during surgery implemented by SN. (*B*) Postoperative CB-CT 3-dimensional view. (*C*) Scientific evaluation of condyle position and bone healing by SN tools. (*D*) The authors' condyle and mandible positioning plate (produced by Medartis, Switzerland) for fixation of mandible position during imaging and navigation of the lower jaw as well as for condyle positioning during orthognathic surgery.

delayed reconstruction (**Figs. 9** and **10**). In delayed reconstruction it is helpful to look for suitable vessels (CT angiography) and plan the bone reconstruction with SN. During surgery, time could be saved by navigation of vessels and by calculating the amount of time required for reconstruction.

Table 4 provides an overview of advanced SN cases with corresponding figures and case descriptions.

Another way to treat cases of volume deficiency of the orbit is to calculate it and to replace the loss by a suitable hydrocolloid osmotic expander (**Fig. 15B**), whereby the authors now have 12 years of experience.[17]

Of course, inherent alterations and syndromes, as well as difficult orthognathic cases, cleft palate patients, or cases of craniofacial syndromes can also benefit from advanced SN, but are not addressed in this article.

REAL-TIME IMAGE-GUIDED SURGICAL NAVIGATION: INFLUENCE ON THE AUTHORS AND SCIENTIFIC CAPABILITY

In 2005 we began using SN. Three years later, we obtained our first CB-CT (Newtom 3G) in the OR for intraoperative imaging. All this has improved the quality of our surgery.

Our first cases were with supraforaminal osteotomy[18] in orthognathic surgery of the mandible. SN helped plan the osteotomy line above the foramen of the mandible to prevent a gap between the proximal and distal segment. This goal could be achieved by performing the osteotomy in a predicted angle to the occlusal plane indicated during surgery by SN (**Fig. 20A**). After performing fewer than 10 cases we realized that this could be accomplished sufficiently without SN, so this practice was stopped. These cases were all reevaluated with the help of postoperative CB-CT

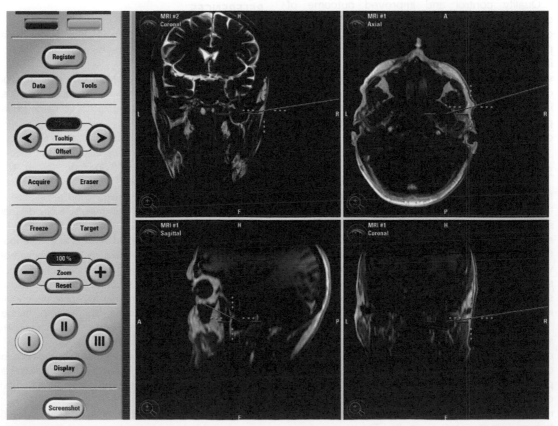

Fig. 21. SN used to guide the injection of botulin toxin to lateral pterygoid muscle in a case of myopathia and disc dislocation of the TMJ. In addition, one can determine the depth of the needle tip (*red indicated on the left toolbar*).

(see **Fig. 20**B) and SN tools (see **Fig. 20**C) as scientific work (see **Fig. 20**D).

The use of SN has led us to develop a transmucosal osteosynthesis plate (**Fig. 16**A, C).

SN has helped us to perform closed bone reposition and to avoid the mandible nerve and roots of teeth during osteosynthesis (see **Fig. 16**B). This technique is used only for complex cases.[19]

For 3 years we have used SN for injection of botulin toxin into the lateral pterygoid muscles for persistent muscle spasm and dystonia. This technique is very helpful in delivering this expensive drug into a central position inside the muscles (**Fig. 21**).

Lastly, SN has led to the development of a navigable temporomandibular joint (TMJ) arthroscope with integrated working channel[19] produced and offered by Karl Storz Company, Tuttlingen, Germany (www.karlstorz.de). This arthroscope could help in avoiding complications during TMJ puncture, or give additional information during surgical treatment of high condyle fractures of the mandible. A correlation of MRI and the arthroscopic position in the joint could be of scientific interest.

Quality control and improved outcome of surgery are the main advantages of SN. We are convinced that SN can help to change our surgical procedures and approaches and lead to further improvements. Standard values and standard skull libraries for various age groups and gender could be established with SN. The appropriate integration of today's innovative technologies promises to become the most important aspect of improving the quality and safety of our surgery.

SUMMARY

Modern navigational systems guide us through the human body and can help to manage the impossible. Close cooperation with the radiologist is necessary to obtain appropriate medical imaging for use with SN. Everything is navigable, but only with proper imaging. This article aims to give support to reconstructive and maxillofacial surgeons who are beginning to use real-time image-guided SN.

Currently available SN systems support the surgeon in multiple ways: searching, locating, marking, saving, removing, verifying, guiding, decision making, looking in hidden regions, transposition and reposition, (re)shaping, documenting, collecting data and experiences, percolating information, and comparing and controlling preoperative and postoperative results. The surgeon can make the right decisions, avoid mistakes, minimize the surgical trauma, and increase the surgical

accuracy with SN. SN makes it possible to create anatomic 3D libraries for special demands and further surgical progress. Last but not least, SN is suitable in resident training as well as in advanced surgical training for the practitioner.

In this article a large number of routine and advanced SN applications are reported for reconstructive and maxillofacial surgery, such as tumor surgery, traumatology, transplantation, (dental) implantation, and endoscopic surgery.

In the future it will be up to the surgeon to reconsider surgical procedures and to decide which cases are suitable for SN. The decision to use SN is influenced by the amount of surgical experience with the systems.

In the authors' opinion, the use of SN can improve surgical outcomes in a wide variety of cases.

ACKNOWLEDGMENTS

Thank you, Prof Dr Patrick Louis, for dedication of the issue. Thank you, all of our colleagues, for their great assistance.

REFERENCES

1. Spiegel EA, Wycis HT, Marks M. Stereotactic apparatus for operations on the human brain. Science 1947;106:349–50.
2. Watanabe E, Watanabe T, Manaka S, et al. 3D digitizer (Neuronavigator): new equipment for computed tomography-guided stereotactic surgery. Surg Neurol 1987;27:543–7.
3. Schramm A, Gellrich NC, Schmelzeisen R. Navigational surgery of the facial skeleton. Berlin, Heidelberg (Germany), New York: Springer; 2007. p. 47.
4. Dekomien C, Roeschies B, Winter S. System architecture for intraoperative ultrasound registration in image-based medical navigation. Biomed Tech (Berl) 2012;57(4):229–37.
5. Mischkowski RA, Zinser MJ, Ritter L, et al. Intraoperative navigation in the maxillofacial area based on 3D imaging obtained by a cone-beam device. Int J Oral Maxillofac Surg 2007;36:687–94.
6. Pillai P, Sammet S, Ammirati M. Application accuracy of computed tomography-based, image-guided navigation of temporal bone. Neurosurgery 2008;63(4):326–32 [discussion: 332–3].
7. Zhang W, Wang C, Shen G, et al. A novel device for preoperative registration and automatic tracking in cranio-maxillofacial image guided surgery. Comput Aided Surg 2012;17(5):259–67.
8. Caversaccio M, Langlotz F, Nolte LP, et al. Impact of a self-developed planning and self-constructed navigation system on skull base surgery: 10 years experience. Acta Otolaryngol 2007;127(4):403–7.

9. Dixon BJ, Daly MJ, Chan H, et al. Augmented image guidance improves skull base navigation and reduces task workload in trainees: a preclinical trial. Laryngoscope 2011;121(10):2060–4.

10. Lucas C, Kaduk WM, Podmelle F, et al. Navigierte Mund-Kiefer-Gesichtschirurgie und zahnärztliche Operationen mit intraoperativer DVT-Kontrolle. Quintessenz 2010;61(8):963–5.

11. Strauss G, Koulechov K, Röttger S, et al. Evaluation of a navigation system for ENT with surgical efficiency criteria. Laryngoscope 2006;116(4):564–72.

12. Collyer J. Review. Stereotactic navigation in oral and maxillofacial surgery. Br J Oral Maxillofac Surg 2010; 48:79–83.

13. Zheng GS, Su YX, Liao GQ. Mandible reconstruction assisted by preoperative virtual surgical simulation. Oral Surg Oral Med Oral Pathol Oral Radiol 2012; 113(5):604–11.

14. Tavassol F, Kokemüller H, Müller-Tavassol C, et al. A quantitative approach to orbital decompression in Graves' disease using computer-assisted surgery: a compilation of different techniques and introduction of the "temporal cage". J Oral Maxillofac Surg 2012;70(5):1152–60.

15. Santo G. Korrektur des Exophthalmus bei Morbus Basedow assoziierter Ophthalmopathie durch en bloc Teilresektion der lateralen und inferioren Orbitawand—eine klinische Untersuchung. Inauguraldissertation. Gießen. 2008. p. 29–40.

16. Wang X, Lin Y, Yu H, et al. Image-guided navigation in optimizing surgical management of craniomaxillofacial fibrous dysplasia. J Craniofac Surg 2011; 22(5):1552–6.

17. Kaduk WM, Schriewer A, Podmelle F. Treatment of orbital deficiency with Hydrogel expanders. J Cranio-Maxillofac Surg 2008;36:88.

18. Kaduk WM, Podmelle F, Louis PJ. Revisiting the supraforaminal horizontal oblique osteotomy of the mandible. J Oral Maxillofac Surg 2012;70(2):421–8.

19. Kaduk WM, Podmelle F. Advantages and new possibilities by implementation of the first TMJ arthroscope with integrated working channel into endoscopic surgery. Bruges (Belgium): Medimond; 2010. p. 347–51.

Index

Note: Page numbers of article titles are in **boldface** type.

Oral Maxillofacial Surg Clin N Am 25 (2013) 335–339
http://dx.doi.org/10.1016/S1042-3699(13)00054-X

Moving?

Make sure your subscription moves with you!

To notify us of your new address, find your **Clinics Account Number** (located on your mailing label above your name), and contact customer service at:

Email: journalscustomerservice-usa@elsevier.com

800-654-2452 (subscribers in the U.S. & Canada)
314-447-8871 (subscribers outside of the U.S. & Canada)

Fax number: 314-447-8029

Elsevier Health Sciences Division
Subscription Customer Service
3251 Riverport Lane
Maryland Heights, MO 63043

*To ensure uninterrupted delivery of your subscription, please notify us at least 4 weeks in advance of move.

Moving?

Make sure your subscription moves with you!

To notify us of your new address, find your Clinics Account **Number** (located on your mailing label above your name), and contact customer service at:

Email: journalscustomerservice-usa@elsevier.com

800-654-2452 (subscribers in the U.S. & Canada)
314-447-8871 (subscribers outside of the U.S. & Canada)

Fax number: 314-447-8029

Elsevier Health Sciences Division
Subscription Customer Service
3251 Riverport Lane
Maryland Heights, MO 63043

Printed and bound by CPI Group (UK) Ltd, Croydon, CR0 4YY

03/10/2024

01040347-0002